Inflammatory Myocardial Diseases

Edited by David C. Gaze

Published in London, United Kingdom

Inflammatory Myocardial Diseases
http://dx.doi.org/10.5772/intechopen.1003311
Edited by David C. Gaze

Contributors
Abena Agyekum, Adedayo Adeboye, Aiswarya Pillai, Alicia M. Maceira, Derek Geeslin, Effat Davoudi-Monfared, Emad Hakami, Ernest Tsiaze, Fidan Natig Gasimova, Kai Shiang Lin, Gerrit Hellige, Gift Echefu, Gonzalo J. Prado Bustamante, Guliyeva Ilkana Makh, Gulnara Sadig Nur-Mammadova, Gulustan Hamid Babayeva, Inna Bukharovich, Ismail Raslan, Jan Herzberg, Kaveh Hedayati Emami, Khalid Hussein, Kian Alipasandi, Leman Kamaladdin Babayeva, Maghrur Yashar Mammadov, Mahi L. Ashwath, Marquis Griffin, Mayuresh Chaudhari, Mohamed Laimoud, Mosleh Alanazi, Nana Osei, Nisha Arenja, Parviz Gunduz Niftiyev, Rehan Qureshi, Rozana Sadraldin, Sarah Keller, Stasa Krasic, Vladislav Vukomanovic, Vusala Niyat Atakishiyeva

First published in London, United Kingdom, 2025 by IntechOpen
IntechOpen is the global imprint of INTECHOPEN LIMITED, registered in England and Wales, registration number: 11086078, 167-169 Great Portland Street, London, W1W 5PF, United Kingdom

For EU product safety concerns: IN TECH d.o.o., Prolaz Marije Krucifikse Kozulić 3, 51000 Rijeka, Croatia, info@intechopen.com or visit our website at intechopen.com.

British Library Cataloguing-in-Publication Data
A catalogue record for this book is available from the British Library

Inflammatory Myocardial Diseases
Edited by David C. Gaze
p. cm.

This title is part of the Cardiology and Cardiovascular Medicine Book Series, Volume 8
Topic: Cardiovascular Diseases and Health
Series Editor: Kaan Kırali
Topic Editor: Mahi L. Ashwath

Print ISBN 978-0-85014-897-8
Online ISBN 978-0-85014-896-1
eBook (PDF) ISBN 978-0-85014-898-5
ISSN 3033-361X

IntechOpen Book Series

Cardiology and Cardiovascular Medicine

Volume 8

Aims and Scope of the Series

Today, since molecular science on structural causes of oncological pathologies and their molecular treatments are developing at an unbelievable rate, the primary medical cause of death in the twenty-first century will be cardiovascular disease. Neither pandemics that threaten all humanity nor deterioration in the ecosystem will be able to change this fact. Especially, this century seems poised to witness an incredible struggle against atherosclerotic disease, which develops in the arterial walls and results in narrowing and occlusion of the arterial lumen. In addition to this disease, there has been an increasing prevalence of heart rhythm problems, deterioration of heart valves due to aging, and heart failure. Serious vascular pathologies such as stenosis and occlusion, dissection and rupture, and aneurysmal enlargement are also major concerns. Medical and invasive treatment methods may work to save human lives, but they will never provide a real solution. All kinds of medical, technological, and genetic engineering developments obtained in these processes have not yet been sufficient to alleviate or eliminate cardiovascular disease. This book series, Cardiology and Cardiovascular Medicine, includes three topics. The first, Cardiovascular Diseases and Health, reviews important cardiovascular diseases and the developments in their prognosis. The second topic, Cardiovascular Electrophysiology, illuminates the abnormal functioning of the cardiac conduction system, which is caused by all heart pathologies and negatively affects prognosis. The third topic in this series, Cardiovascular Surgery, details treatment for cardiovascular pathologies and how to regulate normal physiological functions with percutaneous or extracorporeal interventions.

Meet the Series Editor

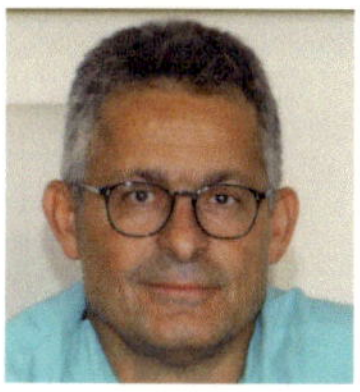

After completing his studies at the Medicine Faculty of Istanbul University in 1990, Prof. Kaan Kırali fulfilled his mandatory medical service and commenced his residency training at Koşuyolu Heart and Research Hospital in 1992. Following five years of assistant education, he pursued further training in England and the USA in 1998. Specializing in laparoscopic and minimally invasive cardiac surgery, he earned the titles of consultant cardiovascular surgeon in 1998, Assistant Professor in 1999, Associate Professor in 2002, and Chief in 2005 at the same hospital. Prof. Kırali also developed an interest in preventive medicine, obtaining an MSc in Public Health from Istanbul University in 2000. Over the past two decades, he has concentrated his scientific pursuits on cardiovascular repairs requiring specialized experience. With his expertise in coronary artery surgery, minimally invasive cardiac surgery, valve repair, and aortic root surgery, he has established new methods for awake coronary bypass revascularization, a new surgical approach for AVR during first and re-operations, aortic valve-sparing procedure, and radiofrequency ablation. Notably, he pioneered awake complete coronary artery bypass grafting (CABG) with bilateral internal mammary arteries (BIMA) and played a crucial role in advancing aortic root surgery with a new aortotomy incision, simplifying aortic valve interventions. Since the year 2000, Prof. Kırali has expanded his interests to heart transplantation, and in recent years, to left ventricular assist devices. He has served as the head of the transplantation department since 2015 and currently continues his work as the director of Koşuyolu High Specialization Education and Research Hospital in Istanbul, Turkey. In his prolific career, he has authored numerous papers in SCI journals, contributed to various book chapters, and served as an editor and reviewer for multiple academic journals. Additionally, he has edited several international books in the field of cardiovascular medicine.

Meet the Volume Editor

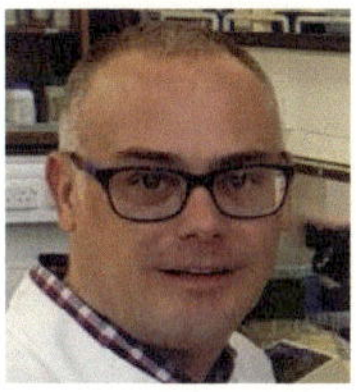

Dr. David C. Gaze is Senior Lecturer in Chemical Pathology, Director of Employability, and Course Leader for the MSc Biomedical Science programme at the University of Westminster, London, UK. His academic research interests include cardiovascular pathology; in particular, the development and clinical utility of cardiac biomarkers for the detection of cardiovascular diseases. Dr. Gaze has authored and co-authored more than 150 peer-reviewed papers and 200 abstracts. He has contributed five book chapters to cardiovascular textbooks as well as authored a textbook on cardiac troponin. He is a peer reviewer for twenty-five medical journals and writes regularly for the scientific forum The Conversation. Dr. Gaze is the commissioning editor for review articles for the Annals of Clinical Biochemistry & Laboratory Medicine and is Deputy Director of Scientific Affairs at the Association for Laboratory Medicine (formerly, the Association for Clinical Biochemistry and Laboratory Medicine), United Kingdom.

Contents

Preface

Myocarditis and pericarditis are inflammatory conditions of the heart that can lead to significant morbidity and mortality if not detected and managed promptly. These conditions are often challenging to diagnose due to their nonspecific clinical presentation and variable disease course. In recent years, the use of cardiac biomarkers has emerged as a valuable tool for the early detection and risk stratification of patients with myocarditis and pericarditis, including cardiac troponin, B-type natriuretic peptide (BNP), and C-reactive protein (CRP). These, along with the clinical presentation and advanced imaging, aid the clinician in diagnosing these diseases.

Cardiac inflammatory diseases (CID) are a group of conditions that cause inflammation within the heart's structure. There are many types of CID's which are categorised in **Table 1**. CID's include pericarditis, myocarditis, and endocarditis. The prevalence of CID's appears to be higher in males than females and affects all age groups. In some

Cause Category	Pericarditis	Myocarditis	Endocarditis
Infectious Causes	Viral (e.g., Coxsackievirus, HIV)	Vial (e.g., Coxsackievirus, adenovirus)	Bacterial (e.g., *Staphylococcus aureus*, *Streptococcus viridans*)
	– Bacterial (e.g., tuberculosis, pneumococcus)	Bacterial (e.g., *Corynebacterium diphtheriae*, *Borrelia*)	Fungal (e.g., *Candida*, *Aspergillus*)
	Fungal (e.g., *Histoplasma capsulatum*)	Parasitic (e.g., *Trypanosoma cruzi*)	Rarely viral (in immunocompromised patients)
Autoimmune / Inflammatory	Systemic lupus erythematosus (SLE)	Rheumatic fever	Rheumatic heart disease
	Rheumatoid arthritis	Sarcoidosis	Systemic lupus erythematosus (SLE)
	Post-myocardial infarction (Dressler's syndrome)	Autoimmune myocarditis	
Post-surgical / Trauma	Following cardiac surgery	Cardiac trauma	Prosthetic valve implantation (risk factor)
	Chest radiation therapy		
Toxic / Drug-induced	Drug-induced lupus (e.g., hydralazine, isoniazid)	Chemotherapy (e.g., anthracyclines)	Intravenous drug use (as a predisposition to infection)
		Alcohol or cocaine-induced toxicity	
Idiopathic	Most common form (often presumed viral)	Frequently idiopathic, presumed viral	Rarely idiopathic; usually a pathogen is identified

Table 1.
Categorisation of cardiac inflammatory diseases.

cases, the disease is self-limiting, resulting in full recovery, however, in other affected individuals, a chronic pathophysiology of the disease can occur. Identifying the primary cause of CID's is critical for successful intervention and reduction in morbidity and mortality. The aetiology of CID's is complex and can be initiated by a large variety of infectious agents such as viruses and bacteria, fungi and parasites and non-infectious causes such as autoimmune diseases; pharmacological intervention including traditional chemotherapy and immune checkpoint inhibitors; environmental toxin exposure; substance abuse such as alcohol or other illicit drugs.

Historical perspective

In the 1750s, the collection and description of findings relating to different organs, médecine sémiotique [semiotic medicine; relating to signs and symbols] emerged as the underlying basis of disease classification. The first descriptions of 'inflammations of the heart', commonly referred in many historic publications as 'carditis'; occurred in 1749 by the French physician Jean-Baptiste de Sénac (1693–1770), living in Versailles, in his work 'Traité des maladies du Coeur'. In 1761, in his essay 'De Sedibus et Causis Morborum,' Giovanni Battista Morgagni (1682–1771) described cardiac anatomical findings suggestive of myocardial fibrosis. The father of vaccination, the British physician Edward Jenner (1749–1823), discovered the relationship between cardiac involvement and rheumatic fever. This description of rheumatic heart disease was sent to a medical journal in London but was lost and never published. In Paris, 1806, Jean-Nicolas Corvisart-Desmarets (1755–1821) produced a monograph entitled 'Essai sur les maladies et des lesions organiques du Coeur et des gros vaisseaux' which documented all pathology, symptoms and therapies known at the time relating to diseases of the heart. The Scottish anatomist and surgeon Allan Burns (1781–1813) produced the first descriptive book of heart diseases in Great Britain in 1809 entitled 'The most frequent and important disease of the heart'. Rudolf Ludwig Carl Virchow (1821–1902), the father of modern pathology, then discriminated between inflammation of the parenchyma and interstitial tissues and was the first to use the term chronic myocarditis (**Figure 1**).

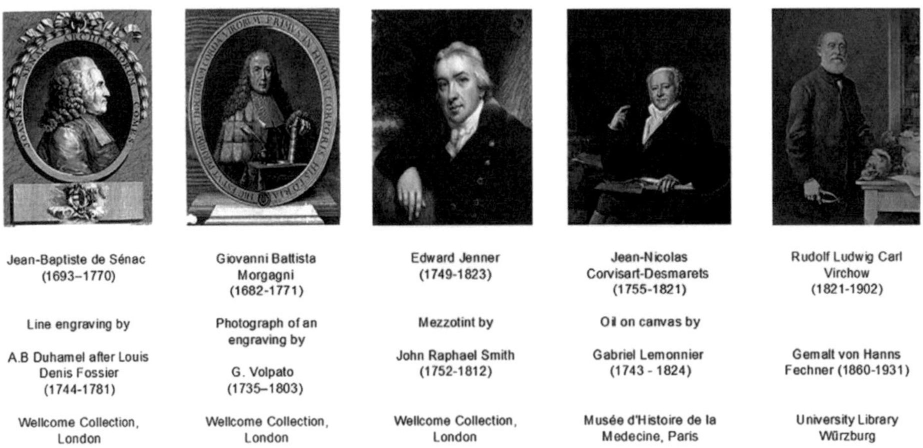

Figure 1.
Notable Anatomists, Physicians and Pathologists first describing 'inflammations of the heart' [carditis]. Images in public domain.

The 1930s defined disease as 'cor hypertonicum' due to electrocardiography, and in 1937, it was differentiated into disease of the heart muscle caused by coronary heart disease by Paul Dudley White (1886–1973) in 'Heart Disease', published by Macmillan, New York (White 1931). In the 1940's links to bacterial and viral agents causing myocarditis were made, including Streptococcus and Coxackie virus. Modern viral agents such as SARS-CoV-19 are also known as a causative agent of severe myocardial inflammation.

There are many diagnostic modalities used to diagnose CID's which assess structural anatomy of the heart, contractility and function along with biochemical markers of cardiac pathology (**Table 2**).

Modality	Clinical utility and/or examples
Biochemical testing	
Blood culture	Identification of pathogenic organism
Cardiac markers	IL-6, CRP, CK/CK-MB, myoglobin, Cardiac Troponin, Natriuretic peptides,
Inflammatory markers	FBC, ESR, IL-6 CRP
Cardiac autoantibodies	b-1 adrenergic receptors (β1-AR), cardiac myosin, cardiac troponin I, cardiac myosin binding protein-C (cMyBP-C), Na/K-ATPase.
Imaging techniques	
Electrocardiogram (ECG)	Electrical activity and contractility
Echocardiogram (echo)	Ultrasonic imaging to establish blood flow, structural wall indicators and contractility.
Cardiac computer tomography (cardiac CT)	Visualisation of ASCVD, plaque formation and extent of coronary calcification.
Cardiac magnetic resonance imaging (c-MRI)	Magnetic fields and radio waves to generate structural image of cardiac function.
Chest X ray (CXR)	Basic imaging technique to identify cardiac shape and size.
Invasive procedural diagnostics	
Endomyocardial biopsy (EMB)	Surgical resection of myocardial tissue for histological analysis. Considered the gold standard for myositis.
Cardiac catheterisation	Visualisation of ASCVD

Table 2.
Diagnostic modalities used to detect cardiac inflammatory diseases.

This book provides a comprehensive review of Inflammatory Myocardial Diseases. It is organized into three sections: (1) Pathobiology of Myocardial Inflammatory Diseases; (2) Imaging for Inflammatory Myocardial Diseases; and (3) Interventions for Inflammatory Myocardial Diseases. Chapters address topics including inflammatory diseases in rheumatological patients; acute and recurrent pediatric pericarditis;

clinical detection methods; imaging methods including cardiac magnetic resonance in scleroderma; extracorporeal membrane oxygenation for fulminant myocarditis complicated with cardiogenic shock; and surgical interventions.

Dr. David C. Gaze
Biomedical Sciences,
School of Life Sciences,
University of Westminster,
London, United Kingdom

Dedication

Dedicated to Martin John Brealey in his 50th year

Section 1

Pathobiology of Myocardial Inflammatory Diseases

Chapter 1

Inflammatory Heart Disease in Patients with Rheumatological Profile

Fidan Natig Gasimova, Gulustan Hamid Babayeva, Gulnara Sadig Nur-Mammadova, Leman Kamaladdin Babayeva, Guliyeva Ilkana Makhaddin, Vusala Niyat Atakishiyeva, Maghrur Yashar Mammadov and Parviz Gunduz Niftiyev

Abstract

Rheumatic diseases are among the most severe immune-inflammatory diseases and are characterized by a chronic progressive course with damage to many organs and systems of the body, leading to the loss of professional and social skills, disability in working age, and a decrease in the life expectancy of patients. Depending on the leading mechanism of immune activation, they are conventionally divided into two main categories: autoimmune and autoinflammatory. Rheumatic diseases, as a result of chronic systemic inflammation, often lead to damage to the cardiovascular system, which can vary from asymptomatic or mild to severe and life-threatening, being a significant cause of morbidity and mortality in this category of patients. In this case, multispectral damage can be observed: from changes in the myocardium, pericardium, valves, and conduction system, to the development of premature atherosclerosis, and as a consequence, to the occurrence of coronary heart disease at a younger age, and in some cases, the occurrence of vasculitis is possible. In this chapter, the authors presented a broad overview of the main groups of rheumatological diseases and the characteristics of cardiovascular damage in this group of patients. It is always necessary to remember the need for multidisciplinary management of rheumatological patients, given the diversity and high risks of disability and mortality in the presence of cardiovascular lesions.

Keywords: rheumatological diseases, cardiovascular lesions, myocarditis, pericarditis, atherosclerosis, vasculitis

1. Introduction

Immunoinflammatory rheumatic diseases (RD) are a group of diseases that are among the most complex and difficult to diagnose and treat in modern medicine.

These diseases have a chronic progressive course, which means that inflammatory processes in the body do not stop, but, on the contrary, worsen over time, leading to damage to many organs and systems. This not only significantly worsens the quality of life of patients, but can also lead to a complete loss of their professional and social functions. In some cases, the disease ends in disability at working age, which is a significant social problem [1]. In addition, rheumatic diseases can significantly reduce the life expectancy of patients, making them more vulnerable to various infections and cardiovascular complications.

One of the key characteristics of these diseases is their ability to affect not only the joints, as is often assumed, but also other vital organs and systems, which makes them systemic in nature. At the same time, depending on which mechanism of activation of the immune system dominates in the pathogenesis of the disease, RDs are divided into two main categories: autoimmune and autoinflammatory. Autoimmune diseases occur when the body's immune system begins to attack its own tissues, mistaking them for foreign, while autoinflammatory diseases are associated with hyperactivation of inflammatory processes, but without the participation of an autoimmune reaction.

Rheumatic diseases, as a result of chronic systemic inflammation, often have a negative impact on the cardiovascular system (CVS), which is one of the most significant aspects determining the severity of the disease and its prognosis. Cardiac lesions in RD can manifest themselves in a variety of forms, ranging from asymptomatic changes and mild disorders that do not cause immediate concern, to severe cardiovascular catastrophes such as heart failure, myocardial infarction, and other acute conditions. These complications are one of the main causes of morbidity and mortality in patients with rheumatic diseases.

As part of cardiovascular lesions in RD, changes can occur in various structures of the heart, including the myocardium (heart muscle), valves, pericardium (heart lining), and the cardiac conduction system. For example, chronic inflammation can lead to myocarditis—inflammation of the heart muscle, which impairs its ability to effectively contract and pump blood. This, in turn, can cause heart failure and even cardiogenic shock in severe cases. Damage to the heart valves can lead to their deformation and insufficiency, which disrupts normal blood circulation and requires surgical intervention. Inflammation of the pericardium (pericarditis) can also cause pain and difficulty in the normal functioning of the heart.

In addition, rheumatic diseases often contribute to the development of premature atherosclerosis, a condition in which fatty and calcium deposits are deposited in the walls of arteries, narrowing the vessels and reducing their elasticity. Atherosclerosis causes a chronic lack of oxygen in the tissues, which is especially dangerous for the heart muscle. This process can lead to the development of coronary heart disease (CHD)—a condition in which, due to insufficient blood supply, the heart muscle suffers from a lack of oxygen and nutrients. CHD, in turn, increases the risk of myocardial infarction, arrhythmia, and chronic heart failure. Importantly, with RD, atherosclerosis develops much earlier than in the general population and more often affects younger age groups [2].

A feature of these diseases is that inflammation in the body can spread to the vessels, which can lead to the development of vasculitis—inflammation of the walls of blood vessels. This condition disrupts normal blood flow and can lead to thrombosis, ischemia, and even tissue necrosis, which significantly worsens the patient's condition.

The extended spectrum of cardiovascular lesions in patients with rheumatological diseases is presented in **Table 1**.

Myocardial	Pericardial	Valvular	Vascular	Electrical
Congestive heart failure	Pericardial effusion	Libman-Sacks vegetation	Atherosclerosis	Sudden cardiac death
Left ventricular hypertrophy	Pericarditis	Valvular regurgitation	Arterial stiffness	Ventricular arrythmia
Diastolic dysfunction		Valvular nodule	Vasculitis	Supraventricular tachycardia
Myocardial fibrosis			Thrombosis	Atrioventricular block
Amyloidosis				

Table 1.
Some of cardiovascular manifestations of rheumatic diseases.

Thus, the interaction between rheumatic diseases and cardiovascular pathologies is an important area for research and clinical practice. Patients with RD require a comprehensive approach to treatment, since it is necessary not only to control the inflammatory process in joint and other tissues, but also to actively monitor the state of the cardiovascular system, preventing the development of life-threatening complications. It is also important that such patients are under constant supervision of specialists—cardiologists, rheumatologists, and other doctors, which will allow timely adjustment of treatment and improve the prognosis of the disease.

2. Damage to the cardiovascular system in rheumatoid arthritis

The most typical and common representative of immunoinflammatory diseases is rheumatoid arthritis (RA) [1].

Cardiovascular diseases (CVD) are recognized as the leading cause of mortality in patients with RA, accounting for almost 40% [3]. In recent years, it has been found that in patients suffering from RA, life expectancy is reduced by 7–10 years, and the risk of developing CV pathologies increases by 50% [4]. Cardiac symptoms can be caused both by the direct inflammatory process in the membranes of the heart and by the early development of atherosclerosis [5, 6]. The risk of CVD increases in the presence of traditional risk factors, such as high cholesterol, smoking, arterial hypertension (HTN), decreased physical activity, use of non-steroidal anti-inflammatory drugs (NSAIDs), glucocorticoids (GC), and the influence of inflammatory cytokines on the vascular endothelium [7].

In RA, CVD risk factors are observed long before the appearance of clinical signs; subsequently, chronic inflammation, characteristic of RA, contributes to the development of atherosclerosis [8].

The key role in this process is played by the severity of RA: high disease activity, the presence of extra-articular manifestations, severe functional joint insufficiency, seropositivity for rheumatoid factor (RF) and antibodies to cyclic citrullinated peptide (ACCP), and the use of GCs [9, 10].

Patients suffering from RA are highly susceptible to the development of all forms of coronary artery disease, heart failure (HF), pericarditis, myocarditis, atrial fibrillation, valvular heart disease, and cardiac amyloidosis [11]. In patients with RA, the risk of myocardial infarction (MI) and stroke increases by two times, and this risk is almost three times higher in patients suffering from this disease for 10 years or more [3]. Based on the above, RA itself is a risk factor for the development of CVD and its complications, and cardiac lesions in these patients have pronounced clinical manifestations [12]. In this disease, all membranes of the heart are involved in the pathological process: myocardium, pericardium, endocardium, as well as the aorta and coronary arteries of the heart. In RA, the most common manifestation of cardiovascular (CV) pathology is pericarditis, which occurs in 4% of patients and, as a rule, is asymptomatic [11]. Patients with RA are 10 times more likely to develop pericardial effusion than patients without RA [13].

Exudative or adhesive pericarditis is much more common, which is detected at autopsy in 50% of cases. It usually manifests itself as asymptomatic effusions into the pericardial cavity, determined by echocardiography (Echo-CG), which is detected in approximately 30% of patients. These effusions are rarely large enough to cause cardiac tamponade, but if prolonged, they can lead to constrictive pericarditis. Constrictive pericarditis requires pericardiectomy because this condition involves fibrosis that does not respond to immunosuppressive therapy [14]. Rheumatoid pericarditis is determined, as a rule, in patients with high inflammatory activity and usually in patients with multiple systemic manifestations [5]. In most patients, pericardial effusion develops after the onset of arthritis, but there are cases where RA was diagnosed after pericarditis [15]. Pericarditis in RA is prone to recurrence.

Exudative pericarditis is clinically manifested by chest pain, pericardial friction noise, increased heart size, muffled heart sounds, inversion of the terminal part of the ventricular complex on electrocardiography (ECG), pericardial separation, and other symptoms detected by echocardiography.

Rarely, but the development of right ventricular failure is possible. Sometimes repeated evacuation of fluid from the pericardium is required. Pericardial effusion exhibits low glucose levels and elevated concentrations of immunoglobulins, total protein, and lactate dehydrogenase [5]. Immune complexes and RF may also be present in the pericardial fluid, but their presence does not confirm that pericarditis is caused specifically by RA [2].

The use of biological agents, widely used in the treatment of severe RA, is currently considered one of the "cornerstones" of therapy for RA associated with the development of pericardial effusion. These treatment complications mainly occur within 4 months of starting biological anti-inflammatory antirheumatic drugs (bDMADRs) such as infliximab and etanercept [16]. In particular, purulent pericardial effusion has been reported in patients receiving infliximab and etanercept [17, 18].

Myocarditis in RA, unlike pericarditis, is less common. According to the results of autopsies, myocarditis was found in 19% of patients with RA, mainly in females with active arthritis, but in most patients myocarditis is clinically asymptomatic [11]. Myocarditis usually manifests and is diagnosed during periods of maximum activity of the main rheumatoid process, which corresponds to the next pronounced exacerbation of the articular syndrome. Interstitial or granulomatous myocarditis occurs, ending in the development of small focal cardiosclerosis. Interstitial myocarditis occurs subclinically and does not lead to pronounced hemodynamic disturbances. On the contrary, granulomatous myocarditis, caused by the formation of rheumatoid nodules in the heart muscle, may be accompanied by persistent disturbances in heart rhythm and conduction, but even in this case, there is no significant increase in heart size or a significant decrease in cardiac output [5].

Endocarditis in RA is observed much less frequently than pericarditis. Pathological studies demonstrate frequent involvement of the endocardium, in particular the valve apparatus, in the form of nonspecific inflammatory changes in the leaflets and valve ring, as well as specific granulomas.

With rheumatoid endocarditis, valvulitis is also possible, which leads to deformation of the valves and severe insufficiency of the affected valve, most often the mitral valve, which requires surgical correction of the defect. Mitral insufficiency is common and aortic insufficiency is less common. As for mitral stenosis and aortic stenosis, this is a privilege of rheumatic heart disease and practically does not occur in RA. Aortitis caused by the development of rheumatoid nodules in the aortic arch (granulomatous aortitis) is extremely rare. Cardiac conduction abnormalities, cardiomyopathy, coronary artery occlusion, and aortic regurgitation have been described but are rare. Chronic inflammation in RA contributes to the accelerated development of atherosclerosis, increasing the risk of coronary events such as myocardial infarction (MI) and angina. Traditional CVD risk factors, systemic inflammation, immunological activity, and the influence of antirheumatic drugs play an important role in the progression of atherosclerosis in RA [19]. In RA, inflammation is considered a key factor, increasing the risk of CVD by 1.5–2 times compared with the general population [20, 21].

Atherosclerosis and RA share many common inflammatory mechanisms: Inflammatory processes in the synovial membranes of joints are similar to those that lead to instability of atherosclerotic plaques. Proinflammatory cytokines, such as α-tumor necrosis factor (α-TNF), interleukin-1 (IL-1), and interleukin-6 (IL-6), play a central role in both the development of RA and atherosclerosis [22]. Overproduction of these cytokines in inflamed synovial fluid leads to the activation of macrophages in atherosclerotic plaques, which partly explains the progression of atherosclerosis and the development of CV complications [23]. Autoimmune inflammation acts as a key risk factor for the development of both clinical and subclinical manifestations of atherosclerosis. This explains why chronic arthritis is often considered a natural model for studying atherosclerosis. The accelerated development of atherosclerosis can actually be considered a systemic manifestation of RA [1].

3. Damage to the cardiovascular system in ankylosing spondylitis

Seronegative spondyloarthritis (SSpA) is a group of inflammatory RDs with common clinical and etiological features, including axial and peripheral inflammatory arthritis, enthesitis, extra-articular manifestations, and a close association with the presence of the human leukocyte antigen HLA-B27 [24]. The SSpA group includes ankylosing spondylitis (AS), psoriatic arthritis (PsA), reactive arthritis, as well as arthritis associated with inflammatory bowel disease, undifferentiated spondylitis, and juvenile AS. A characteristic feature of all SSpA is the absence of RF in the blood serum of patients. Ankylosing spondylitis is the most common disease in the SSpA group. It is a chronic inflammatory disease that typically occurs most often in young men, primarily affecting the spine and sacroiliac joints and, to a lesser extent, the peripheral joints. CVS lesions are detected in approximately 2–10% of patients with AS, although this figure can reach 30% [25, 26]. The risk of developing cardiac complications increases with the patient's age, duration of AS, the presence of HLA-B27, and damage to peripheral joints [27]. There are three types of inflammatory heart diseases associated with AS, which include aortic regurgitation and aortitis, conduction abnormalities, and myocardial damage affecting left ventricular (LV) ejection fraction [28]. CV manifestations usually occur with a long course of AS, but can also occur at an earlier time. Some cardiac syndromes in AS, such as aortitis and aortic insufficiency, conduction disorders, myocarditis, valvulitis, are associated with disease activity and can occur at any stage [29]. Manifestations of cardiovascular complications in late, advanced stages of AS often lead to the development of irreversible cardiac structural changes [30, 31].

Damage to the cardiovascular system plays a key role in the clinical manifestation of AS, as this has a decisive influence on the prognosis of the disease and approaches to its treatment.

The following cardiac syndromes occur with AS:

- damage to the aorta and its structures—aortitis, periaortitis, aortic dissection, and aortic insufficiency;
- conduction disturbances with the development of atrioventricular (AV) block;
- pericarditis with threat of cardiac tamponade; myocarditis with the possible development of left ventricular (LV) dysfunction;
- valve defects—aortic insufficiency, mitral insufficiency, and stenosis with possible subsequent valve replacement.

Aortic damage is one of the most common cardiovascular complications in AS. It is characterized by inflammatory changes in the adventitia (aortitis), and degenerative and atherosclerotic changes in the intima-media complex, which leads to fibrosis, dilation of the ascending aorta and arch, narrowing and obliteration of the vasa vasorum, and perivascular infiltration [32, 33].

The morphological basis of aortitis is made up of changes occurring in the wall of both the aorta itself and the vasa vasorum, namely:

- intimal proliferation;
- fibrosis and thickening of the adventitia;
- focal destruction of elastic tissue by inflammatory cells;
- perivascular infiltration by inflammatory cells and obliterating endarteritis vasa vasorum.

A characteristic feature of the inflammatory process in AS associated with HLA-B27 is occlusion of the vasa vasorum [34]. Aortitis in AS usually covers a small area of the aorta, including the root and ascending part. Aortitis is often accompanied by valvulitis of the aortic valve, which leads to fibrosis, thickening, and retraction of the leaflets. Developing aortic regurgitation is caused by both aortic dilatation and valve insufficiency [32].

The development of relative aortic insufficiency in patients with AS is most often associated with expansion of the aortic root [35]. In this disease, the most commonly affected structures are the ascending section and root of the aorta, the leaflets of the aortic and mitral valves, as well as the zone of transition of the posterior wall of the base of the aorta into the anterior mitral leaflet, where a ridge-like thickening of the endocardium is formed, represented by post-inflammatory fibrous tissue. This phenomenon is called the "subaortic bump", and is considered specific to AS and other SpA [36]. In patients with AS, the incidence of conduction disorders is higher compared to the general population [25, 37]. This is explained by the fact that in AS, during the period of exacerbation of inflammation, the cardiovascular system is often involved in the pathological process, which leads to arrhythmias against the background of myocarditis and endocarditis [38, 39]. With a decrease in inflammation, disorders that appeared during high AS activity may disappear [40]. However, relief of inflammation is often accompanied by the development of connective tissue in the myocardium, including its subendocardial part, which can lead to chronic conduction and rhythm disturbances. These disorders do not disappear without constant medical or surgical intervention [39, 41, 42].

One of the most common cardiac manifestations of AS is AV block. According to various sources, the frequency of AV blockade in AS ranges from 15 to 20%. Various conduction disorders, including AV and intraventricular blocks, occur in almost 1/3 of patients. About 7% of patients suffer from sinus bradycardia, which may be associated with dysfunction of the sinus node due to pathological changes in the wall of the artery supplying the node and the myocardium of the right atrium. Most patients have a first-degree block or incomplete block of the left bundle branch.

Complete heart block, requiring pacemaker implantation, occurs in 1–9% of male patients with AS, 20% of whom are HLA-B27 positive. In women, the frequency of detection of the gene was not noted [2]. According to numerous studies, in AS, in addition to the main risk factors for CVD, cardiac conduction disturbances are observed, which are more common in males, mainly with higher disease activity [43]. Patients with AS also experience frequent occurrence of bradycardia and ECG changes in the form of prolongation of the QT and PQ intervals, which leads to an increased risk of developing atrial fibrillation and AV block of the first degree. In turn, atrial fibrillation increases the risk of developing heart failure and stroke by five times and, in general, the risk of mortality by two times [44–46].

There are two main hypotheses explaining the etiology of conduction disturbances in patients with AS: The first theory suggests that inflammation causes damage to the interventricular septum, while the second associates these disturbances with AV node dysfunction, which occurs due to impaired conduction of impulses from the sinus node. These processes contribute to the appearance of supraventricular extrasystoles and the formation of AV blockades [47, 48].

According to Goulenok et al., routine ECG testing in patients with AS often does not reveal CV disorders. However, if patients with AS have symptoms such as shortness of breath, fatigue, and decreased exercise tolerance, an ECG should be performed to assess possible rhythm and conduction disturbances [46]. The proportion of patients with AS who have coronary artery disease and hypertension is the same both among those who have cardiac conduction disorders and among those who do not have such disorders [45]. According to the AS treatment protocol, patients require long-term, continuous use of NSAIDs, which may contribute more to the development of IHD in this category of patients than the course of the disease itself. Since patients with more severe forms of AS are more likely to take relatively high doses of NSAIDs, their likelihood of developing CHD is significantly higher. This is explained by the fact that the use of COX-2 inhibitors has a direct correlation with the occurrence of ischemic heart disease [47, 48]. Pericarditis with AS is rare—less than 1% of cases. As a rule, it is adhesive and occurs with mild clinical symptoms; it is diagnosed using Echo-CG or X-ray examination by the presence of pleuropericardial adhesions [5].

4. Damage to the cardiovascular system in psoriatic arthritis

Psoriatic arthritis is a chronic progressive systemic disease associated with psoriasis (Ps), characterized by the development of peripheral arthritis, dactylitis, multiple enthesitis, and spondyloarthritis with the localization of the pathological process mainly in musculoskeletal tissues [49]. PsA is a multifactorial disease in which many organs and systems of the body are involved in the pathological process, and various metabolic disorders are observed, which allows us to consider this pathology as a multisystem disease [50].

In PsA, cardiac damage is of primary importance among visceral pathologies, which occurs in every 3-rd patient.

Currently, large registries and cohort observations have obtained information about the high prevalence of traditional CV risk factors, such as smoking, dyslipidemia, and abdominal obesity, which contribute to the development of fatal MI and acute cerebrovascular accident in people with PsA, which reduces the life expectancy of patients compared with general population [51]. In addition, the development of a wide range of CVDs is noted, primarily metabolic syndrome (MS), hypertension, acute coronary syndrome, and thromboembolism [52]. Thus, in a prospective study conducted by Bengtsson et al., in an analysis of the Swedish National Register, it was shown that patients with PsA are at high risk of developing acute coronary syndrome and strokes [53, 54].

The occurrence of cardiovascular pathology in patients with PsA is associated both with chronic systemic inflammation and autoimmune disorders, which form the basis of the pathogenesis of these diseases, and with the side effects of antirheumatic therapy [55].

Systemic inflammation that occurs in PsA is accompanied by an increase in the level of pro-inflammatory cytokines such as α-TNF, IL-2, IL-6, IL-8, and IL-17, which affect angiogenesis, adipogenesis, regulation of insulin production, activation of inflammatory cells, and platelet adhesion [56, 57]. As is known, high levels of α-TNF lead to reversible endothelial dysfunction, increased expression of adhesion molecules, and activation of invasion by dendritic cells of vessel walls [58, 59]. An increase in the level of IL-6 and IL-2 is accompanied by a pronounced disturbance of microcirculation, increased thrombus formation, and, ultimately, the formation of an atherosclerotic plaque. Thus, when conducting positron emission computed tomography (PECT) in patients with moderate and severe Ps, signs of generalized systemic inflammation were found in the heart, aortic wall, liver, skin, joints, and ligaments, including in patients without clinical signs of arthritis [54, 60].

Thus, the combination of traditional CVD risk factors and systemic inflammation in PS and PsA appears to explain their high prevalence and increased cardiovascular risk in these diseases compared to the general population [61]. This is due to the fact that many of the inflammatory mediators and cell adhesion molecules, the concentrations of which increase in PsA, can directly contribute to the development of endothelial dysfunction, which leads to the occurrence of CVD [62, 63]. This fact is confirmed by the information that in patients with PsA and without CV risk factors or clinical manifestations of the disease, signs of endothelial dysfunction were found [64]. Thus, the relative risk of MI increases with increasing severity of PS and PsA, and in men over 30 years of age, there is a threefold increase in this risk [65]. In addition, studies have shown a correlation between the risk of developing CVD and the severity of PsA, as well as an increase in the incidence of peripheral vascular diseases and cerebrovascular disorders [66, 67].

Among the cardiovascular pathologies in patients with PsA, the most common development is myocarditis, which is usually observed against the background of high laboratory activity and is manifested by a moderate expansion of the borders of the heart, a weakening of the first sound, the appearance of a third sound, moderate systolic murmur, tachycardia not consistent with fever, rhythm and conduction disturbances, diffuse changes in the myocardium according to ECG data, prolongation of the QT interval. To identify myocarditis, it is not so much these changes that are important, but their close relationship with exacerbations of the disease and positive dynamics under the influence of the therapy. Pericarditis is usually adhesive, has a blurred clinical picture, and is identified by the presence of pleuropericardial adhesions. In rare cases, pericardial effusion has been observed [68].

Aortitis often occurs in PsA. A detailed Echo-CG study of two groups of patients, one of which consisted of patients with PsA without damage to the axial skeleton and the second with stage III-IV sacroiliitis and/or AS, revealed significant differences in the condition of the aorta [68].

Aortic dilatation occurred significantly more often in patients with PsAS than in patients with only peripheral arthritis. When the spine was affected, Echo-CG signs of thickening of the aortic wall were more often observed. In some cases, foci of thickening up to 5–9 mm are noted on the posterior wall of the aorta at a distance of 2–3 cm from its root (subaortic bump), as is observed in AS. In PsA, fibrosis of the ascending aortic arch is observed, spreading to the aortic valves, the ostia of the coronary arteries, and the interatrial septum, which is more typical for psoriatic spondylitis.

Particular attention is drawn to the localization of inflammatory processes in the endocardium. A comprehensive analysis of clinical and instrumental data, including ultrasound examination of the heart, revealed organic defects, such as combined mitral disease, combined mitral-aortic defects, as well as isolated aortic insufficiency. Determining the etiology of heart defects presents significant difficulties due to the prevailing opinion that combined mitral-aortic defects, especially mitral stenosis, are characteristic of rheumatic carditis. In some cases, a combination of PsA and rheumatic heart disease is possible. In some patients without a history of RDs, heart defects developed against the background of psoriatic rashes, erosive arthritis and/or AS, and in these cases, valve damage can be considered a consequence of psoriatic endocarditis [68].

5. Damage to the cardiovascular system in systemic lupus erythematosus

Systemic lupus erythematosus (SLE) is a chronic autoimmune disease with multi-system involvement and unknown etiology, characterized by a wide range of clinical manifestations and an unpredictable course [49]. It should be noted that over the past decades, due to the increase in the effectiveness of therapy, mortality from all causes in SLE has decreased significantly, while mortality from CVD remains at a high level and they remain the leading cause of death in these patients [69, 70]. The prevalence of CVD in patients with SLE is more than 50%, which is significantly higher than that in the general population [71, 72].

The heart is one of the most commonly affected organs in patients with SLE, which can affect all its anatomical structures, including the pericardium, myocardium, endocardium, coronary arteries, valves, and conduction system, which can ultimately lead to end-stage heart failure CV continuum [73]. In addition to pericarditis and myocarditis, coronary heart disease is quite common and is recognized as one of the main causes of mortality, especially in elderly patients and in those with long-standing SLE [74]. SLE is associated with an increased risk of accelerated atherosclerosis and CV events such as CAD, stroke, and peripheral artery disease [75], which occur in both early and late stages of the disease, with younger patients at significantly greater risk compared with their peers of the same age [76].

The increased incidence of CVD in patients with SLE is explained by a combination of traditional risk factors, as well as factors directly related to disease activity and therapy. In addition, antiphospholipid antibodies (aPL), hyperhomocysteinemia, and the proatherogenic effects of chronic systemic inflammation play a significant role [77, 78].

Pericarditis is the most common clinical manifestation of cardiac damage, the prevalence of which in SLE, according to some autopsy data, is about 62% [79]. Pericarditis in SLE, along with pleurisy, is included in the classification criteria of the disease. Lupus pericarditis occurs predominantly in women in approximately 92% of cases, which is mainly due to the predominance of SLE in women [80].

The development of lupus pericarditis is usually accompanied by the appearance of pain behind the sternum and/or in the precardiac and/or epigastric region, which intensifies with breathing, bending the body forward, coughing, and swallowing. The pain is quite variable in nature, intensity, and duration. Cases of asymptomatic pericardial effusions are not uncommon. Effusions are usually mild, and although moderate-to-large effusions may occur, serious complications such as cardiac tamponade are rare in patients without renal failure. In renal failure, it is difficult to distinguish pericarditis caused by uremia from pericarditis associated with SLE. Pericardial fluid typically presents as an exudate containing LE cells, antinuclear antibodies, immune complexes, low complement levels, as well as a predominance of neutrophils, increased protein content, and normal or decreased glucose concentrations [81]. These characteristics are similar to those of bacterial pericarditis, so it is important to rule out infection [2]. With long-term SLE and recurrent pericarditis, massive adhesions develop. Pericardial friction rub is detected in 8–29% of patients with lupus pericarditis, which is associated with the short duration of this phenomenon. Instrumental methods, in particular ECG, play an important role in the diagnosis and assessment of the dynamics of lupus pericarditis. ECG changes similar to those with pericarditis of other origins are recorded in 52–75% of patients. In the acute phase, ST segment elevation is observed in all standard leads, as well as in aVL, aVF, and V2-V6. After a few days, the ST segment usually returns to the baseline, after which T wave flattening and inversion may be observed in those leads where ST segment elevation was previously detected.

Complications such as constrictive pericarditis or cardiac tamponade are extremely rare (<1%), tamponade occurs mainly in patients with drug-induced lupus [82, 83]. Typically, the development of tamponade is observed with high activity of SLE and more often in children and young adults. With cardiac tamponade, high pressure in the pericardial cavity prevents diastolic filling of the ventricles, which is clinically manifested by a condition characterized, on the one hand, by low cardiac output, and on the other, by increased central venous pressure. Although lupus myocarditis is uncommon in SLE, it is a serious complication due to its effects on the conduction system and cardiac function [84]. Subclinical manifestations of cardiac dysfunction detected by echocardiography are much more common than pronounced clinical manifestations [82]. In SLE, myocardial dysfunction usually has a multicomponent nature and is associated with a combination of ischemic heart disease, hypertension, renal failure, and valvular defects. Systolic dysfunction and wall damage caused by myocarditis are reversible thanks to immunosuppressive therapy and control of SLE activity.

Clinical manifestations of myocarditis in SLE are very diverse and nonspecific: fever, shortness of breath, chest pain, tachycardia, arrhythmia, edema. Clinically manifested myocarditis associated with dysfunction (systolic and/or diastolic) of the LV myocardium is called inflammatory cardiomyopathy [85]. Biopsy performed to diagnose cardiomyopathy in patients with SLE demonstrates small areas of myocardial fibrosis, rare interstitial mononuclear cell infiltrates, and myocyte necrosis with the deposits of immune complexes and complement [2]. In patients with myocarditis caused by lupus, ECG changes are varied and do not have specific signs. Among them are sinus tachycardia, which does not correspond to the degree of fever, nonspecific changes in the ST segment, various conduction disorders, including AV block up to complete transverse block. Excitability disorders may also occur, which may manifest as atrial fibrillation, atrial flutter, and ventricular tachyarrhythmias.

In lupus myocarditis, echocardiography reveals an increase in the size of the heart chambers, a decrease in the parameters of global LV systolic function, impaired LV diastolic function, segmental disturbances in the movement of the ventricular walls, an increase in the thickness of the LV walls, and the formation of intracardial thrombi [86].

Endocarditis in SLE, although considered a common cardiac manifestation, is much more commonly detected at autopsy than in clinical practice. Non-bacterial vegetations (Libman-Sacks) are found in 15–60% of patients during autopsy studies [2]. Libman-Sacks endocarditis is a non-infectious lesion that occurs concomitantly with SLE and antiphospholipid syndrome, affecting the heart valves, especially the mitral valve, causing stenosis or regurgitation [87]. Endocarditis develops due to the accumulation of sterile fibrin-containing vegetations on the heart valves, which is considered a manifestation of hypercoagulability associated with antiphospholipid antibodies [5]. In addition to autoantibodies to aPL, the presence of Libman-Sacks endocarditis is associated with neutrophil extracellular traps, which contain lupus autoantigens, such as histones and (ds)deoxyribonucleic acid DNA [88].

Echo-CG studies demonstrated a high prevalence of valvular abnormalities, which was observed in more than 50% of patients [89]. Valvular abnormalities manifest as clusters (classic Libman-Sacks vegetations), diffuse leaflet thickening, valvular regurgitation, and, infrequently, stenosis. Valvular regurgitation is more common than stenosis and is observed mainly in patients with thickened leaflets. Diffuse or focal thickening of the cusps of the mitral and aortic valves is observed. Vegetations are most common on the mitral valve, followed by the aortic valve. They are usually located on the atrial side of the mitral valve and the arterial side of the aortic valve. Complications of endocarditis are uncommon; vegetations rarely cause embolic phenomena. Valvular lesions may develop, resolve, persist, or worsen, regardless of disease activity. Fibrosis of the valve leaflets can lead to regurgitation associated with valvular insufficiency [90–93]. Valvular insufficiency and, less commonly, stenosis can contribute to the development of heart failure and arrhythmias, particularly atrial fibrillation, which is secondary to structural abnormalities in the atrium due to changes in pressure and hemodynamic compromise.

High cardiovascular risk in SLE is most often associated with the accelerated development of atherosclerosis, and less often with thrombosis, embolism, vasospasm, and coronaritis. Patients with SLE have twice as many atherosclerotic plaques in the coronary and femoral arteries compared with other RDs [94]. The peak prevalence of CVD associated with atherosclerosis in patients with SLE occurs at the age of 40–50 years, while in the general population it is at 65–74 years [95].

The progression of atherosclerosis in SLE is due not only to the increased frequency of all traditional risk factors, but also to the influence of specific factors associated with the disease itself: high activity, the presence of irreversible changes in the cardiovascular system, nephritis, neuropsychiatric disorders, positivity for aPL antibodies, a large cumulative dose of GC [96]. In SLE, immune complex deposition is thought to cause initial intimal damage, followed by accelerated development of atherosclerosis in patients with traditional risk factors [97].

6. Damage to the cardiovascular system in antiphospholipid syndrome

Antiphospholipid syndrome (APS) is a systemic autoimmune disease characterized by arterial, venous, or microvascular thrombosis, pregnancy morbidity, or nonthrombotic manifestations in patients with persistent antiphospholipid antibodies (aPL) [98].

Cardiac involvement in APS is multifactorial, with thrombosis as well as immune-mediated damage playing an important role [99]. The clinical manifestations of cardiac damage in APS are quite diverse against the background of both secondary and primary APS, while no significant differences in CVS damage were found in APS against the background of SLE and primary APS. The most common cardiac manifestations are valvulopathies, which can range from valvular thickening and nonbacterial thrombotic endocarditis (Libman-Sacks endocarditis) to regurgitation and severe valve damage, as well as CAD. Valvulopathies and CAD are the key cardiac manifestations in APS, while others less common include myocardial dysfunction, pulmonary hypertension (PH), and intracardiac thrombi. Older age is also a significant risk factor for cardiac manifestations in patients with primary APS [100].

- Damage to the CVS can be conditionally divided into pathology of the valvular apparatus of the heart, coronary arteries and myocardium:
    - Heart valve pathology:
    - Pseudo-infectious endocarditis with vegetations.
    - Insufficiency and/or stenosis of the mitral, aortic, and/or tricuspid valves.
    - Thickening, fibrosis, and calcification of valve leaflets.
- Damage to the coronary arteries:
    - acute MI;
    - unstable angina;
    - *restenosis after coronary artery bypass surgery;*
    - *restenosis after percutaneous transluminal coronary angioplasty.*

- Myocardial damage (cardiomyopathy).

  Other heart pathologies: intracardiac thrombi;

  - cerebrovascular disorders due to cardiogenic embolism;
  - arterial hypertension (AH);
  - pulmonary hypertension (PH).

According to the study, the frequency of CV pathology in patients with APS includes the following indicators: thickening or dysfunction of the heart valves—in 11.6% of patients, MI—in 5.5%, angina pectoris—in 2.7%, cardiomyopathy—in 2.9%, retrocoronary shunts—in 1.1%, and intracardiac thrombi—in 0.4% [5]. Heart valve damage in patients with antibodies to aPL in the blood deserves special attention. Valvular damage is the earliest and most common cardiac manifestation of APS [101, 102]. Valvular involvement may manifest as thickening, vegetation formation (also called Libman-Sacks endocarditis), and thrombotic masses on the valves. This pathology is often accompanied by arterial thrombosis and can be observed in the early stages of the disease, sometimes even before the onset of thrombosis or obstetric complications [103, 104]. Valvular lesions in APS are manifested by thickening of the valve by more than 3 mm, mainly in the proximal or middle part of the leaflets, as well as the presence of characteristic nodules on the atrial side of the mitral valve or the vascular side of the aortic valve. The mitral valve is most commonly affected, followed by the aortic valve [105–108].

aPL-associated damage to the heart valves is characterized by the presence of aPL in the blood (laboratory criterion for APS) in combination with detected damage (according to Echo-CG) and / or valve regurgitation, and / or stenosis of the mitral and / or aortic valve, and/or combined disorders.

Valve examination can be performed with/without transesophageal echocardiography.

Indicators of valve damage are:

- their thickening >3 mm;
- local thickening of the valve leaflet in the proximal or middle part;
- irregular nodules on the atrial surface of the mitral valve and/or on the ventricular surface of the aortic valve.

Despite the high incidence of heart valve involvement in APS, there is little information about the outcome of this pathology, except for the predominance of thromboembolic complications. APS rarely develops severe heart failure requiring surgical intervention [109, 110]. Information about the outcomes of valve replacement for APS is reduced mainly to the description of isolated clinical cases. A study by Bercun and colleagues [109] looked at 10 patients who underwent heart valve replacement over a 13-year period (7 mitral valves, 2 aortic valves, and 1 both mitral and aortic valves). Histomorphological analysis of these valves revealed uneven tissue thickening, varying degrees of destruction of the collagen layer and signs of chronic inflammation. In 9 of 12 cases, neovascularization was detected, and in 5, calcification of varying degrees was detected. Vegetations ranging from microscopic to round and warty were present in almost all cases. Histological examination showed that they consist of fibrin thrombi with minimal inflammatory infiltrate [111, 112].

Venous thromboembolism is one of the most common manifestations of APS with a very high risk of recurrence. APS-associated pulmonary embolism (PE) often leads to chronic thromboembolic PH, which is a common non-valvular cardiac manifestation of APS [113, 114]. The presence of PH alone in patients worsens the prognosis. Over time, right ventricular dilatation, isolated tricuspid valve regurgitation, and right ventricular failure may lead to secondary PH.

Various pathogenetic mechanisms, such as recurrent leg venous embolism, *in situ* thrombosis, embolization from the right heart chambers, and immune-mediated pulmonary vascular injury leading to endothelin-1-associated vascular remodeling, can lead to the development of chronic thromboembolic PH [115–118].

Diffuse cardiomyopathy in APS is less common. However, several studies describe a possible histopathological association between dilated cardiomyopathy and the presence of aPL antibodies in the absence of traditional risk factors [101, 102, 119–121]. In such cases, autopsy reveals widespread microthrombosis of small myocardial arterioles and microinfarction zones around the affected arterioles, which leads to significant myocardial necrosis. Histopathological studies did not reveal evidence of vasculitis, supporting the hypothesis that aPL causes thrombotic effects directly and not through damage to the vascular walls [122].

Cardiac surgery due to cardiovascular disease in APS is a serious problem. Unexplained thrombosis in cardiac patients should alert cardiac surgeons to APS for more aggressive antithrombotic therapy and careful follow-up monitoring.

7. Damage to the cardiovascular system in systemic scleroderma

Systemic scleroderma (SSc) is a progressive disease in which generalized damage to connective tissue occurs, and thickening and hardening of the skin with fibrosis and degenerative changes in internal organs happens.

Cardiac manifestations in SSc range from clinically asymptomatic manifestations to overt signs of CVD, which may be associated with increased morbidity and mortality. In most cases, cardiac damage in SSc occurs in the late stages of the disease, is usually asymptomatic, and is mainly detected during instrumental studies [14, 123]. In SSc, all three layers of the heart are affected: the myocardium in 83–90% of cases, the endocardium in 18–35%, and the pericardium in 13–21%. Multisegmental disturbances of myocardial perfusion both at rest and during exercise, myocardial fibrosis, and focal cardiosclerosis leading to progressive chronic heart failure are often observed [124].

Damage to the heart, especially the myocardium, occupies a leading place among the visceral signs of SSc both in frequency and significance, which is the main cause of sudden death in patients.

Cardiac pathology is based on the processes of fibrosis characteristic of the disease, damage to small vessels, and microcirculation disorders (with the main coronary arteries intact), leading to the development of ischemic zones and non-coronarogenic cardiosclerosis [5]. Ventricular myocardial fibrosis is a cause of LV systolic and diastolic dysfunction [125]. An enlarged heart, rhythm and conduction disturbances, infarct-like changes on the ECG, and a decrease in myocardial contractile function are often observed. Conduction abnormalities occur in 1/5 of patients with systemic sclerosis [126]. Often, cardiac conduction damage is manifested by prolongation of the P-Q interval, first-degree AV block, and disruption of intraventricular conduction, mainly in the form of blockade of the anterior branch of the left bundle branch [127]. Autopsy data have shown that the conduction system is relatively protected from the myocardial changes observed in patients with SSc, suggesting that conduction abnormalities are a consequence of myocardial damage rather than the conduction tissue itself [126].

Rhythm disturbances in CVD are manifested by polytopic supraventricular tachycardia and group extrasystoles. There is evidence in the literature that ventricular arrhythmia is an independent predictor of mortality, reflecting the severity of heart disease in patients with SSc [128]. In patients with SSc, supraventricular arrhythmias are less common (approximately 30%) than ventricular arrhythmias (67%) [129]. Atrial fibrillation has been found in approximately 1/3 of patients with diffuse SSc, particularly in patients with LV diastolic dysfunction associated with left atrial mechanical overload and elevated brain natriuretic peptide (BNP) levels [130]. Interestingly, the prevalence and severity of ventricular arrhythmias did not correlate with clinical symptoms and objective signs of the disease [131]. Daily ECG monitoring, Echo-CG, and myocardial scintigraphy contribute to the early diagnosis of heart damage, identification of perfusion defects, prognostically unfavorable forms of myocardial instability, and latent HF. Damage to the valve apparatus due to damage to the endocardium can lead to the formation of scleroderma, most often mitral heart disease. In some patients, mitral valve prolapse is detected [5].

Damage to the pericardium in the form of adhesive and rarely exudative pericarditis occurs in 70–80% of patients, usually asymptomatic [132, 133]. Echo-CG reveals thickening of the membrane and a small amount of fluid. It is extremely rare to find significant pericardial effusion, which can lead to cardiac tamponade. Morphologically, in some cases, a picture of serous-fibrinous pericarditis is revealed [5]. Clinical symptoms of heart damage can manifest themselves in the form of discomfort or prolonged dull pain in the pericardium, tachycardia and arrhythmia, and shortness of breath. Clinically apparent myocarditis is rare, which is in contrast to autopsy data, which often shows focal or diffuse myocardial fibrosis and linear necrosis of cardiomyocytes [124]. It is believed that myocardial damage in SSc is caused by microvascular abnormalities such as transient spasm of the coronary arteries, leading to repeated focal ischemia [134, 135].

Endocardial damage in systemic scleroderma is characterized by marginal sclerosis and shortening of the mitral valve chordae with the development of its prolapse and mitral regurgitation [124].

The development of pancarditis is possible—damage to the myocardium, pericardium, and endocardium with a characteristic predominance of fibrosis. Heart damage in this pathology in most cases develops gradually, over 4–6 years, but the process steadily progresses, leading to chronic heart failure. In 30% of cases, cardiac damage becomes the direct cause of death in patients with scleroderma [124].

Pulmonary arterial hypertension (PAH) is one of the most common cardiac complications of systemic sclerosis, with a prevalence of 12% [126, 136]. PAH associated with systemic sclerosis has a high mortality rate, with a median survival of only 3 years [137]. PAH is a late complication of this pathology, occurring approximately 20 years after the onset of the disease. PAH associated with systemic sclerosis is initially indolent with few symptoms until right ventricular function deteriorates. In the early stages of the disease, patients may experience symptoms of fatigue, dizziness, and shortness of breath on exertion [137]. As the disease progresses, they typically experience progressive dyspnea and may experience syncope on exertion, tachycardia, and chest pain. Physical examination reveals increased right ventricular pressure and right ventricular failure; tricuspid regurgitation murmur; jugular venous dilatation; and lower extremity edema [138].

8. Damage to the cardiovascular system in dermatomyositis/polymyositis

Dermatomyositis (DM) and polymyositis (PM) are rare idiopathic inflammatory myopathies (IIMs) clinically characterized by symmetrical proximal muscle weakness due to inflammatory cell infiltrates in skeletal muscle and involvement of the endomysial in PM or perimysial layers of skeletal muscle in DM [49]. An increasing number of studies show that the risk of CVD in patients with IIM is much higher than in the general population [139]. In clinical studies, the incidence of cardiac injury in DM varies widely (from 9 to 72%) [140]. Among patients with IIM, cardiovascular disease is the leading cause of mortality. Previous studies have found that about 10–20% of patient deaths can be associated with CV events, such as ischemic heart disease, heart failure, and myocarditis with the development of complete heart block [139, 141]. It has been found that death due to CVDs most often occurs an average of 5 years after the main course of the disease [142].

According to the EuroMyositis registry, clinically significant cardiac damage in the form of pericarditis, myocarditis, various arrhythmias, and sinus tachycardia was detected in 9% of patients with PM/DM [143].

Patients with inflammatory myopathies may experience myocardial damage, which is an unfavorable prognostic factor and one of the most common causes of patient mortality [142, 144]. However, its recognition in clinical practice is often difficult, partly because the process is slow, insidious, and initially asymptomatic [145]. One of the most commonly reported clinical cardiac manifestations in PM/DM is congestive HF, which can occur due to myocarditis and is accompanied by serious complications such as pulmonary edema, tachyarrhythmias, or sudden cardiac death [146]. Myocarditis can also lead to LV dysfunction and restrictive cardiomyopathy. Other pathophysiological mechanisms contributing to LV diastolic dysfunction include increased chamber stiffness due to ongoing fibrotic transformation of the myocardium, as well as possible disturbances in calcium regulation, which ultimately leads to clinically significant symptomatic HF [147]. Symptoms of myocarditis in MI include chest pain, fatigue, shortness of breath, palpitations, and fever [148].

In MD/PM, myocarditis may manifest on the ECG as a variety of rhythm and conduction abnormalities, including atrial and ventricular arrhythmias, bundle branch block, AV block, prolonged PR interval, ventricular premature beats, left atrial abnormalities, abnormal Q waves, and nonspecific ST segment changes. In some cases, patients have required permanent pacemakers, and there have been cases where conduction abnormalities were fatal [149, 150]. Cases of dilated cardiomyopathy in patients with IIM have also been described. Most often, echocardiography reveals diastolic dysfunction, decreased LV contractile function, and mitral valve prolapse [139, 151]. Pericarditis, pericardial effusion, and cardiac tamponade are rare in patients with IIM. However, with high activity of clinical and laboratory parameters, constrictive pericarditis can develop, although it is not typical for patients with inflammatory myopathies and its frequency is approximately 10% [125, 150].

In addition to inflammatory myocardial diseases, cardiovascular lesions in patients with DM/PM may be associated with vascular changes in the heart.

Cases of vasculitis, small vessel smooth muscle cell proliferation, medial sclerosis, and cardiac microvascular disease with vasospasm resulting in decreased capillary blood flow have been reported [152, 153]. This so-called small vessel disease is characterized by narrowing of the lumen due to smooth muscle hyperplasia with minimal or absent intimal proliferation, which, in turn, can manifest itself with clinical symptoms such as arrhythmia and angina pectoris [150]. It should be noted that symptoms of heart damage can be associated both with coronary atherosclerosis and with the use of high doses of GCs (steroid myocardial dystrophy). In patients with inflammatory myopathies, the risk of developing coronary artery disease was 2.19 times higher compared to individuals without this pathology [154, 155]. Inflammatory myopathies, like other chronic inflammatory diseases, contribute to the development of atherosclerosis. Inflammatory cytokines, oxidative stress, and endothelial cell activation enhance vasculopathy, and chronic endothelial dysfunction and systemic inflammation may accelerate the development of atherosclerosis in patients with DM [156–158]. Moreover, systemic inflammation associated with autoimmune disease may also promote hypercoagulability, which is another important predisposing risk factor for the development of CAD [141]. In addition, imbalance of autoimmune cells and dysregulation of the immune system in patients with CAD lead to abnormal proliferation of B lymphocytes and their differentiation into plasma cells and the production of higher levels of myositis-associated autoantibodies, which have a direct link to cardiac damage [159]. It is well known that traditional CVD risk factors such as hypertension, diabetes mellitus, and dyslipidemia were more prevalent in patients with IIM compared with the general population, and they may influence the progression of atherosclerosis by inducing an inflammatory response. Numerous studies have demonstrated that the combination of traditional CV risk factors and the use of GCs increase the total risk of developing CHD in patients with IIM [160, 161].

9. Damage to the cardiovascular system in systemic vasculitis

Systemic vasculitis (SV) is a heterogeneous group of diseases, the main morphological feature of which is generalized damage to the vascular wall (arteries, veins, and capillaries of various sizes) with secondary involvement of the corresponding organs and tissues in the pathological process [49]. Most types of vasculitis are systemic in nature and manifest themselves with a varied clinical picture, which requires a multidisciplinary approach. According to the etiology, the causes of SV may be different; vasculitis can be either an independent disease or a secondary condition caused by other autoimmune diseases, and may also be associated with other triggers such as medications, infections, or malignancies [162]. Most cases of coronary vasculitis occur as part of systemic (primary) vasculitides, which are classified according to the type and size of vessels involved, as well as the cellular component involved in tissue infiltration. According to the classifications of the American College of Rheumatology and the International Consensus Conference in Chapel Hill, the following categories of vasculitis are distinguished [163]:

- Vasculitis of large vessels: Giant cell (temporal) arteritis, Takayasu's arteritis (AT);
- Vasculitis of medium-sized vessels: Polyarteritis nodosa (PAN), Kawasaki disease (KD);
- Small vessel vasculitis:

Vasculitis associated with antineutrophil cytoplasmic antibodies (ANCA-associated vasculitis): granulomatosis with polyangiitis (Wegener's), eosinophilic granulomatosis with polyangiitis (Churgia-Stross), microscopic polyangiitis

- Immune complex vasculitis of small vessels: IgA vasculitis (Schönlein-Henoch), essential cryoglobulinemic vasculitis, cutaneous leukocytoclastic angiitis

- Variable vasculitis: Behçet's disease, Cogan syndrome.

Clinically significant cardiac lesions are rare in SV but can pose a serious threat to life [164]. Since many symptoms of cardiovascular disease may not appear in the initial stages of the disease, it is necessary to regularly monitor such patients.

The relationship between systemic vasculitis and CVD can be twofold:

1. direct damage to the heart, either due to the disease itself or treatment associated mainly with the use of GCs;

2. caused by inflammation and endothelial dysfunction [165].

Regarding inflammation in the myocardium and small vessels, it can contribute to cardiac ischemia and myocardial remodeling. This occurs under the influence of various inflammatory cytokines, such as IL-6, IL-17, and α-TNF, which influences cardiac tissue [166]. With vasculitis, all tissues of the heart can be affected—from the myocardium to the epicardium, endocardium, conduction system, and coronary arteries. However, CV manifestations caused by vasculitis should be distinguished from those that may occur during GC therapy and immunosuppressants [167].

Myocarditis caused by vasculitis varies widely from 25 to 70% of cases. It is caused by necrotizing vasculitis, the presence of granulomas, or fibrosis. In eosinophilic granulomatous polyangiitis (EGPA), eosinophil infiltration is considered a possible cause, and cardiac magnetic resonance imaging (MRI) is important for early detection of myocardial inflammation, especially in patients with atypical presentation [168]. In Kawasaki disease, myocarditis is detected in almost 50% of patients [169].

Pericardial involvement occurs in 22% of patients with EGPA, 8% of patients with Wegener's granulomatosis, and 27% of patients with polyarteritis nodosa and, if untreated, can lead to the development of constrictive pericarditis [164].

Endocardial involvement is quite rare, but in some cases, it can lead to valve deformation. Arrhythmias (mainly supraventricular), AV block, or bundle branch block may also result from myocarditis, ischemia, or heart failure [164]. With vasculitis, pulmonary hypertension is one of the rare complications. Damage to the coronary arteries can be identified in connection with coronary arteritis, which leads to the formation of thrombosis, dissection and aortic stenosis and often to MI. This complication is observed in 50% of patients with polyarteritis nodosa. It is also widespread in Kawasaki disease, occurring in 20% of untreated cases, and can be easily diagnosed by echocardiography and MRI [169]. MRI also helps to assess the condition of the coronary arteries and promptly detect MI [170].

9.1 Damage to the cardiovascular system in giant cell arteritis

Giant cell arteritis (GCA), temporal angiitis, and Horton's disease are rare forms of systemic vasculitis affecting large vessels. Giant cell arteritis (GCA) mainly affects people over 50 years of age and is most common among people aged 70 to 80 years [171]. Approximately 27–56% of GCA cases have a common association and pathogenetic roots with polymyalgia rheumatica (PM) [172]. This disease has a number of similarities with Takayasu's arteritis. In both GCA and AT, the aorta and its main branches are involved and are histopathologically indistinguishable from each other. Although the prevalence of coronary artery disease in GCA is considered relatively low [173], large cohort studies have shown that patients with GCA are at greater risk of developing vascular events; in particular, the incidence of acute myocardial infarction is two times higher than in patients without it, especially in early time period after diagnosis [174]. GCA, often granulomatous, usually affects the aorta and/or its major branches, including the branches of the vertebral and carotid arteries.

The risk of death from CVD is higher in patients with GCA than in the general population [175, 176]. Li et al. found that patients with GCA had a higher risk of vascular events, which included peripheral vascular disease, stroke, venous thromboembolism, and aortic dissection and aneurysm [177].

GCA is characterized by damage to the aorta and its branches, and in particular the brachiocephalic trunk, superficial temporal, carotid, subclavian, and femoral arteries [178]. Cardiac injury in GCA occurs in less than 5% of cases and includes aortic regurgitation due to aortic aneurysm, epicardial coronary artery disease (coronaritis), pericarditis, and myocarditis [179–181]. Typical clinical signs of GCA include headache, predominantly in the temporal region, low-grade fever, weight loss of more than 2 kg, night sweats, fatigue, blurred vision, symptoms of polymyalgia rheumatica, and other systemic manifestations. Physical examination reveals pain sensitivity, thickening of the superficial temporal arteries with or without decreased pulsation, weakened pulse, and decreased blood pressure (BP) in the upper extremities [182]. The disease does not affect life expectancy, except in those patients who have aortic dissection.

9.2 Damage to the cardiovascular system in Takayasu arteritis

Takayasu arteritis (AT), called pulseless disease, is an immunoinflammatory disease that causes damage to the aorta and its major vessels, particularly the renal, carotid, and subclavian arteries [183].

AT most often affects young women and affects large vessels, including the aortic arch, its proximal branches, and the pulmonary arteries. A peculiar lesion of the coronary bed has been established in patients with AT—in almost 90% of cases, damage to the mouth of the coronary vessels was noted [184]. In AT, the pathological process involves predominantly the proximal segments of the coronary arteries, while the distal sections remain undamaged. These complications arise from coronaritis associated with disease activity. In some cases, the disease may manifest as isolated coronary artery stenosis, leading to clinical manifestations of acute coronary syndrome. This onset of the disease is more often observed in men with nonspecific aortoarteritis [185]. Most patients also suffer from subclavian stenosis, resulting in weakened or absent radial pulses [186]. Aortic regurgitation associated with the enlargement of the aortic root is a fairly common complication in patients with AT, occurring in 7–11% of cases [184, 187].

A study by Ren et al., which included 103 patients with AT, found that 64% had valvular insufficiency, 62% of patients had aortic regurgitation, 61% had mitral valve disease, 54.6% had tricuspid valve disease, and 6.1% have pulmonary insufficiency [188]. Valvular damage in patients with AT can lead to myocardial remodeling, impaired LV function, and increased afterload, which can ultimately cause HF, which becomes the leading cause of death among patients with this disease [189]. In patients with AT, coronary artery involvement is limited [184]. The underlying mechanism of this lesion involves inflammatory-induced intimal proliferation and subsequent fibrous vasoconstriction. Narrowing of the coronary arteries, caused by inflammation of the aorta or coronary vessels, occurs in 10–45% of patients and can lead to the development of angina, which has serious consequences. Patients often improve with immunosuppressive therapy [190]. Inflammation that occurs in the artery wall can lead to narrowing of the lumen of the vessel and destruction of the elastic lamina, causing an aortic aneurysm.

Arterial hypertension in AT, according to various studies, occurs in 35–50% of cases, which is renovascular and is caused by the involvement of the renal arteries and/or the development of coarctation of the aorta [191]. The central nature of hypertension associated with ischemia of the vasomotor center due to carotid vasculitis is also possible. As a result of hypertension, coronaritis, and aortic regurgitation, patients often develop HF. Coronaritis can lead to myocardial hibernation with a diffuse decrease in contractility, as well as to MI with local damage to myocardial tissue [185]. Analyzing pathological changes in the heart with vasculitis of large vessels, it should be noted that the main complications in these patients are lesions of the large coronary arteries, which lead to clinical manifestations in the form of angina, MI, and HF.

9.3 Damages of the cardiovascular system in polyarteritis nodosa

Polyarteritis nodosa (PAN) is a disease from the group of systemic necrotizing vasculitis with predominant involvement of medium and small arteries with the formation of aneurysms and secondary damage to organs and systems [185].

Cardiovascular manifestations of PAN include coronary artery disease, cardiomyopathy associated with vasculitis, myocarditis, and myocardial ischemia. In a study by Schrader et al., 50% of patients with PAN had evidence of coronary arteritis at autopsy [192]. Most often, coronary artery aneurysms occur in the proximal and central segments of the right coronary artery, and then the initial segments of the left anterior descending and left circumflex arteries [193]. The most common coronary angiographic finding in PAN is the development of multiple aneurysms [194]. One of the common manifestations of CV complications in vasculitis is hypertension, usually associated with damage to the renal arteries. Damage to the coronary vessels is more often complicated by MI, including its painless form, even in the absence of atherosclerotic damage. Cases of transmural MI without angiographic signs of coronary artery damage have also been described, indicating a significant role of vasospasm against the background of the inflammatory process [195].

Congestive HF may be a complication of hypertension or result from myocardial infarction caused by vasculitis. In the vast majority of patients, hypertension is characterized by consistently high blood pressure levels, and in approximately 1/3 of cases, the disease occurs in a malignant form. A characteristic feature of hypertension in PAN is a sharp increase in blood pressure, which occurs against the background of widespread damage to the walls of peripheral vessels due to an active inflammatory process or due to vascular sclerosis with the formation of multiple aneurysms. The rapid development of high hypertension limits the ability of target organs to adapt to a sharp increase in pressure. With the progression of vasculitis, hypertension leads to dilatation of the cavities of the heart, subsequently causing chronic heart failure, and plays an important role in the development of acute hemorrhagic cerebrovascular accidents [185].

The prognosis in some cases is determined by the severity and duration of hypertension. Prognostic studies in PAN have found that patients with cardiac lesions have lower survival rates. Thus, the five-year survival rate among patients with PAN who have cardiac or renal lesions is 38%, while among patients without such lesions, this figure reaches 78% [196].

9.4 Damages of the cardiovascular system in Kawasaki disease

Kawasaki disease (KD) is a systemic medium-vessel vasculitis in children, primarily affecting infants and children under 5 years of age [197]. Cardiovascular complications are a major cause of morbidity and are responsible for virtually all deaths due to coronary vasculitis associated with hypercoagulability, leading to MI and sudden death [198]. The following cardiovascular pathologies occur in patients with KD: coronary artery aneurysms, myocarditis, pericarditis with pericardial effusion and cardiac tamponade, endocarditis, cardiomyopathy, and valvular lesions [199].

Myocarditis is the most common non-coronary complication of KD and is observed in 50–70% of patients in the acute phase [198, 200]. Myocarditis in KD often results from acute or subacute inflammation of the myocardial interstitial tissue and is usually concentrated around the coronary vessels. Myocardial inflammation peaks by the 10th day of illness and gradually subsides by the end of the 3rd week, in contrast to coronary vasculitis and coronary artery anomalies, which usually develop after the 10th day of illness. At this stage, inflammation of the small myocardial arteries is observed, including perivasculitis [201, 202].

Clinically, myocarditis in KD may manifest as unexplained tachycardia, congestive heart failure, hemodynamic instability, and arrhythmias [203, 204].

Pericarditis with pericardial effusion is also common in the acute phase of the disease, affecting approximately 25% of patients [198]. Valvular lesions occur in approximately 1% of patients and may occur due to papillary muscle dysfunction, rupture of chordae tendineae, or valvulitis, leading to the development of mitral regurgitation [198, 205]. Slight dilatation of the aortic root is also common in the acute phase and may be associated with aortic regurgitation [206].

Coronary artery aneurysms are one of the main complications of KD, which can develop in 15–25% of untreated children, usually in the subacute phase, classified as small (internal diameter < 5 mm), medium (5–8 mm), or giant (>8 mm) [200, 205, 207]. Aneurysms are often multiple and occur in the proximal parts and at bifurcations of the coronary arteries [208]. Coronary artery lesions can progress differently: Aneurysms in the right coronary artery are more prone to massive thrombosis, while aneurysms in the left coronary artery are more prone to progressive focal stenosis. Aneurysm size is a prognostic factor: Giant aneurysms (>8 mm) are associated with a higher risk of rupture, thrombosis, and stenosis, which can lead to MI and death [209]. Giant aneurysms usually do not regress.

9.5 Damage to the cardiovascular system in ANCA-associated vasculitis

ANCA-associated vasculitis is a systemic necrotizing vasculitis of small vessels associated with the production of antineutrophil cytoplasmic antibodies (ANCA) that are represented in most cases by three nosological forms: granulomatosis with polyangiitis (GPA), eosinophilic granulomatosis with polyangiitis (EGPA), and microscopic polyangiitis (MPA) [210].

One of the main complications and causes of mortality in patients with ANCA-associated vasculitis, especially in the active phase of the disease, are lesions of the cardiovascular system [211, 212]. The pathogenesis of ANCA-associated vasculitis is based on systemic inflammation, which leads to platelet activation and endothelial dysfunction, which, in turn, increases the risk of not only CV events, but also venous thrombotic complications, including pulmonary embolism and deep venous thromboembolism, thrombosis, most of which occur during treatment of active disease, with an incidence of 8–10% [211, 213]. Involvement of the cardiovascular system in ANCA-associated vasculitis is quite common and can be the result of various mechanisms, mainly both direct involvement of the heart in the process of vasculitis and increased susceptibility to coronary artery disease [214]. Cardiac damage is a severe complication that typically occurs in a significant proportion of patients with EGPA, but only in a small number of patients with GPA and MPA [215–217]. It is no coincidence that cardiac involvement has been identified as an independent predictor of all-cause and CV mortality in patients with EGPA and GPA [215, 218, 219]. Moreover, the presence of cardiac symptoms at initial examination further increases the risk of death in these patients.

The incidence of cardiac damage in EGPA varies significantly, ranging from 15–55%, being the main cause of death in these patients [2]. Among CV complications, eosinophilic myocarditis is the most common, but restrictive or dilated cardiomyopathy, pericarditis, coronaritis, valvular defects, arrhythmias, elevated troponin-1 levels, LV dysfunction, and intracardiac thrombosis may also occur [220]. Myocardial damage may occur due to extensive tissue infiltration leading to fibrosis and/or due to coronary or small vessel vasculitis and subsequent myocardial ischemia. Most often, biopsy reveals eosinophilic infiltrates in tissues, and granulomas can also be found in the epicardium and myocardium. Patients may rapidly develop myocardial dysfunction with HF, which may be reversible with timely and aggressive treatment. Congestive HF is observed in 15–30% of cases and, as a rule, is quite severe [2]. The clinical phenotype of EGPA is highly variable, but in general, depending on the presence of ANCA, it can be divided into two main subgroups.

In ANCA-negative patients, eosinophilic manifestations predominate, such as pulmonary infiltrates, cardiac involvement, and gastrointestinal disease, while in ANCA-positive patients, vasculitic manifestations such as glomerulonephritis, purpura, and peripheral neuropathy are more common [221, 222]. Therefore, ANCA status may serve as an important prognostic factor for the development of cardiac complications and survival assessment [223]. Over the past decades, the prognosis for patients with EGPA has improved significantly, with 10-year survival increasing from 81 to 92% [224, 225]. It should be noted that up to 50% of deaths associated with this disease are due to cardiac damage [215, 226].

Clinically significant cardiac damage is rare in GPA. Thus, among North American patients with GPA followed for more than 8 years, the incidence of cardiac symptoms was 3.3% [227]. Cardiac lesions such as pericardial effusion, cardiomyopathy, heart failure, conduction defects, and valvular disease have been described in patients with GPA and MPA, with pericarditis and supraventricular arrhythmias being the most common cardiac manifestations, occurring in 1 to 6% of patients.

Intracardiac thrombosis is a rare event, occurring in less than 1% of patients [181, 228]. The results of the studies showed that 21% of patients with GPA had valve lesions (aortic valve—in 57.1%, mitral valve—in 14.3%), which manifested themselves in the form of chronic necrotic granulomas, severe lymphoplasmacytic inflammation, fibrous changes with hyalinosis, and microscopic neutrophilic abscesses involving the central annulus fibrosus [229]. Arrhythmias associated with GPA, although rare, include atrial tachycardia, fibrillation, and flutter [230]. Several cases of atrioventricular block have also been noted [231, 232].

In rare cases, GPA causes coronaritis, which can lead to severe cardiomyopathy. Coronary vasculitis does not have specific clinical manifestations, but it must be taken into account that they can lead to myocardial ischemia and acute HF [233]. The prevalence of HF in MPA ranges from 6.8 to 17.6%. A study in a Dutch population found a high prevalence of coronary ectasia and aneurysm among patients with MPA, suggesting that coronaritis with necrotic changes and wall weakening may be an integral component of MPA, contributing to increased CV risk in these patients [234].

Although overt clinical symptoms are rare, recent studies indicate that subclinical forms may be much more common and often go undetected.

9.6 Damage to the cardiovascular system in Behçet's disease

Behçet's disease (BD) is a systemic vasculitis characterized by damage to blood vessels of any type and caliber, manifested by multisystem damage to internal organs and systems. Cardiac pathology is one of the most severe manifestations of BD, which is associated with a poor prognosis [235] and is a major cause of morbidity and approximately 20% of mortality in such patients [236]. The prevalence of CV lesions in BD ranges from 7 to 46%, with venous lesions (29%) being more common than arterial lesions (8–18%) [237].

Heart pathology is more often diagnosed in young men (86.5% of cases). Some of the most common symptoms of heart damage are pericarditis, myocarditis, rhythm disturbances, including ventricular tachycardia, and cardiac conduction, ischemic, non-ischemic, or inflammatory cardiomyopathy, manifested by systolic and/or diastolic dysfunction of the LV, endocarditis with the development of valve insufficiency (aortic valve insufficiency, less commonly mitral regurgitation), endomyocardial fibrosis, intracardiac thrombosis, coronaritis with or without MI, congestive heart failure, cardiac aneurysms, stenoses of the coronary arteries, or sinus of Valsalva [238, 239].

In patients with BD, MI is observed in 17% of cases, despite the absence of visible changes in the coronary arteries on angiography. This is associated with thickening of the vascular intima, which contributes to the development of MI.

It is believed that microvascular dysfunction associated with focal fibrinoid deposition and fibroblast proliferation in small coronary arteries may be responsible for myocardial ischemia and subsequent endomyocardial fibrosis and lead to coronary events in these patients [240]. In BD, aneurysms, stenoses, and occlusions of the coronary arteries are the most common causes of CAD, but sometimes intact coronary aneurysms are observed in patients with MI. Although coronary aneurysms are rare in patients with BD, they most often present as an acute coronary syndrome, although in some cases they may be asymptomatic [241]. A retrospective study by Vural et al. showed an increased prevalence of angina (31%), acute coronary syndrome (8%), and arrhythmias (8%) in patients with BD [242]. Coronary artery aneurysms predominantly form in their proximal sections and can be either single or multiple [243, 244]. In BD, the formation of aneurysms of the interatrial septum is rarely observed; however, aneurysms of the sinus of Valsalva can develop, which occur in the active phase of BD and are more often diagnosed after their rupture [245]. There is information in the literature about a decrease in the size of aneurysms and their resolution after immunosuppressive therapy [239].

Coronary artery disease is a rare but potentially dangerous complication of BD [244], and can manifest as angina (both stable and unstable), arrhythmias, myocardial infarction, and even sudden cardiac death [238, 244]. The anterior interventricular branches of the left and right coronary arteries are most often affected, followed by the circumflex branch and trunk of the left coronary artery.

Patients with BD who exhibit CVS lesions generally have a poor prognosis. However, the situation may improve with the use of oral anticoagulants, immunosuppressive drugs, and colchicine. An analysis of survival in BD at 5 years showed that in patients with cardiac involvement it was 83.6%, while in those without cardiac involvement it was 95.8% ($p = 0.03$) [243].

10. Damage to the cardiovascular system due to gout

An equally important pathology predisposing to CVD is gout, the prevalence of which tends to increase worldwide [246].

Gout is an inflammatory crystal arthropathy characterized by hyperuricemia and intra-articular deposition of monosodium urate crystals [247]. Both gout and subclinical hyperuricemia are associated with adverse CV outcomes. Hyperuricemia, as a cardinal sign of gout, is associated with endothelial dysfunction and increases the incidence of both coronary artery disease and stroke [248]. According to some authors, almost half of patients with gout have coronary artery disease, and ECG signs of damage to the myocardium and coronary vessels are more common in chronic gout and are more pronounced. Patients have hidden coronary insufficiency and a decrease in the functional capacity of the myocardium.

Gout is known to be associated with systemic inflammation. The most important among the markers of systemic inflammation is C-reactive protein (CRP), an increased level of which is considered as a predictor of an increased risk of developing CVD both in the population and in RDs [249, 250]. CRP levels often increase in both acute gouty arthritis and chronic gout.

According to two large prospective studies, indicators of chronic inflammation, such as high CRP levels and arthritis severity, were even more significant in predicting all-cause and CV mortality than traditional risk factors for CAD [251].

Metabolic syndrome (MS) is a combination of various metabolic disorders, each of which is an independent risk factor for CVD. The frequency of MS in patients with gout was three times higher than in the general population—62.8% in patients with gout and 25.4% without this disease [252]. Hyperuricemia has a close relationship with various components of MS, especially with hypertension, which is detected in 20–50% of patients with gout, while gouty arthritis is detected among 20–40% of patients with hypertension [253]. With gout, diastolic and mean blood pressure levels increase to a greater extent. The combination of hypertension aggravates the course of each of these conditions. On the one hand, the presence of hypertension causes disruption of microcirculation, and, as a consequence, tissue ischemia, which can lead to the development of hyperuricemia due to two mechanisms: the breakdown of ATP into adenine and xanthine and increased production of xanthine oxidase, as well as excessive formation of lactate, which blocks secretion urate in the renal tubules. On the other hand, hypertension leads to a decrease in renal blood flow and stimulation of urate reabsorption [243]. Patients with a combination of gout and hypertension, compared to patients without it, are characterized by a more severe course of gout and a relatively high concentration of uric acid in the blood. In patients with gout and hypertension, there is a direct correlation between uric acid levels and the stage and severity of hypertension [244].

There is evidence that hyperuricemia, even in the absence of gout, can cause an increase in blood pressure, which is associated with the following mechanisms: direct stimulation of the renin-angiotensin system in the kidneys; inhibition of vascular synthesis of NO, which is a potential vasodilator; stimulating the proliferation of smooth muscle cells in the vascular wall, thereby increasing vasoconstriction; and kidney damage (interstitial nephritis or tubular damage), indirectly leading to the development of hypertension [245, 246].

Studies have shown that in hyperuricemia and hypertension, an increase in blood uric acid levels of 1 mg/dL is associated with an increase in the incidence of CVD by 10%, which is equivalent to an increase in systolic blood pressure (SBP) of 10 mmHg. Art. or an increase in cholesterol levels of 20 mg/dL [247]. For a more detailed analysis of the relationship between uric acid and CV risk in various populations, numerous studies have been conducted, which have revealed that hyperuricemia is a risk factor not only for hypertension and diabetes, but also for heart disease, atrial fibrillation, MI, HF, cerebrovascular events, and chronic kidney disease [248–250]. A systematic review and meta-analysis found a significant positive association between uric acid levels and the risk of CV mortality, with a stronger association found in women compared to men [251]. In addition, hyperuricemia plays a significant role in the progression of coronary atherosclerosis, and in men suffering from gout, it is detected two times more often than in persons without it. In patients with gout, type IV hyperlipoproteinemia predominates, with an increase in the β-fraction of lipoproteins, triglycerides, and total cholesterol. Under conditions of hyperuricemia, peroxidation of low-density lipoproteins (LDL) increases and the production of free radicals increases, which leads to increased oxidative stress and may contribute to increased atherosclerotic processes. The influence of uric acid on the processes of platelet adhesion and aggregation, the damaging effect of xanthine oxide on the endothelium, and increased production of cytokines (α-TNF, a marker of nonspecific inflammation), which, along with other factors, can increase the risk of atherothrombosis, including coronary artery thrombosis, are also considered [252]. Research shows that elevated uric acid levels are closely associated with the development of carotid atherosclerosis, stroke, preeclampsia, and vascular dementia [249]. In addition, hyperuricemia activates the renin-angiotensin system, reduces the activity of nitric oxide synthesis, stimulates the proliferation of smooth muscle cells of blood vessels, and contributes to the development of insulin resistance [253]. Metabolic disorders that occur in gout due to hyperuricemia, such as obesity, lipid, and carbohydrate metabolism disorders, are closely related to atherosclerosis and are considered independent risk factors for CVD. In 2000, WHO included gout in the list of diseases that are closely associated with obesity, such as hypertension, coronary atherosclerosis, and type 2 diabetes. Gout can be considered a metabolic disease, which is confirmed by numerous studies that have revealed a high prevalence of comorbid pathology, in particular CVD, among patients with gouty arthritis. This fact undoubtedly obliges us to regard gout as a general medical problem, which is characterized by a high risk of fatal CV events associated with atherosclerosis.

11. Conclusion

Thus, it should be noted that in almost all RDs, lesions of the cardiovascular system are observed, which are associated primarily with systemic inflammation, damaging not only all the membranes of the heart (endocardium, myocardium, pericardium), but also the coronary vessels. As a result, complications are identified in the form of multiple valve defects, cardiac rhythm, and conduction disturbances, as well as various clinical manifestations of coronary artery disease. CVS lesions can serve as a marker reflecting the severity and mortality rate in this category of patients.

Acknowledgements

The authors acknowledge the use of generative artificial intelligence bot (ChatGPT) to polish the language of the manuscript and avoid any possible grammatical mistakes.

Conflict of interest

The authors have declared that there is no conflict of interest.

Author details

Fidan Natig Gasimova[1], Gulustan Hamid Babayeva[1*], Gulnara Sadig Nur-Mammadova[1], Leman Kamaladdin Babayeva[2], Guliyeva Ilkana Makhaddin[3], Vusala Niyat Atakishiyeva[4], Maghrur Yashar Mammadov[5] and Parviz Gunduz Niftiyev[6]

1 Department of Therapy, Azerbaijan State Advanced Training Institute for Doctors named after A. Aliyev, Baku, Azerbaijan

2 Department of Therapy, Absheron Central Hospital, Baku, Azerbaijan

3 City Polyclinic No. 7, Baku, Azerbaijan

4 Department of Therapy, Binagadi Medical Centre, Baku, Azerbaijan

5 Department of Rheumatology, General Clinical Hospital of the Ministry of Defense of Azerbaijan, Baku, Azerbaijan

6 Department of Cardiology, West Hospital, Baku, Azerbaijan

*Address all correspondence to: ghbabayeva@gmail.com

References

[1] Popkova TV, Novikova DS, Nasonov EL. Cardiovascular diseases in rheumatoid arthritis: New data. Scientific and Practical Rheumatology. 2016;**54**(2):122-128. DOI: 10.14412/1995-4484-2016-122-128

[2] Villa-Forte A, Mandell BF. Cardiovascular disorders and rheumatic disease. Revista Española de Cardiología. 2011;**64**(9):809-817. DOI: 10.1016/j.rec.2011.05.013

[3] Dhawan SS, Quyyumi AA. Rheumatoid arthritis and cardiovascular disease. Current Atherosclerosis Reports. 2008;**10**(2):128-133. DOI: 10.1007/s11883-008-0019-x

[4] Rebrov AP. Rheumatoid arthritis and heart damage - Is it really relevant? Emergency Cardiology and Cardiovascular Risks. 2021;**5**(2):c.1406-c.1410. DOI: 10.51922/2616-633X.2021.5.2.1406

[5] Badokin VV. Rheumatology. Clinical Lectures. Publishing House LitTerra; 2014. p. 592

[6] Gupta A, Fomberstein B. Evaluating cardiovascular risk in rheumatoid arthritis. Journal of Musculoskeletal Medicine. 2009;**26**(8):481-494

[7] Ralston SH, Penman ID, Strachan MWJ, Hobson R. Davidson's Principles and Practice of Medicine. 23rd ed. Elsevier; 2021. p. 544 c

[8] Popkova TV, Novikova DS, Nasonov EL. Cardiovascular risk factors in rheumatic diseases: Connection with inflammation. Research Institute of Rheumatology RAMS. 2010;**12**(2):112-118. Available from: https.consilium.orscience.ru/2075-1753/article/view/93176

[9] Avalos I, Rho YH, Chung CP, et al. Atherosclerosis in rheumatoid arthritis and systemic lupus erythematosus. Clinical and Experimental Rheumatology. 2008;**26**(Suppl. 51):5-13

[10] Dessein PH, Joffe BI. When is a patient with rheumatoid arthritis at risk for cardiovascular disease? The Journal of Rheumatology. 2006;**33**:201-203

[11] Ali RA, Halabi H, Almoallim H. Cardiovascular diseases and rheumatology. In: Skills in Rheumatology. Singapore: Springer; 2021. DOI: 10.1007/978-981-15-8323-0_16

[12] DeMizio DJ, Geraldino-Pardilla LB. Autoimmunity and inflammation link to cardiovascular disease risk in rheumatoid arthritis. Rheumatology and Therapy. 2020;**7**(1):19-33. DOI: 10.1007/s40744-019-00189-0

[13] Corrao S, Messina S, Pistone G, et al. Heart involvement in rheumatoid arthritis: Systematic review and meta-analysis. International Journal of Cardiology. 2013;**167**(5):2031-2038. DOI: 10.1016/j.ijcard.2012.05.057

[14] West S. Rheumatology Secrets. In: Kolfenbach J, editor. 4th ed. Elsevier; 2019. p. 784. ISBN: 9780323641869

[15] Levy PY, Corey R, Berger P, Habib G, et al. Etiologic diagnosis of 204 pericardial effusions. Medicine. 2003;**82**(6):385-391. DOI: 10.1097/01.md.0000101574.54295.73

[16] Edwards MH, Leak AM. Pericardial effusions on anti-TNF therapy for rheumatoid arthritis-A drug side effect

or uncontrolled systemic disease? Rheumatology. 2009;**48**(3):316-317. DOI: 10.1093/rheumatology/ken463

[17] Harney S, O'Shea FD, FitzGerald O. Peptostreptococcal pericarditis complicating anti-tumour necrosis factor alpha treatment in rheumatoid arthritis. Annals of the Rheumatic Diseases. 2002;**61**(7):653-654. DOI: 10.1136/ard.61.7.653

[18] Sweet DD, Isac G, Morrison B, Fenwick J, Dhingra V. Purulent pericarditis in a patient with rheumatoid arthritis treated with etanercept and methotrexate. Canadian Journal of Emergency Medical Care. 2007;**9**(1):40-42

[19] Choy E, Sattar N. Interpreting lipid levels in the context of high-grade inflammatory states with a focus on rheumatoid arthritis: A challenge to conventional cardiovascular risk actions. Annals of the Rheumatic Diseases. 2009;**68**(4):460-469. DOI: 10.1136/ard.2008.101964

[20] Fomicheva OA, Popkova TV, Krugly LB, Gerasimova EV, Novikova DS, Pogorelova OA, et al. Factors of progression and development of atherosclerosis in rheumatoid arthritis. Cardiology. 2021;**61**(1):12-21. DOI: 10.18087/cardio.2021.1.n1331

[21] Arida A, Protogerou A, Kitas G, Sfikakis P. Systemic inflammatory response and atherosclerosis: The paradigm of chronic inflammatory rheumatic diseases. International Journal of Molecular Sciences. 2018;**19**(7):1890. DOI: 10.3390/ijms19071890

[22] Brennan FM, McInnes IB. Evidence that cytokines play a role in rheumatoid arthritis. Journal of Clinical Investigation. 2008;**118**(11):3537-3545. DOI: 10.1172/JCI36389

[23] Ramji DP, Davies TS. Cytokines in atherosclerosis: Key players in all stages of disease and promising therapeutic targets. Cytokine & Growth Factor Reviews. 2015;**26**(6):673-685. DOI: 10.1016/j.cytog-fr.2015.04.003

[24] Khaidarova YM, Kurmanova GM, Omarova KS, Abdrakhmanova AE. Diagnostic criteria for seronegative spondyloarthritis: Stages of development and optimization. Comparative Analysis. Review. Bulletin of KAZNMU. 2022;**2**(61):151-175. DOI: 10.53065/kaznmu.2022.67.22.010. ISSN Online: 2524-0692

[25] Ozkan Y. Cardiac involvement in ankylosing spondylitis. Journal of Clinical Medical Research. 2016;**8**(6):427-430. DOI: 10.14740/jocmr2488w

[26] Kazmierczak J, Peregud-Pogorzelska M, Biernawska J, et al. Cardiac arrhythmias and conduction disturbances in patients with ankylosing spondylitis. Angiology. 2007;**58**(6):751-756. DOI: 10.1177/0003319707299208

[27] Ulusoy V, Ates A, Cicekcioglu H, et al. Third-degree heart block developing in a female patient with HLA-B27 positive ankylosing spondylitis. Rheumatology International. 2006;**26**(8):779-780

[28] Bhattad P, Kulkarni M, Patel PD, et al. Cardiovascular morbidity in ankylosing spondylitis: A focus on inflammatory cardiac disease. Cureus. 2022;**14**(6):e25633. DOI: 10.7759/cureus.25633

[29] Vasilenko EA, Mazurov VI, Gaidukova IZ, al. The influence of IL-17 on the pathogenesis and risks of developing cardiovascular diseases in spondyloarthritis. Breast Cancer. 2020;**11**:39-42

[30] Rebrov AP, Gaidukova IZ, Poddubny DA. Cardiovascular pathology in patients with ankylosing spondylitis. Scientific and Practical Rheumatology. 2012;**2**:100-105

[31] Derakhshan MH, Goodson NJ, Packham JC, et al. Increased risk of hypertension associated with spondyloarthritis disease duration: Results from the ASAS-COMOSPA study. The Journal of Rheumatology. 2019;**46**(7):701-709. DOI: 10.3899/jrheum.180538

[32] Godzenko AA, Bochkova AG, Mukhortova OV, Aslanidi IP, et al. Aortitis in ankylosing spondylitis: Diagnostic and treatment possibilities. Rheumatology Science and Practice. 2013;**51**(4):451-455

[33] Gupta BK, Panwar RB, Kabra PK, et al. Ankylosing spondylitis in association with mitral stenosis, mitral regurgitation, and aortic regurgitation: A case report and review of the literature. Echocardiography. 2003;**20**(3):275-277. DOI: 10.1046/j.1540-8175.2003.03025.x

[34] Roifman I, Beck PL, Anderson TJ, et al. Chronic inflammatory diseases and cardiovascular risk: A systematic review. The Canadian Journal of Cardiology. 2011;**27**:174-182. DOI: 10.1016/j.cjca.2010.12.040

[35] Looi JL, Pui K, Hart H, et al. Valvulitis and aortitis associated with ankylosing spondylitis: Early detection and monitoring response to therapy using cardiac magnetic resonance imaging. International Journal of Rheumatic Diseases. 2011;**14**(4):e56-e58. DOI: 10.1111/j.1756-185X.2011.01650.x

[36] Bulkley BH, Roberts WC. Ankylosing spondylitis and aortic regurgitation. Description of the characteristic cardiovascular lesion from study of eight necropsy patients. Circulation. 1973;**48**:1014-1027

[37] Klingberg E, Svealv BG, Tang MS, et al. Aortic regurgitation is common in ankylosing spondylitis: Time for routine echocardiography evaluation? The American Journal of Medicine. 2015;**128**(11):1244-1250.e1. DOI: 10.1016/j.amjmed.2015.04.032

[38] Rakhimova MB. Rhythm and conduction disturbances in patients with ankylosing and psoriatic spondylitis. Central Asian Journal of Medical and Natural Sciences. 2023;**04**:c.17-c.25. ISSN: 2660-4159. Available from: http:cajmns.centralasianstudies.org

[39] Vasina LV, Petrishchev NN, Vlasov TD. Markers of endothelial dysfunction. Regional Blood Circulation and Microcirculation. 2017;**16**(1):c.4-c15. DOI: 10.24884/1682-6655-2017-16-1-4-15

[40] Nargiza A. Quality of life in patients with ankylosing spondyloarthritis after covid-19. Journal of Biomedicine and Practice. 2022;7(2):95-101. DOI: 10.5281/zenodo.6589065

[41] Ahmed S, Zimba O, Gasparyan AY. COVID-19 and the clinical course of rheumatic manifestations. Clinical Rheumatology. 2021;**40**(7):2611-2619. DOI: 10.1007/s10067-021-05691-x

[42] Sari I, Okan T, Akar S, Cece H. Impaired endothelial function in patients with ankylosing spondylitis. Rheumatology. 2006;**45**(3):283-286. DOI: 10.1093/rheumatology/KEI145

[43] Bengtsson K, Klingberg E, Deminger A, Wallberg H. Cardiac conduction disturbances in patients with ankylosing spondylitis: Results from a 5-year follow-up cohort study. RMD

Open. 2019;**5**:e001053. DOI: 10.1136/rmdopen-2019-001053

[44] Longo B, Kirchner LA, Simioni J, et al. Electrocardiographic changes in spondyloarthritis and use of anti-TNF-α drugs: A retrospective study with 100 patients. einstein (Sao Paulo). 2019;**17**:eAO4539. DOI: 10.31744/einstein_journal/2019AO4539

[45] Forsblad-d'Elia H, Wallberg H, Klingberg E, et al. Cardiac conduction system abnormalities in ankylosing spondylitis: A cross-sectional study. BMC Musculoskeletal Disorders. 2013;**14**:237. DOI: 10.1186/1471-2474-14-237

[46] Goulenok TM, Meune C, Gossec L, et al. Usefulness of routine electrocardiography for heart disease screening in patients with spondyloarthropathy or rheumatoid arthritis. Joint, Bone, Spine. 2010;**77**(2):146-150. DOI: 10.1016/j.jbspin.2010.01.001

[47] Yildirir A, Aksoyek S, Calguneri M, Aytemir K. QT dispersion as a predictor of arrhythmic events in patients with ankylosing spondylitis. Rheumatology. 2000;**39**(8):875-879. DOI: 10.1093/rheumatology/39.8.875

[48] Essers I, Stolwijk C, Boonen A, et al. Ankylosing spondylitis and risk of ischaemic heart disease: A population-based cohort study. Annals of Rheumatology Disease. 2016;**75**:203-209. DOI: 10.1136/annrheumdis-2014-206147

[49] Nasonov EL. Russian clinical recommendations. In: Rheumatology. Moscow: GEOTARM Media; 2019;. p. 464c

[50] Barilo AA, Smirnova SV, Smolnikova MV. Immunity indicators in patients with psoriatic arthritis depending on age. Medical Immunology. 2019;**21**(1):c.69-c.76. DOI: 10.15789/1563-0625-2019-1-69-76

[51] Armstrong EJ, Harskamp CT, Armstrong AW. Psoriasis and major adverse cardiovascular events: A systemic review and meta-analysis of observational studies. Journal of the American Heart Association. 2013;**2**(2):e000062. DOI: 10.1161/JAHA.113.000062

[52] Markelova EI, Korotaeva TV, Novikova DS, et al. Prevalence of metabolic syndrome in patients with psoriatic arthritis: Its relationship with inflammation and subclinical atherosclerosis. Scientific and Practical Rheumatology. 2016;**54**(App. 1):c.20-c.24. DOI: 10.14412/1995-4484-2016-1S-20-24

[53] Bengtsson K, Forsblad-d'Elia H, Lie E, et al. Are ankylosing spondylitis, psoriatic arthritis and undifferentiated spondyloarthritis associated with an increased risk of cardiovascular events? A prospective nationwide population-based cohort study. Arthritis Research & Therapy. 2017;**18;19**(1):102. DOI: 10.1186/s13075017-1315-z

[54] Batkaeva NV, Korotaeva TV, Batkaev EA. The structure of cardiovascular comorbidity in patients with severe forms of psoriasis: Data from a retrospective analysis of a hospital cohort. Scientific and Practical Rheumatology. 2017;**55**(5):493-499. DOI: 10.14412/1995-4484-2017-493-499

[55] Gazi IF, Boumpas DT, Mikhailidis DP, et al. Clustering of cardiovascular risk factors in rheumatoid arthritis: The rationale for using statins. Clinical and Experimental Rheumatology. 2007;(25):102-111

[56] Ding HS, Yang J, Jang J, et al. Interleukin-17 contributes to

cardiovascular diseases. Molecular Biology Reports. 2012;**39**(7):7473-7478. DOI: 10.1007/s11033-012-1580-5

[57] Davidovici BB, Sattar N, Prinz JC, et al. Psoriasis and systemic inflammatory diseases: Potential mechanistic links between skin disease and comorbid conditions. The Journal of Investigative Dermatology. 2010;**130**:1785-1796. DOI: 10.1038/jid.2010.103

[58] Kunder EV. The role of cytokines in the development of systemic and local inflammation in psoriatic arthritis. Cytokines and Inflammation. 2010;**9**(1):C.25-C.28

[59] Smirnova SV, Smolnikova MV. Immunopathogenesis of psoriasis and psoriatic arthritis. Medical Immunology. 2014;(2):c.127-c.138. DOI: 10.15789/1563-0625-2014-2-127-138

[60] Mehta NN, Yi Y, Saboury B, et al. Systemic and vascular inflammation in patients with moderate to severe psoriasis as measured by [18F]-Fluorodeoxyglucose positron emission tomography-computed tomography (FDG-PET/CT). Archives of Dermatology. 2011;**147**(9):1031-1039. DOI: 10.1001/archdermatol.2011.119

[61] Gladman DD, Ang M, Su L, et al. Cardiovascular morbidity in psoriatic arthritis. Annals of the Rheumatic Diseases. 2009;**68**(7):1131-1135. DOI: 10.1136/ard.2008.094839

[62] Olisova OY, Garanyan LG. Epidemiology, etiopathogenesis and comorbidity in psoriasis - new facts. Russian Journal of Skin and Venereal Diseases. 2017;**20**(4):214-219. DOI: 10.18821/1560-9588-2017-20-4-214-219

[63] Deanfield JE, Halcox JP, Rabelink TJ. Endothelial function and dysfunction testing and clinical relevance. Circulation. 2007;**115**(10):1285-1295. DOI: 10.1161/circulationaha.106.652859

[64] Azfar RS, Gelfand JM. Psoriasis and metabolic disease: Epidemiology and pathophysiology. Current Opinion in Rheumatology. 2008;**20**(4):416-422. DOI: 10.1097/bor.0b013e3283031c99

[65] Olisova OY, Garanyan LG. Comorbidities in psoriasis. Russian Journal of Skin and Venereal Diseases. 2016;**19**(6):346-348. DOI: 10.18821/1560-9588-2016-19-6-346-3484

[66] Abuabara K, Azfar RS, Shin DB, et al. Cause-specific mortality in patients with severe psoriasis: A population-based cohort study in the UK. The British Journal of Dermatology. 2010;**163**(3):586-592. DOI: 10.1111/j.1365 2133.2010.09941.x

[67] Ryan C, Kirby B. Psoriasis is a systemic disease with multiple cardiovascular and metabolic comorbidities. Dermatologic Clinics. 2015;**33**(1):41-55. DOI: 10.1016/j.det.2014.09.004

[68] Badokin VV, Kotelnikova GP. Heart damage in patients with psoriatic arthritis. Therapeutic Archive. 2004;**76**(5):c.56-c.61

[69] Arshinov AV, Levshin NY, Maslova IG. Cardiovascular complications in systemic lupus erythematosus: Mechanisms of accelerated development of atherosclerosis, diagnosis, correction possibilities. Scientific and Practical Rheumatology. 2017;**55**(3):304-310. DOI: 10.14412/1995-4484-2017-304-310

[70] Björnadal L, Yin L, Granath F, et al. Cardiovascular disease a hazard despite

improved prognosis in patients with systemic lupus erythematosus: Results from a Swedish population based study 1964-95. The Journal of Rheumatology. 2004;**31**(4):713-719

[71] Amaya-Amaya J, Sarmiento-Monroy JC, Caro-Moreno J, et al. Cardiovascular disease in Latin American patients with systemic lupus erythematosus: A cross-sectional study and a systematic review. Autoimmune Diseases. 2013;**2013**:20. Article ID 794383. DOI: 10.1155/2013/794383

[72] McMahon M, Skaggs B. Pathogenesis and treatment of atherosclerosis in lupus. Rheumatic Diseases Clinics of North America. 2014;**40**(3):475-495. DOI: 10.1016/j.rdc.2014.04.003

[73] Kim CH, Al-Kindi SG, Jandali B, et al. Incidence and risk of heart failure in systemic lupus erythematosus. Heart. 2017;**103**(3):227-233. DOI: 10.1136/heartjnl-2016-309561

[74] Miner JJ, Kim AH. Cardiac manifestations of systemic lupus erythematosus. Rheumatic Diseases Clinics of North America. 2014;**40**(1):51-60. DOI: 10.1016/j.rdc.2013.10.003

[75] Aviña-Zubieta JA, To F, Vostretsova K, et al. Risk of myocardial infarction and stroke in newly diagnosed systemic lupus erythematosus: A general population-based study. Arthritis Care & Research (Hoboken). 2017;**69**:849-856. DOI: 10.1002/acr.23018

[76] Jha SB, Rivera AP, Flores MG, et al. Systemic lupus erythematosus and cardiovascular disease. Cureus. 2022;**14**(2):e22027. DOI: 10.7759/cureus.22027

[77] Symmons DP, Gabriel SE. Epidemiology of CVD in rheumatic disease, with a focus on RA and SLE. Nature Reviews Rheumatology. 2011;**7**(7):399-408. DOI: 10.1038/nrrheum.2011.75

[78] Wajed J, Ahmad Y, Durrington PN, Bruce IN. Prevention of cardiovascular disease in systemic lupus erythematosus: Proposed guidelines for risk factor management. Rheumatology (Oxford). 2004;**43**(1):7-12. DOI: 10.1093/rheumatology/keg436

[79] Alghareeb R, Hussain A, Maheshwari MV, et al. Cardiovascular complications in systemic lupus erythematosus. Cureus. 2022;**14**(7):e26671. DOI: 10.7759/cureus.26671

[80] Buppajamrntham T, Palavutitotai N, Katchamart W. Clinical manifestation, diagnosis, management, and treatment outcome of pericarditis in patients with systemic lupus erythematosus. Journal of the Medical Association of Thailand. 2014;**97**(12):1234-1240

[81] Dein E, Douglas H, Petri M, et al. Pericarditis in lupus. Cureus. 2019;**11**(3):e4166. DOI: 10.7759/cureus.4166

[82] Doria A, Iaccarino L, Sarzi-Puttini P, et al. Cardiac involvement in systemic lupus erythematosus. Lupus. 2005;**14**(9):683-686. DOI: 10.1191/0961203305lu2200oa

[83] Roman MJ, Salmon JE. Cardiovascular manifestations of rheumatologic diseases. Circulation. 2007;**116**(20):2346-2355. DOI: 10.1161/circulationaha.106.678334

[84] Wijetunga M, Rockson S. Myocarditis in systemic lupus erythematosus. The American Journal of Medicine. 2002;**113**:419-423. DOI: 10.1016/s0002-9343(02)01223-8

[85] Tereshchenko SN, Zhirov IV, Masenko VP, et al. Diagnosis and treatment of myocarditis. Eurasian Journal of Cardiology. 2019;**3**:4-33

[86] Panafidina TA, Popkova TV, Kondratyeva LV. Frequency and structure of heart damage in systemic lupus erythematosus. Doctor Ru. 2022;**21**(2):72-79. DOI: 10.31550/1727-2378-2022-21-2-72-79

[87] Sharma J, Lasic Z, Bornstein A, Cooper R, Chen J. Libman-Sacks endocarditis as the first manifestation of systemic lupus erythematosus in an adolescent, with a review of the literature. Cardiology in the Young. 2013;**23**:1-6. DOI: 10.1017/S1047951112001023

[88] Appelgren D, Dahle C, Knopf J, et al. Active NET formation in Libman-Sacks endocarditis without antiphospholipid antibodies: a dramatic onset of systemic lupus erythematosus. Autoimmunity. 2018;**51**(6):310-318. DOI: 10.1080/08916934.2018.1514496

[89] Grimaldi A, De Gennaro L, Vermi A, et al. Cardiac valve involvement in systemic diseases: A review. Clinical Cardiology. 2013;**36**(3):117-124. DOI: 10.1002/clc.22099

[90] Moyssakis I, Tektonidou MG, Vasilliou VA, et al. Libman-Sacks endocarditis in systemic lupus erythematosus: Prevalence, associations, and evolution. The American Journal of Medicine. 2007;**120**:636-642. DOI: 10.1016/j.amjmed.2007.01.024

[91] Ibrahim AM, Siddique MS. Libman-Sacks endocarditis. In: StatPearls [Internet]. Treasure Island (FL): StatPearls Publishing; 2025 Jan. 2023. PMID: 30422459. Bookshelf ID: NBK532864

[92] Mohammadi KY, Avesta L, Habibzadeh A, Hemmati M. Libman-Sacks endocarditis in patients with systemic lupus erythematosus with secondary antiphospholipid syndrome. Caspian Journal of Internal Medicine. 2019;**10**(3):339-342. DOI: 10.22088/cjim.10.3.339

[93] Tektonidou MG, Kravvariti E, Protogerou A, et al. Subclinical atherosclerosis in systemic lupus erythematosus: Comparable risk with diabetes mellitus and rheumatoid arthritis. Autoimmunity Reviews. 2017;**16**(3):308-312. DOI: 10.1016/j.autrev.2017.01.009

[94] Reiss AB, Jacob B, Ahmed S, et al. Understanding accelerated atherosclerosis in systemic lupus erythematosus: Toward better treatment and prevention. Inflammation. 2021;**44**(5):1663-1682. DOI: 10.1007/s10753-021-01455-6

[95] Tselios K, Gladman DD, Su J, et al. Evolution of risk factors for atherosclerotic cardiovascular events in systemic lupus erythematosus: A longterm prospective study. The Journal of Rheumatology. 2017;**44**(12):1841-1849. DOI: 10.3899/jrheum.16112

[96] Zeller CB, Appenzeller S. Cardiovascular disease in systemic lupus erythematosus: The role of traditional and lupus related risk factors. Current Cardiology Reviews. 2008;**4**(2):116-122. DOI: 10.2174/157340308784245775

[97] Barbhaiya M et al. ACR/EULAR antiphospholipid syndrome classification criteria. Annals of the Rheumatic Diseases. 2023;**82**:1258-1270. DOI: 10.1136/ard-2023-224609

[98] Kolitz T, Shiber S, Sharabi I, et al. Cardiac manifestations of antiphospholipid syndrome with focus on its primary form. Frontiers in

Immunology. 2019;**10**:941. DOI: 10.3389/fimmu.2019.00941

[99] Djokovic A, Stojanovich L, Kontic M, et al. Association between cardiac manifestations and antiphospholipid antibody type and level in a cohort of Serbian patients with primary and secondary antiphospholipid syndrome. The Israel Medical Association Journal : IMAJ. 2014;**16**:162-167

[100] Paule R, Morel N, Le Guern V, Fredi M, et al. Classification of primary antiphospholipid syndrome as systemic lupus erythematosus: Analysis of a cohort of 214 patients. Autoimmunity Reviews. 2018;**17**:866-872. DOI: 10.1016/j.autrev.2018.03.011

[101] Kaplan SD, Chartash EK, Pizzarello RA, Furie RA. Cardiac manifestations of the antiphospholipid syndrome. American Heart Journal. 1992;**124**:1331-1338. DOI: 10.1016/0002-8703(92)90420-Z

[102] Roldan CA. Valvular and coronary heart disease in systemic inflammatory diseases: Systemic disorders in heart disease. Heart. 2008;**94**:1089-1101. DOI: 10.1136/hrt.2007.132787

[103] Tenedios F, Erkan D, Lockshin MD. Cardiac manifestations in the antiphospholipid syndrome. Rheumatic Diseases Clinics of North America. 2006;**32**:491-507. DOI: 10.1016/j.rdc.2006.05.008

[104] Kahan A, Coghlan G, McLaughlin V. Cardiac complications of systemic sclerosis. Rheumatology. 2009;**48**(Suppl. 3):45-48. DOI: 10.1093/rheumatology/kep110

[105] Cervera R, Tektonidou MG, Espinosa G, et al. Task force on catastrophic antiphospholipid syndrome (APS) and non-criteria APS manifestations (I): Catastrophic APS, APS nephropathy and heart valve lesions. Lupus. 2011;**20**:165-173. DOI: 10.1177/0961203310395051

[106] Reshetnyak TM, Seredavkina NV, Nasonov EL. Heart damage in antiphospholipid syndrome. Consilium Medicum. 2008;(11):115-122

[107] Shostak NA, Klimenko AA. Systemic scleroderma: Modern classification and treatment methods. General Medicine. 2009;**4**:c.4-c12

[108] Mazurov VI. Clinical Rheumatology. 3rd ed. Revised and expanded. Guide for doctors. M.: E-noto. 2021. p. 696 c

[109] Bercun Y, Elami A, Meir K, et al. Increased morbidity and mortality in patients with antiphospholipid syndrome undergoing valve replacement surgery. The Journal of Thoracic and Cardiovascular Surgery. 2004;**127**(2):414-420. DOI: 10.1016/j.jtcvs.2003.07.016

[110] Mani P, Gonzalez D, Chatterjee S, Faulx MD. Cardiovascular complications of systemic sclerosis: What to look. Cleveland Clinic Journal of Medicine. 2019;**86**(10):685-695. DOI: 10.3949/ccjm.86a.1810

[111] Vaccaro F, Caccavo D, Roumpedaki E, De Vincentis G, et al. Dilated cardiomyopathy due to thrombotic microangiopathy as the only manifestation of antiphospholipid syndrome: A case report. International Journal of Immunopathology and Pharmacology. 2008;**21**:237-241. DOI: 10.1177/0394632008 02100128

[112] Wang Q, Shang Y, Li S, et al. Complete heart block in systemic sclerosis: A case report and literature review. Medicine (Baltimore). 2018;**97**(46):e13226. DOI: 10.1097/MD.0000000000013226

[113] Lang IM. Chronic thromboembolic pulmonary hypertension — Not so rare after all. The New England Journal of Medicine. 2004;**350**:2236-2238. DOI: 10.1056/NEJMp048088

[114] De Luca G, Bosello SL, Gabrielli FA, et al. Prognostic role of ventricular ectopic beats in systemic sclerosis: A prospective cohort study shows ECG indexes predicting the worse outcome. PLoS One. 2016;**11**(4):e0153012. DOI: 10.1371/journal.pone.0153012

[115] Chen Y, Chen G, Zhu C, et al. Severe systemic lupus erythematosus in emergency department: A retrospective single-center study from China. Journal of Clinical Rheumatology. 2011;**30**:1463-1469. DOI: 10.1007/s10067-011-1826-y

[116] Kampolis C, Tektonidou M, Moyssakis I, et al. Evolution of cardiac dysfunction in patients with antiphospholipid antibodies and/or antiphospholipid syndrome: A 10-year follow-up study. Seminars in Arthritis and Rheumatism. 2014;**43**:558-565. DOI: 10.1016/j.semarthrit.2013.07.016

[117] Seferović PM, Ristić AD, Maksimović R, et al. Cardiac arrhythmias and conduction disturbances in autoimmune rheumatic diseases. Rheumatology (Oxford). 2006;**45**(Suppl. 4):iv39-iv42. DOI: 10.1093/rheumatology/kel315

[118] Lee K-I, Manuntag LJ, Kifayat A, Manuntag SE, et al. Cardiovascular manifestations of systemic sclerosis: An overview of pathophysiology, screening modalities and treatment options. Cardiology in Review. 2023;**31**(1):22-27. DOI: 10.1097/CRD.0000000000000420

[119] Tektonidou MG, Ioannidis JP, Moyssakis I, et al. Right ventricular diastolic dysfunction in patients with anticardiolipin antibodies and antiphospholipid syndrome. Annals of the Rheumatic Diseases. 2001;**60**:43-48. DOI: 10.1136/ard.60.1.43

[120] Vacca A, Meune C, Gordon J, et al. Scleroderma clinical trial consortium cardiac subcommittee. Cardiac arrhythmias and conduction defects in systemic sclerosis. Rheumatology (Oxford). 2014;**53**(7):1172-1177. DOI: 10.1093/rheumatology/ket377

[121] Parks JL, Taylor MH, Parks LP, Silver RM. Systemic sclerosis and the heart. Rheumatic Diseases Clinics of North America. 2014;**40**:87-102. DOI: 10.1016/j.rdc.2013.10.007

[122] Cannarile F, Valentini V, Mirabelli G, et al. Cardiovascular disease in systemic sclerosis. Annals of Translational Medicine. 2015;**1**:8-19. DOI: 10.3978/j.issn.2305-5839.2014.12.12

[123] Dimitroulas T, Giannakoulas G, Karvounis H. Micro- and macrovascular treatment targets in scleroderma heart disease. Current Pharmaceutical Design. 2014;**20**(4):536-544. DOI: 10.2174/13816128113199990555

[124] Allanore Y, Meune C. Primary myocardial involvement in systemic sclerosis: Evidence for a microvascular origin. Clinical and Experimental Rheumatology. 2010;**28**(5 Suppl. 62):S48-S53

[125] Morrisroe K, Stevens W, Sahhar J, et al. Epidemiology and disease characteristics of systemic sclerosis-related pulmonary arterial hypertension: Results from a real-life screening program. Arthritis Research & Therapy. 2017;**19**(1):42. DOI: 10.1186/s13075-017-1250-z

[126] Chaisson NF, Hassoun PM. Systemic sclerosis-associated pulmonary arterial

hypertension. Chest. 2013;**144**(4):1346-1356. DOI: 10.1378/chest.12-2396

[127] Chatterjee S. Pulmonary hypertension in systemic sclerosis. Seminars in Arthritis and Rheumatism. 2011;**41**(1):19-37. DOI: 10.1016/j.semarthrit.2010.08.004

[128] Gupta R, Wayangankar SA, Targoff IN, Hennebry TA. Clinical cardiac involvement in idiopathic inflammatory myopathies: A systematic review. International Journal of Cardiology. 2011;**148**:261-270. DOI: 10.1016/j.ijcard.2010.08.013

[129] Zhang L, Wang G, Ma L, et al. Cardiac involvement in adult polymyositis or dermatomyositis: A systematic review. Clinical Cardiology. 2012;**35**(11):686. DOI: 10.1002/clc.22026.691

[130] Qin L, Li F, Luo Q, Chen L, Yang X, Wang H. Coronary heart disease and cardiovascular risk factors in patients with idiopathic inflammatory myopathies: A systemic review and meta-analysis. Frontiers in Medicine (Lausanne). 14 Jan 2022;**8**:808915. DOI: 10.3389/fmed.2021.808915. eCollection 2021. PMID: 35096896. PMCID: PMC8795615

[131] Dankó K, Ponyi A, Constantin T, et al. Long-term survival of patients with idiopathic inflammatory myopathies according to clinical features: A longitudinal study of 162 cases. Medicine (Baltimore). 2004;**83**:35-42. DOI: 10.1097/01.md.0000109755.65914.5e

[132] Lilleker JB, Vencovsky J, Wang G, et al. The EuroMyositis registry: An international collaborative tool to facilitate myositis research. Annals of the Rheumatic Diseases. 2018;**77**:30-39. DOI: 10.1136/annrheumdis-2017-211868

[133] Diederichsen LP, Simonsen JA, Diederichsen AC, et al. Cardiac abnormalities assessed by non-invasive techniques in patients with newly diagnosed idiopathic inflammatory myopathies. Clinical and Experimental Rheumatology. 2015;**33**:706-714

[134] Sen G, Scully P, Gordon P, Sado D. Advances in the diagnosis of myocarditis in idiopathic inflammatory myopathies: An overview of diagnostic tests. Rheumatology. 2024;**63**(7):1825-1836. DOI: 10.1093/rheumatology/keae029

[135] Ammirati E, Moslehi JJ. Diagnosis and treatment of acute myocarditis. JAMA. 2023;**329**(13):1098-1113. DOI: 10.1001/jama.2023.3371

[136] Trybuch A, Tarnacka B. Cardiac involvement in polymyositis and dermatomyositis: Diagnostic approaches. Reumatologia. 2023;**61**(3):202-212. DOI: 10.5114/reum/168362

[137] Lampejo T, Durkin SM, Bhatt N, Guttmann O. Acute myocarditis: A etiology, diagnosis and management. Clinical Medicine (Northfield IL). 2021;**21**:e505-e510. DOI: 10.7861/clinmed.2021-0121

[138] Gonzales LL, Gamez-Nava JI, Sanchez L, et al. Cardiac manifestations in dermato-polymyositis. Clinical and Experimental Rheumatology. 1996;**14**:373-379

[139] Lundberg IE. The heart in dermatomyositis and polymyositis. Rheumatology. 2006;**45**:18-21. DOI: 10.1093/rheumatology/kel311

[140] Liu XH, Feng XJ, Shi JY, et al. The quest for diagnostic approaches of cardiac involvement in polymyositis and dermatomyositis. Annals of Palliative Medicine. 2020;**9**(4):2256-2270. DOI: 10.21037/apm-19-650

[141] Stern R, Godbold JH, Chess Q, Kagen LJ. ECG abnormalities in polymyositis. Archives of Internal Medicine. 1984;**144**:2185-2189

[142] Haupt HM, Hutchins GM. The heart and cardiac conduction system in polymyositis-dermatomyositis: A clinicopathologic study of 16 autopsied patients. The American Journal of Cardiology. 1982;**50**:998-1006

[143] Lai YT, Dai YS, Yen MF, Chen LS, et al. Dermatomyositis is associated with an increased risk of cardiovascular and cerebrovascular events: A Taiwanese population-based longitudinal follow-up study. The British Journal of Dermatology. 2013;**168**:1054-1059. DOI: 10.1111/bjd.12245

[144] Rai SK, Choi HK, Sayre EC, Aviña-Zubieta JA. Risk of myocardial infarction and ischaemic stroke in adults with polymyositis and dermatomyositis: A general population-based study. Rheumatology (Oxford). 2016;**55**:461-469. DOI: 10.1093/rheumatology/kev336

[145] Ungprasert P, Suksaranjit P, Spanuchart I, et al. Risk of coronary artery disease in patients with idiopathic inflammatory myopathies: A systematic review and metanalysis of observational studies. Seminars in Arthritis and Rheumatism. 2014;**44**(1):63-67. DOI: 10.1016/j.semarthrit.2014.03.004

[146] Frostegård J. Atherosclerosis in patients with autoimmune disorders. Arteriosclerosis, Thrombosis, and Vascular Biology. 2005;**25**:1776-1785. DOI: 10.1161/01.ATV.0000174800.78362.ec

[147] Abou-Raya A, Abou-Raya S. Inflammation: A pivotal link between autoimmune diseases and atherosclerosis. Autoimmunity Reviews. 2006;**5**:331-337. DOI: 10.1016/j.autrev.2005.12.006

[148] Betteridge Z, Tansley S, Shaddick G, et al. Frequency, mutual exclusivity and clinical associations of myositis autoantibodies in a combined European cohort of idiopathic inflammatory myopathy patients. Journal of Autoimmunity. 2019;**101**:48-55. DOI: 10.1016/j.jaut.2019.04.001

[149] Fardet L, Fève B. Systemic glucocorticoid therapy: A review of its metabolic and cardiovascular adverse events. Drugs. 2014;**74**:1731-1745. DOI: 10.1007/s40265-014-0282-9

[150] Cavagna L, Monti S, Caporali R, et al. How I treat idiopathic patients with inflammatory myopathies in the clinical practice. Autoimmunity Reviews. 2017;**16**:999-1007. DOI: 10.1016/j.autrev.2017.07.016

[151] Chakravarty K, Ong VH, Denton CP. Secondary vasculitis in autoimmune connective tissue diseases. Current Opinion in Rheumatology. 2016;**28**:60-65. DOI: 10.1097/bor.0000000000000241

[152] Jennette JC, Falk RJ, Bacon PA, et al. 2012 revised International Chapel Hill consensus conference nomenclature of vasculitides. Arthritis and Rheumatism. 2013;**65**(1):1-11. DOI: 10.1002/art.37715

[153] Pagnoux C, Guillevin L. Cardiac involvement in small and medium-sized vessel vasculitide. Lupus. 2005;**14**(9):718-722. DOI: 10.1191/0961203305lu2207oa

[154] Cohen Tervaert JW. Cardiovascular disease due to accelerated atherosclerosis in systemic vasculitides. Best Practice & Research. Clinical Rheumatology. 2013;**27**(1):33-44. DOI: 10.1016/j.berh.2012.12.004

[155] Ali AM, Yakupoglu HY, Fuchs TA, Larsen TH, et al. Cardiac involvement in systemic and local vasculitides: The value

of noninvasive multimodality imaging. Current Problems in Cardiology. 2023;**48**(8):101718. DOI: 10.1016/j.cpcardiol. 2023.101718

[156] Mavrogeni S. Cardiac involvement in small and medium-sized vasculitides. Journal of the ESC Council for Cardiology Practice. 2007;**6**(14)

[157] Mavrogeni S, Tsirogianni AK, Gialafos EJ, Manoussakis MN. Detection of myocardial inflammation by contrast-enhanced MRI in a patient with Churg-Strauss syndrome. International Journal of Cardiology. 2007;**131**(2):54-55. DOI: 10.1016/j.ijcard.2007.05.101

[158] Mavrogeni S, Papadopoulos G, et al. Magnetic resonance angiography is equivalent to X-ray coronary angiography for the evaluation of coronary arteries in Kawasaki disease. Journal of the American College of Cardiology. 2004;**43**(4):649-652. DOI: 10.1016/j.jacc.2003.08.052

[159] Mavrogeni S, Papadopoulos G, Douskou M, et al. Magnetic resonance angiography, function and viability evaluation in patients with Kawasaki disease. Journal of Cardiovascular Magnetic Resonance. 2006;**8**(3):493-498. DOI: 10.1080/10976640600604773

[160] Camellino D, Matteson EL, Buttgereit F, Dejaco C. Monitoring and long-term management of giant cell arteritis and polymyalgia rheumatica. Nature Reviews Rheumatology. 2020;**16**:481-495. DOI: 10.1038/s41584-020-0458-5

[161] Salvarani C, Cantini F, Hunder GG. Polymyalgia rheumatica and giant-cell arteritis. Lancet. 2008;**372**:234-245. DOI: 10.1016/S0140-6736(08)61077-6

[162] Mednick Z, Farmer J, Khan Z, Warder D, Hove MT. Coronary arteritis: An entity to be considered in giant cell arteritis. Canadian Journal of Ophthalmology. 2016;**51**:e6-e8. DOI: 10.1016/j.jcjo.2015.09.011ю

[163] Tomasson G, Peloquin C, Mohammad A, et al. Risk for cardiovascular disease early and late after a diagnosis of giant-cell arteritis: A cohort study. Annals of Internal Medicine. 2014;**160**:73-80. DOI: 10.7326/M12-3046

[164] Brekke LK, Fevang BS, Diamantopoulos AP, et al. Survival and death causes of patients with giant cell arteritis in Western Norway 1972-2012: A retrospective cohort study. Arthritis Research & Therapy. 2019;**21**:154. DOI: 10.1186/s13075-019-1945-4

[165] Lee YH, Song GG. Overall and cause-specific mortality in giant cell arteritis: A meta-analysis. Zeitschrift für Rheumatologie. 2018;**77**:946-951. DOI: 10.1007/s00393-018-0440-7

[166] Li L, Neogi T, Jick S. Giant cell arteritis and vascular disease-risk factors and outcomes: A cohort study using UK clinical practice research datalink. Rheumatology (Oxford). 2017;**56**(5):753-762. DOI: 10.1093/rheumatology/kew482

[167] Hellmich B, Agueda A, Mont S, et al. 2018 update of the EULAR recommendations for the management of large vessel vasculitis. Annals of the Rheumatic Diseases. 2020;**79**:19-30. DOI: 10.1136/annrheumdis-2019-215672

[168] Kushnir A, Restaino SW, Yuzefpolskaya M. Giant cell arteritis as a cause of myocarditis and atrial fibrillation. Circulation. Heart Failure. 2016;**9**(2):e002778. DOI: 10.1161/circheartfailure.115.002778

[169] Tiosano S, Adler Y, Azrielant S, et al. Pericarditis among giant cell

arteritis patients: From myth to reality. Clinical Cardiology. 2018;**41**(5):623-627. DOI: 10.1002/clc.22927

[170] Miloslavsky E, Unizony S. The heart in vasculitis. Rheumatic Diseases Clinics of North America. 2014;**40**:11-26. DOI: 10.1016/j.rdc.2013.10.006

[171] Dzhus M, Mostbauer H. Cardiovascular lesions in giant cell arteritis. Reumatologia. 2022;**60**(6):399-407. DOI: 10.5114/reum.2022.123670

[172] Vats V, Patel K, Sharma DD, Almansouri NE. Exploring cardiovascular manifestations in vasculitides: An in-depth review. Cureus. 2023;**15**(8):e44417. DOI: 10.7759/cureus.44417

[173] Endo M, Tomizawa Y, Nishida H, et al. Angiographic findings and surgical treatments of coronary artery involvement in Takayasu arteritis. The Journal of Thoracic and Cardiovascular Surgery. 2003;**125**:570-577

[174] Strizhakov LA, Krivosheev OG, Semenkova EN, Kogan EA. Cardiological aspects of systemic vasculitis. Concilium Modicum. 2008;**10**(11):c.135-c.142

[175] Weyand CM, Goronzy JJ. Immune mechanisms in medium and large-vessel vasculitis. Nature Reviews Rheumatology. 2013;**9**(12):731-740. DOI: 10.1038/nrrheum.2013.161

[176] Arima M, Kanoh T, Kawano Y, et al. Isolated coronary ostial stenosis associated with coronary vasospasm. Japanese Circulation Journal. 2000;**64**:985-987

[177] Ren Y, Du J, Guo X, et al. Cardiac valvular involvement of Takayasu arteritis. Clinical Rheumatology. 2021;**40**(2):653-660. DOI: 10.1007/s10067-020-05290-2

[178] An X, Han Y, Zhang B, et al. Takayasu arteritis presented with acute heart failure: Case report and review of literature. European Journal of Heart Failure. 2017;**4**:649-654. DOI: 10.1002/ehf2.12174

[179] Yokokawa T, Kunii H, Kaneshiro T, Ichimura S, et al. Regressed coronary ostial stenosis in a young female with Takayasu arteritis: A case report. BMC Cardiovascular Disorders. 2019;**19**:79. DOI: 10.1186/s12872-019-1066-7

[180] Johnston SL, Rock RJ, Gompels MM. Takayasu arteritis: A review. Journal of Clinical Pathology. 2002;**55**(7):481-486

[181] Schrader ML, Hochman JS, Bulkley BH. The heart in polyarteritis nodosa: A clinicopathologic study. American Heart Journal. 1985;**109**:1353-1359

[182] Wi J, Choi HH, Lee CJ, et al. Acute myocardial infarction due to polyarteritis nodosa in a young female patient. Korean Circulation Journal. 2010;**40**(4):197-200. DOI: 10.4070/kcj.2010.40.4.197

[183] Mirza A. Myocardial infarction resulting from nonatherosclerotic coronary artery diseases. The American Journal of Emergency Medicine. 2003;**21**:578-584

[184] Rajani RM, Dalvi BV, D'Silva SA, et al. Acute myocardial infarction with normal coronary arteries in a case of polyarteritis nodosa: Possible role of coronary artery spasm. Postgraduate Medical Journal. 1991;**67**:78-80

[185] Klimenko OV, Semenkova EN, Krivosheev OG. Features of the clinical course, prognostic factors and outcomes of polyarteritis nodosa. Hepatology Forum. 2005;**2**:18-21

[186] Agarwal S, Agrawal DK. Kawasaki disease: Etiopathogenesis and novel treatment strategies. Expert Review of Clinical Immunology. 2017;**13**(3):247-258. DOI: 10.1080/1744666X.2017.1232165

[187] Duarte R, Cisneros S, Fernandez G, et al. Kawasaki disease: A review with emphasis on cardiovascular complications. Insights into Imaging. 2010;**1**(4):223-231. DOI: 10.1007/s13244-010-0035-6

[188] Pilania RK, Jindal AK, Bhattarai D, et al. Cardiovascular involvement in Kawasaki disease is much more than mere coronary arteritis. Frontiers in Pediatrics. 2020;**8**:526969. DOI: 10.3389/fped.2020.526969

[189] Newburger JW, Takahashi M, Gerber MA, et al. Diagnosis, treatment, and long-term management of Kawasaki disease: A statement for health professionals from the committee on rheumatic fever, endocarditis and Kawasaki disease, council on cardiovascular disease in the young, American Heart Association. Circulation. 2004;**110**:2747-2771. DOI: 10.1161/01.CIR.0000145143.19711.78

[190] Dionne A, Dahdah N. Myocarditis and Kawasaki disease. International Journal of Rheumatic Diseases. 2018;**21**:45-49. DOI: 10.1111/1756-185X.13219

[191] Harada M, Yokouchi Y, Oharaseki T, et al. Histopathological characteristics of myocarditis in acute-phase Kawasaki disease. Histopathology. 2012;**61**:1156-1167. DOI: 10.1111/j.1365-2559.2012.04332.x

[192] De Rosa G, Andreozzi L, Piastra M, Castelli B, Rigante D. Acute myocarditis as a revealing clue of complete Kawasaki disease. Reumatismo. 2018;**70**:115-116. DOI: 10.4081/reumatismo.2018.1101

[193] Madhusudan S, Singh S, Rohit M. Late symptomatic myocarditis in Kawasaki disease: An unusual manifestation. Indian Journal of Pediatrics. 2014;**1**:404-405. DOI: 10.1007/s12098-014-1339-1

[194] Chung C, Stein L. Kawasaki disease: A review. Radiology. 1998;**208**:25-33

[195] Ravekes WJ, Colan SD, Gauvreau K, et al. Aortic root dilation in Kawasaki disease. The American Journal of Cardiology. 2001;**87**:919-922. DOI: 10.1016/S0002-9149(00)01541-1

[196] Burns JC. The riddle of Kawasaki disease. The New England Journal of Medicine. 2007;**356**:659-661. DOI: 10.1056/NEJMp068268

[197] Petrunić M, Drinković N, Stern-Padovan R, Mestrović T, Lovrić D. Thoracoabdominal and coronary arterial aneurysms in a young man with a history of Kawasaki disease. Journal of Vascular Surgery. 2009;**50**:1173-1176. DOI: 10.1016/j.jvs.2009.05.025

[198] Suzuki A, Kamiya T, Yasuo O, Kuroe K. Extended long term follow-up study of coronary arterial lesions in Kawasaki disease. Journal of the American College of Cardiology. 1991;**17**:33A. DOI: 10.1016/0735-1097(91)91097-X

[199] Almaani S, Fussner LA, Brodsky S, et al. ANCA-associated vasculitis: An update. Journal of Clinical Medicine. 2021;**10**(7):1446. DOI: 10.3390/jcm10071446

[200] Kronbichler A, Leierer J, Gauckler P, Shin JI. Comorbidities in ANCA-associated vasculitis. Rheumatology (Oxford, England). 2020;**59**(Suppl. 3):i79-ii3. DOI: 10.1093/rheumatology/kez617

[201] Mercuzot C, Letertre S, Daien CI, et al. Comorbidities and health-related quality of life in patients with Antineutrophil cytoplasmic antibody (ANCA) – Associated vasculitis. Autoimmunity Reviews. 2021;**20**(1):102708. DOI: 10.1016/j.autrev.2020.102708

[202] Floyd L, Morris AD, Woywodt A, Dhaygude A. Cardiovascular disease and ANCA-associated vasculitis: Are we missing a beat? Clinical Kidney Journal. 2022;**15**(4):618-623. DOI: 10.1093/ckj/sfac009

[203] Kitching AR, Anders HJ, Basu N, et al. ANCA-associated vasculitis. Nature Reviews Disease Primers. 2020;**6**(1):71. DOI: 10.1038/s41572-020-0204-y

[204] Guillevin L, Cohen P, Gayraud M, et al. Churg-Strauss syndrome. Clinical study and long-term follow-up of 96 patients. Medicine. 1999;**78**:26-37

[205] Guillevin L, Durand-Gasselin B, Cevallos R, et al. Microscopic polyangitis: Clinical and laboratory findings in eighty-five patients. Arthritis and Rheumatism. 1999;**42**:421-430

[206] Reinhold-Keller E, Buege N, Latza U, et al. An interdisciplinary approach to the care of patients with Wegener's granulomatosis. Arthritis and Rheumatism. 2000;**43**:1021-1032

[207] Hazebroek MR, Kemna MJ, Schalla S, et al. Prevalence and prognostic relevance of cardiac involvement in ANCA-associated vasculitis: Eosinophilic granulomatosis with polyangitis and granulomatosis with polyangiitis. International Journal of Cardiology. 2015;**199**:170-179

[208] Guillevin L, Lhote F, Gayraud M, et al. Prognostic factors in polyarteritis nodosa and Churg-Strauss syndrome. A prospective study in 342 patients. Medicine. 1996;**75**:17-28. DOI: 10.1097/00005792-199601000-00003

[209] Bond M, Fagni F, Moretti M, et al. At the heart of eosinophilic granulomatosis with polyangiitis: Into cardiac and vascular involvement. Current Rheumatology Reports. 2022;**24**(11):337-351. DOI: 10.1007/s11926-022-01087-1

[210] Sable-Fourtassou R, Cohen P, Mahr A, et al. Antineutrophil cytoplasmic antibodies and the Churg-Strauss syndrome. Annals of Internal Medicine. 2005;**143**:632-638

[211] Sinico RA, Di Toma L, Maggiore U, et al. Prevalence and clinical significance of antineutrophil cytoplasmic antibodies in Churg-Strauss syndrome. Arthritis and Rheumatism. 2005;**52**:2926-2935. DOI: 10.1002/art.21250

[212] Mavrogeni S, Karabela G, Gialafos E, et al. Cardiac involvement in ANCA (+) and ANCA (−) Churg-Strauss syndrome evaluated by cardiovascular magnetic resonance. Inflammation & Allergy Drug Targets. 2013;**12**(5):322-327. DOI: 10.2174/1871528111312990054

[213] Cohen P, Pagnoux C, Alfred MA, et al. Churg-Strauss syndrome with poor-prognosis factors: A prospective multicenter trial comparing glucocorticoids and six or twelve cyclophosphamide pulses in forty-eight patients. Arthritis and Rheumatism. 2007;**57**(4):686-693. DOI: 10.1002/art.22679

[214] Ribi C, Cohen P, Pagnoux C, et al. Treatment of Churg-Strauss syndrome without poor- prognosis factors: Multicenter, prospective, randomized, open-label study of seventy-two

patients. Arthritis and Rheumatism. 2008;**58**(2):586-594. DOI: 10.1002/art.23198

[215] Bourgarit A, Le Toumelin P, Pagnoux C, et al. Deaths occurring during the first year after treatment onset for polyarteritis nodosa, microscopic polyangiitis, and Churg-Strauss syndrome: A retrospective analysis of causes and factors predictive of mortality based on 595 patients. Medicine. 2005;**84**(5):323-330. DOI: 10.1097/01.md.0000180793.80212.17

[216] McGeoch L, Carette S, Cuthbertson D, et al. Cardiac involvement in granulomatosis with polyangiitis. The Journal of Rheumatology. 2015;**42**(7):1209-1212. DOI: 10.3899/jrheum.141513

[217] Silveira LH. Cardiovascular manifestations of systemic vasculitides. Current Rheumatology Reports. 2020;**22**(10):72. DOI: 10.1007/s11926-020-00952-1

[218] Bayrashevskaya AV, Degtyareva ND, Radenska-Lopovok SG. ANCA-associated vasculitis. Archives of Pathologists. 2022;**84**(1):50-58. DOI: 10.17116/patol20228401150

[219] Lim HE, Lee YH, Ahn JC. Wegener's granulomatosis with progressive conduction disturbances and atrial fibrillation. Heart. 2007;**93**:777. DOI: 10.1136/hrt.2006.090530

[220] Saghabalyan D, Schiller D, Lerch SJ. A 60-year-old with heart failure symptoms due to 1st degree AV-block caused by granulomatosis with polyangiitis (Wegener's granulomatosis). Journal of Cardiology Cases. 2020;**21**:114-118. DOI: 10.1016/j.jccase.2019.11.005

[221] Valente F, Rozen L, Carlier S, Godart P. An uncommon case of complete AV block. BMC Cardiovascular Disorders. 2022;**22**:429. DOI: 10.1186/s12872-022-02866-5

[222] Furuta S, Iwamoto T, Nakajima H. Update on eosinophilic granulomatosis with polyangiitis. Allergology International. 2019;**68**(4):430-436. DOI: 10.1016/j.alit.2019.06.004

[223] Mavrogeni S, Manoussakis MN, Karagiorga TC. Detection of coronary artery lesions and myocardial necrosis by magnetic resonance in systemic necrotizing vasculitides. Arthritis and Rheumatism. 2009;**61**(8):1121-1129. DOI: 10.1002/art.24695

[224] Demirelli S, Degirmenci H, Inci S, et al. Cardiac manifestations in Behcet's disease. Intractable & Rare Diseases Research. 2015;**4**(2):70-75. DOI: 10.5582/irdr.2015.01007

[225] Butt SUR, McNeil J. Complete heart block in a Caucasian woman with Behçet's disease: A case report. Journal of Medical Case Reports. 2016;**10**:102. DOI: 10.1186/s13256-016-0890-y

[226] Gürgün C, Ercan E, Ceyhan C, et al. Cardiovascular involvement in Behçet's disease. Japanese Heart Journal. 2002;**43**:389-398. DOI: 10.1536/jhj.43.389

[227] Desbois AC, Wechsler B, Cluzel P, et al. Cardiovascular involvement in Behçet's disease. La Revue de Médecine Interne. 2014;**35**(2):103-111. DOI: 10.1016/j.revmed.2013.12.002

[228] Ben GI, Belfeki N, Houman MH. Intracardiac thrombus in Behçet's disease. Reumatismo. 2016;**68**(3):148-153. DOI: 10.4081/reumatismo.2016.887

[229] Yurdakul S, Erdemir VA, Yıldırımtürk Ö, et al. Evaluation of

endothelial functions in patients with Behcet's disease without overt vascular involvement. Türk Kardiyoloji Derneği Arşivi. 2012;**40**(6):518-522. DOI: 10.5543/tkda.2012.43078

[230] Meric M, Oztas DM, Ugurlucan M, Tireli E, Dayioglu E. Giant left anterior descending coronary artery aneurysm in a patient with Behçet's disease. Brazilian Journal of Cardiovascular Surgery. 2022;**37**:605-608. DOI: 10.21470/1678-9741-2020-0665

[231] Vural U, Kizilay M, Aglar AA. Coronary involvement in Behçet's disease: What are its risks and prognosis? (Rare cases and literature review). Brazilian Journal of Cardiovascular Surgery. 2019;**34**(6):749-758. DOI: 10.21470/1678-9741-2019-0003

[232] Geri G, Wechsler B, Huong T, Du L, et al. Spectrum of cardiac lesions in Behçet disease. A series of 52 patients and review of the literature. Medicine. 2012;**91**:25-34. DOI: 10.1097/MD.0b013e3182428f4929

[233] Chen H, Zhang Y, Li C, et al. Coronary involvement in patients with Behçet's disease. Clinical Rheumatology. 2019;**38**(10):2835-2841. DOI: 10.1007/s10067-019-04640-z

[234] Owlia MB, Mehrpoor G. Behcet's disease: New concepts in cardiovascular involvements and future direction for treatment. ISRN Pharmacology. 2012;**6**:760484. DOI: 10.5402/2012/760484

[235] Babayeva AR, Kalinina EV, Zvonorenko MS, et al. Cardiovascular and metabolic comorbidity in rheumatic diseases: Focus on hyperuricemia and gout. Russian Medical Inquiry Medical Review. 2023;**7**(3):150-159. DOI: 10.32364/2587-6821-2023-7-3-150-159

[236] Cox P, Gupta S, Zhao SS, Hughes DM. The incidence and prevalence of cardiovascular diseases in gout: A systematic review and meta-analysis. Rheumatology International. 2021;**41**(7):1209-1219. DOI: 10.1007/s00296-021-04876-6

[237] Kim SY, Guevara JP, Kim KM, Choi HK, Heitjan DF, Albert DA. Hyperuricemia and coronary heart disease: A systematic review and meta-analysis. Arthritis Care & Research (Hoboken). Feb 2010;**62**(2):170-180. DOI: 10.1002/acr.20065. PMID: 20191515. PMCID: PMC3156692

[238] Ridker PM. C-reactive protein and the prediction of cardiovascular events among those at intermediate risk: Moving an inflammatory hypothesis toward consensus. Journal of the American College of Cardiology. 2007;**49**(21):2129-2138. DOI: 10.1016/j.jacc.2007.02.052

[239] Nurmohamed MT, Heslinga M, Kitas GD. Cardiovascular comorbidity in rheumatic diseases. Nature Reviews Rheumatology. 2015;**11**(12):693-704. DOI: 10.1038/nrrheum.2015.112

[240] Eliseev MS, Novikova AM, Zhelyabina OV, et al. Assessment of cardiovascular risk in patients with microcrystalline arthritis and rheumatoid arthritis using the ATP III and Reynolds risk score. Scientific and Practical Rheumatology. 2020;**58**(5):512-519. DOI: 10.47360/1995-4484-2020-512-519

[241] Choi HK, Ford ES, Li CY, Curhan G. Prevalence of the metabolic syndrome in patients with gout: The third National Health and nutrition examination survey. American Rheumatism. 2007;**57**(1):109-115. DOI: 10.1002/art.22466

[242] Edwards NL. The role of hyperuricemia and gout in kidney and cardiovascular disease. Cleveland Clinic Journal of Medicine. 2008;**75**:S13-S16. DOI: 10.3949/ccjm.75.suppl5.s13

[243] Johnson RJ, Kang DH, Feig D, et al. Is there a pathogenetic role for uric acid in hypertension and cardiovascular and renal disease? Hypertension. 2003;**41**:1183-1190

[244] Maksudova AN, Halfina TN, Almukhametova AI. At the appointment, a patient with hyperuricemia and chronic kidney disease: Features of management in accordance with Russian recommendations. Therapy No. 3. 2023. pp. 129-135. DOI: 10.18565/therapy.2023.3.129-135

[245] Ouppatham S, Bancha S, Choovichian P. The relationship of hyperuricemia and blood pressure in the Thai army population. Journal of Postgraduate Medicine. 2008;**54**(4):259-562. DOI: 10.4103/0022-3859.43509

[246] Pillinger MH, Goldfarb DS, Keenan RT. Gout and its comorbidities. Bulletin of the NYU Hospital for Joint Diseases. 2010;**68**(3):199-203. PMID: 20969552

[247] Niskanen LK, Laaksonen DE, Nyyssonen K, et al. Uric acid level as a risk factor for cardiovascular and all-cause mortality in middle-aged men: A prospective cohort study. Archives of Internal Medicine. 2004;**164**(14):1546-1551. DOI: 10.1001/archinte.164.14.1546

[248] Saito Y, Tanaka A, Node K, Kobayashi Y. Uric acid and cardiovascular disease: A clinical review. Journal of Cardiology. 2021;**78**:51-57. DOI: 10.1016/j.jjcc.2020.12.013

[249] Feig DI, Kang D, Johnson RJ. Uric acid and cardiovascular risk. The New England Journal of Medicine. 2008;**359**(17):1811-1821. DOI: 10.1056/NEJMra0800885

[250] Borghi C, Agabiti-Rosei E, Johnson RJ, et al. Hyperuricaemia and gout in cardiovascular, metabolic and kidney disease. European Journal of Internal Medicine. 2020;**80**:1-11. DOI: 10.1016/j.ejim.2020.07.006

[251] Rahimi-Sakak F, Maroofi M, Rahmani J, et al. Serum uric acid and risk of cardiovascular mortality: A systematic review and dose-response meta-analysis of cohort studies of over a million participants. BMC Cardiovascular Disorders. 2019;**19**:218. DOI: 10.1186/s12872-019-1215-z

[252] Hink HU, Santanam N, Dikalov S, et al. Peroxidase properties of extracellular superoxide dismutase: Role of uric acid in modulating in vivo activity. Arteriosclerosis, Thrombosis, and Vascular Biology. 2002;**22**:1402-1408

[253] Eliseev MS. Gout. M. GEOTAR-Media; 2019. p. 240 c

Chapter 2

Acute and Recurrent Pediatric Pericarditis

Stasa Krasic and Vladislav Vukomanovic

Abstract

Acute pericarditis belongs to the group of inflammatory pericardial syndromes with or without pericardial effusion, and the diagnosis is confirmed by the presence of two of the four criteria defined by the European Society of Cardiology: (i) chest pain; (ii) pericardial friction; (iii) changes on the electrocardiogram; and (iv) pericardial effusion on echocardiography. The etiology of pericarditis can be divided into infectious and non-infectious, but in most cases, the underlying etiology cannot be identified, and such cases are called "idiopathic." The clinical presentation is determined by the volume of fluid, the rate of accumulation, and the compliance of the myocardium. Anti-inflammatory therapy forms the cornerstone of pericarditis treatment. In acute pericarditis, it is necessary to use ibuprofen as monotherapy, and in case of risk factors, it is necessary to introduce colchicine immediately. Corticosteroids increase the risk of developing recurrent pericarditis. Recurrent pericarditis is the most common complication of acute pericarditis and is defined by the appearance of signs of pericarditis 4–6 weeks after a documented episode of acute pericarditis. It is treated with ibuprofen and colchicine. In the case of corticosteroid-dependent and colchicine-resistant pericarditis, anakinra can be used, even in children.

Keywords: pericarditis, children, etiology, diagnostics, treatment, complications

1. Introduction

Chest pain in the pediatric population is a common cause of visits to the emergency department. Acute chest pain in adults raises concerns about diseases such as myocardial infarction, which require rapid cardiac evaluation to reduce morbidity and mortality. Fortunately, in children and adolescents, fatal heart disease is extremely rare, and chest pain is generally a benign condition. Noncardiac causes of chest pain may be idiopathic but may include musculoskeletal, pulmonary, psychogenic, and gastrointestinal etiologies [1]. Heart diseases cause pain with lower frequency, about 1 to 10% [1–3]. The most common patterns of cardiogenic chest pain are pericarditis, arrhythmias, myocarditis, pulmonary thromboembolism, and sinking coronary artery [1–3].

IntechOpen

Pericarditis is clinically classified as non-exudative, exsudative, exsudative-constrictive, or constrictive pericarditis (CP). Depending on the duration of symptoms and symptoms of the disease, pericarditis can be divided into:

1. Acute pericarditis.

2. Incessant pericarditis—pericarditis with persistent symptoms without a symptom-free interval of 4 to 6 weeks, despite therapy.

3. Recurrent pericarditis—symptoms of pericarditis after a symptom-free interval of 4 to 6 weeks.

4. Chronic pericarditis—inflammation lasts over 3 months [4].

2. Acute pericardities

Acute pericarditis belongs to the group of inflammatory pericardial syndromes with or without pericardial effusion. The reported incidence in the general population of acute pericarditis is 30–150/100,000 per year and accounts for <0.2 to 5% of all emergency department visits for chest pain in children with no prior heart disease [5]. According to the European Society of Cardiology (ESC) recommendations (4), the clinical diagnosis is confirmed by the presence of two of the four criteria: (I) chest pain (85–90% of cases)—typically sharp and pleuritic, the intensity of which decreases when sitting and intensifies when leaning; (II) pericardial friction (≤33% of cases) —a creaking sound best heard with the diaphragm of the stethoscope along the left sternal border; (III) electrocardiogram (ECG) changes (up to 60% of cases)—new diffuse ST-elevation or PR depression in the acute phase; and (IV) pericardial effusion (up to 60% of cases) (**Table 1**) [4].

Depending on the etiology, additional signs and symptoms may be present (fever and leukocytosis or systemic inflammatory disease). Elevated inflammation parameters, C-reactive protein (CRP), erythrocyte sedimentation rate (ESR), and leukocytosis are common findings in patients with acute pericarditis. They may help monitor disease activity and therapy efficacy. Along with pericarditis, there may also be myocarditis, which is indicated by the elevation of the marker of cardiomyocytolysis (troponin) [4, 5]. In case of predominant pericardial inflammation, we talk about myopericarditis; on the contrary, if the myocardial inflammation is predominant, we talk about perimyocarditis.

2.1 Etiology

The etiology of pericarditis can be divided into infectious and non-infectious, but in most cases, the underlying etiology cannot be identified, and such cases are called "idiopathic" [4, 5]. Idiopathic acute pericarditis is of unknown etiology, often of presumed viral etiology, i.e., a condition after a viral infection, with an incidence of 37–68% in the pediatric cohort. Some studies investigate the difference between viral and idiopathic pericarditis by comparing cytokine concentrations in sera and exudates. This study suggested that the pericardial fluid in viral pericarditis exhibits high tumor necrosis factor alpha (TNF-α) and low transforming growth factor beta 1 (TGFβ1) concentrations, in contrast to autoreactive pericarditis [6].

Pericarditis	Definition and diagnostic criteria
Acute	Inflammatory pericardial syndrome, which is confirmed by the existence of two of the four following criteria: 1. Chest pain. 2. Auscultatory registered pericardial friction. 3. ECG changes. 4. Echocardiographically verified effusion. Supporting findings: 5. Elevated positive reactants of the acute phase (ESR, CRP, etc.) 6. Pericardial effusion verified by CT or CMR
Incessant	pericarditis with persistent symptoms without a symptom-free interval of 4 to 6 weeks, despite therapy
Chronic	inflammation of the heart's outer layer that lasts over 3 months
Recurrent	symptoms of pericarditis after a symptom-free interval of 4 to 6 weeks

Abbreviations: CMR – cardiac magnetic resonance; CT – computed tomography; CRP – C-reactive protein; ECG – electrocardiogram; ESR – erythrocyte sedimentation rate.

Table 1.
Definition of and diagnostic criteria for pericarditis.

Infectious pericarditis can be caused by viruses (serous pericarditis), bacteria (purulent pericarditis), tuberculosis bacillus (mainly chronic), fungi, and parasitic. Cardiotropic viruses like Parvovirus-B19, herpes viruses (cytomegalovirus (CMV); Ebstein-Barr virus (EBV); and human herpesvirus 6 (HHV6)), influenza, hepatitis-C virus (HCV), human immunodeficiency virus (HIV), Enterovirus, and Adenovirus species have been described. The most commonly identifiable etiology is viral in origin in developed countries (about 80%), whereas in the developing world, tuberculosis (TB) is the most frequent etiology. On the other hand, bacterial and parasitic infections are rare in developed countries [5].

Non-infectious etiologies include autoimmune pericarditis (systemic inflammatory diseases: mainly systemic lupus erythematosus (SLE), rheumatoid arthritis, Sjögren's syndrome, scleroderma, vasculitis, and mainly Behçet syndrome), autoinflammatory (e.g., familial Mediterranean fever), iatrogenic, drug-related pericarditis (lupus-like syndrome (e.g., due to procainamide, hydralazine, methyldopa, isoniazid, and phenytoin); chemotherapy (e.g., due to anthracyclines), postcardiac injury syndromes (after acute myocardial infarction (MI), percutaneous coronary intervention (PCI), pacemaker implantation, implantable cardioverter defibrillator (ICD) implantation, ablation of arrhythmias, and cardiac or thoracic surgery), metabolic (renal failure, hypothyroidism – myxedema, and as part of anorexia), and during malignant disease (serofibrinous) [7].

Postpericardiotomy syndrome (PPS) is a known complication of any cardiac surgery, with a reported incidence varying widely from 1 to 40%. It is a hypersensitivity reaction characterized by pleural, pericardial, or lung tissue inflammation, followed by cardiac surgery cutdown of pericardial space or myocardial infarction. Pathophysiology research demonstrated antibodies in patients with PPS, thus explaining the syndrome with an autoimmune response. Namely, tissue damage triggers the autoimmune reaction of the pericardium and pleura, mostly occurring between 1 and 6 weeks after the procedure [8]. Some authors have noted that the surgical closure of atrial septal defect (ASD) poses a higher risk for the development of PPS than other operations. Heching et al. found that 28% of patients developed PPS after ASD closure [9].

From 2012 to 2024, in our Institute, 90 patients were treated with acute pericarditis, 56.7% boys and 43.3% girls, average age of 11.4 ±5.4 years. Idiopathic acute pericarditis was the most common (34 patients (pts)), while viral pericarditis was found in 13 patients (viruses: SARS-CoV-2, Parvo-B19, EBV, Adenovirus, Enterovirus). Pericardial affection as part of the Multisystem inflammatory syndrome in children (MIS-C) temporarily associated with SARS-CoV-2 was detected in 15 patients [10, 11]. Autoimmune pericarditis was detected in 19 patients, while postpericardiotomy syndrome was detected in 13 patients (ASD 7/13 pts., ventricular septal defect (VSD) 3/13 pts., modified Blalock-Taussig shunt (MBTS) 1/13 pts., resection of subaortic membrane 1/13 pts., and Tetralogy of Fallot 1/13 pts). Five patients had bacterial pericarditis: *Staphylococcus aureus*, *Haemophilus influenzae*, and tuberculosis (*Mycobacterium tuberculosis* (TBC)). Myocardial involvement was detected in 31 patients: 27 patients had perimyocarditis, while 4 patients had myopericarditis.

2.2 Pathogenesis

Pericardial injury caused by various etiological factors leads to the release of damage-associated molecular patterns (DAMPs) and pathogen-associated molecular patterns (PAMPs). It induces the synthesis of nuclear factor kappa-light-chain-enhancer of activated B cells (NF-κB), which increases the transcription of precursors of inflammatory molecules and cytokines (NOD-like receptor (NLR) family pyrin domain-containing 3 (NLRP3), apoptosis-associated speck-like protein containing a CARD (ASC), pro-caspase-1) that are required to polymerize the NLRP3 inflammasome, ultimately releasing interleukin 1b (IL-1b) and interleukin 18 (IL-18). NF-κB stimulates the synthesis of phospholipase-A2 required to activate the arachidonic acid (AA) pathway and the subsequent synthesis of prostaglandins and thromboxane. The IL-1 receptor (IL-1R) plays a central role because interleukin 1a (IL-1a) functions as an alarm or DAMP released during tissue injury, and IL-1b is released during inflammation and increases inflammatory processes [12].

2.3 Clinical manifestations

The fluid volume determines the clinical presentation of pericardial effusion, the accumulation rate, and the myocardium compliance. In the case of rapid accumulation, even a small amount of effusion can result in cardiac tamponade (CT).

Cardiac tamponade is a life-threatening condition that happens after sudden and/or excessive accumulation of fluid in the pericardial space. The most common causes of tamponade are pericarditis (infection and non-infection), iatrogenic (cardiac invasive procedures and postsurgery), and collagen vascular disease (SLE, scleroderma, dermatomyositis, etc.). The causes of effusion with a high incidence of progression to tamponade include bacterial (*S. aureus*, *Meningococcus*, *H. influenzae*, *Pneumococcus*, *Streptococcus*, *Mycobacterium tuberculosis*, etc.), fungal (*Aspergillus* spp., etc.), human immunodeficiency virus (HIV)-associated infections, bleeding, and cancer involvement. Hypothyroidism could be the cause of CT in childhood [13]. The pericardium has some degree of elasticity, and when the elastic limit is reached, the intrapericardial pressure rises, leading to critical cardiac compression, restriction of ventricular diastolic filling, and impeding cardiac output. Consequently, the classic signs of CT are included in Beck's triad of hypotension, jugular venous distension, and muffled heart sounds. Other clinical signs in a patient with CT include tachycardia, pulsus paradoxus, dyspnea, and orthopnea. Hypotension and bradycardia will appear ultimately before cardiac arrest. Due to specific signs and symptoms, cardiac tamponade is a clinical diagnosis, while an echocardiography examination should confirm the suspicion [14]. Purulent pericarditis may lead to cardiac tamponade and septic shock [15].

Conversely, the slow accumulation of fluid contributes to the development of myocardial tolerance. In certain conditions, such as tuberculous pericarditis, up to 3 liters of fluid can accumulate in the pericardial sac.

The most common symptoms and signs of acute pericarditis are presented in **Table 2** [5].

Patients with acute pericarditis usually have chest pain (>85–90% of cases), which is a consequence of the friction between the layers of the inflamed pericardium. Pericardial pain is the cardinal symptom, and it is sharp chest pain, which may also radiate to the left shoulder, neck, or back and resembles ischemic pain. The pain is typically less severe when sitting up and more severe when lying down or breathing deeply. In contrast, it usually subsides in the upright position and when leaning due to reduced pressure on the parietal pericardium. In the case of increased pericardial effusion, chest pain decreases or disappears. Commonly associated clinical signs and symptoms include intermittent fever, dyspnea, cough, malaise, myalgia, and occasional hiccups. Anamnestic data often indicate a current viral infection, a gastrointestinal or a flu-like syndrome [4].

2.4 Diagnostics

2.4.1 Physical examination

Patients with acute pericarditis often appear uncomfortable or anxious and may have sinus tachycardia and low-grade fever. Auscultation of patients with pericarditis can detect pericardial rub (a pathognomonic sign of pericarditis), which is present in one-third of patients. It is a superficial crackling sound, best heard with the stethoscope's diaphragm along the left sternal border, with the patient leaning forward or resting on elbows and knees. It usually consists of three phases that correspond to the movements of the heart during atrial systole (it is absent in atrial fibrillation), ventricular systole, and the phase of rapid filling of the ventricles—early ventricular diastole. Sometimes, pericardial rub has only two or even one component. A pericardial rub may disappear not only after the resolution of the disease, but also in the case of accumulation of pericardial fluid, which reflects the worsening of the disease. The pericardial rub is a specific sign of acute pericarditis (specificity approximately 100%) [4].

Symptoms	Percent (%)
Chest pain	70–90
Temperature	26
Fatigue	18
Dyspnea	12
Signs of cardiac tamponade	16

Table 2.
Frequency of the most common signs and symptoms of acute pericarditis.

Pulsus paradoxus (PP) is an abnormal drop in systolic blood pressure during inspiration—more than 10 mmHg. Common causes include cardiac tamponade, severe asthma, and chronic obstructive pulmonary disease (COPD). The most accurate PP measurement method is using a manual sphygmomanometer and stethoscope. The initial sounds auscultated are heard only during expiration, and it is important to take note of this pressure. Next, as the cuff pressure is dropped further, the pressure should be noted when Korotkoff sounds are heard during inspiration and expiration. The variation between these two systolic pressures quantifies PP [16]. The sensitivity of PP higher than 10 and 12 mmHg is 98%, while specificity is 70 and 83%, respectively. "Total paradox," also known as "pulse obliteration," is defined as the inspiratory disappearance of the brachial and radial pulses, with the total disappearance of the Korotkoff sounds [17]. Pulsus paradoxus may be absent with tamponade caused by regional right atrial compression [18].

A Kussmaul sign could be seen in patients with constrictive pericarditis. The paradoxical rise in jugular venous pressure or failure to fall on inspiration is related to high right atrial pressure [19].

After carefully taking auto- and hetero-anamnesis data and conducting a physical examination, whereupon acute pericarditis can already be suspected with a high probability, the following should be done:

1. ECG (Recommendation class I, level of evidence C),
2. X-ray of the heart and lungs (Recommendation class I, level of evidence C),
3. Laboratory analyses (Recommendation class I, level of evidence C).
4. Echocardiographic examination (Recommendation class I, level of evidence C) [4].

2.4.2 Electrocardiogram

ECG changes are derived from the epicardium's and adjacent myocardium's inflammation because the parietal pericardium is electrically silent [4]. Sequential changes are seen in only approximately 60% of patients. Evolution is recorded on the ECG during the disease course in a patient with acute pericarditis [20]. At the very beginning of the disease, depression of the PR segment and widespread concave elevation of the ST segment in D1, D2, D3, aVL, aVF, and precordial leads are registered. PR depression and ST elevation are assessed based on the position of the TP segment. In addition, sinus tachycardia may be present on the ECG recording (**Figure 1**) [4, 20].

In the long stage of the disease (1–3 weeks), the ECG gradually normalizes—the PR and ST segments return to the isoelectric line, and flattened T waves are registered. In the third stage, a diffuse inversion of T waves starts from the right and spreads to the left precordial leads (**Figure 2**).

In the last, fourth stage of the disease, there is the normalization of the ECG—the positivity of the T wave, which takes place in the reverse order of the one where it started.

The ECG in acute pericarditis may resemble ST-elevation myocardial infarction (STEMI). The changes indicating acute pericarditis are: (a) appearance of ST elevation less than 5 mm, (b) concavity of the ST segment, (c) diffuseness

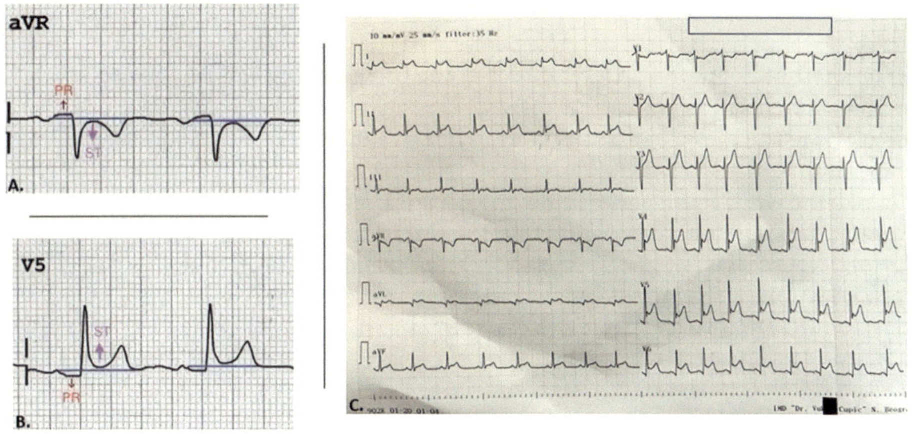

Figure 1.
ECG changes in the first phase of acute pericarditis; PR-segment elevation in aVR (A); ST-segment depression in V5 (B); 12-channel ECG in a patient with acute pericarditis.

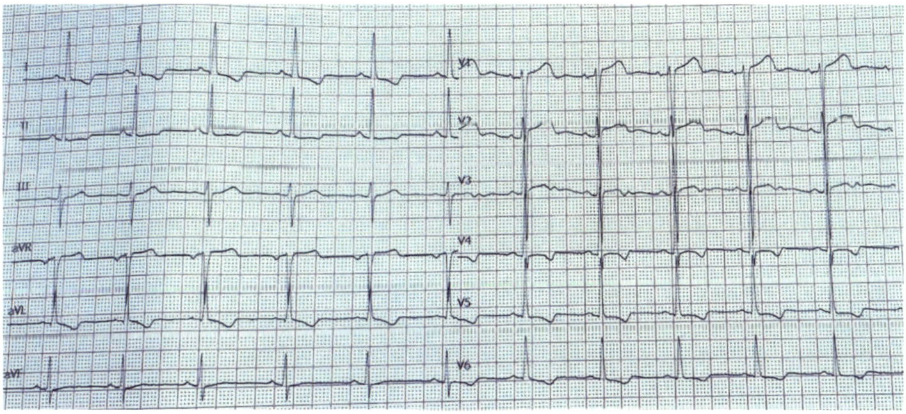

Figure 2.
ECG changes in the third stage of pericarditis—T waves' inversion.

of changes, (d) less pronounced reciprocal depression of the ST segment, (e) elevation of the PR segment in aVR, with reciprocal PR-segment depression in other leads, (f) absence of abnormal Q-waves, and (g) T-wave inversion after ST-segment elevation [13].

ECG changes in acute pericarditis should be distinguished from early repolarization. Namely, in acute pericarditis, the ST-segment elevation and T-wave amplitude ratio in the lead V6 is greater than 0.24 (positive and negative predictive values are 100%). This ECG sign is typical for the differential diagnosis of acute pericarditis and early repolarization. Also, the ratio of ST-segment amplitude to T-wave amplitude ≥0.25 in leads D1, V4, V5, and V6 indicates acute pericarditis [13].

In cardiac tamponade with severe or very severe pericardial effusion, findings on an ECG indicating a large pericardial effusion include low QRS voltage, electrical alternans (changes in the amplitude or morphology of the P, QRS, and ST-T waves from one beat to the next, resulting from cardiac oscillation within the pericardial fluid) [17].

2.4.3 X-ray

The chest radiograph (CXR) is typically the first imaging test performed in patients with potential pericardial disease. Normal pericardial fluid volume in neonates is usually less than 5 milliliters, while in adults, it contains less than 50 mL of serous fluid.

In patients with acute pericarditis, the CXR is usually within normal limits, but if the effusion is larger, the cardiothoracic index is increased. Less than 200 ml of effusions is typically not visible on a CXR [21]. The most sensitive sign of pericardial effusion on CXR is the enlargement of the cardiac silhouette (cardiothoracic ratio (CTR) >50%) (**Figure 3**). This gives rise to a "globular" configuration known as the "water bottle sign."

2.4.4 Biomarkers

Currently, no specific biomarker for pericarditis is available. Elevated concentrations of inflammatory parameters are usually present in patients with acute pericarditis (approximately 80% of patients). Leukocytosis, increased erythrocyte sedimentation rate, and increased C-reactive protein (CRP) are most often registered. CRP is important not only to confirm the suspicion of acute pericarditis but also to monitor the course and activity of the disease and the eventual correction of anti-inflammatory therapy.

Also, cardiospecific proteins, such as troponin I, must be administered to patients with pericarditis. Elevated troponin values are found in about 30% of cases of acute pericarditis. If pericardial inflammation is dominant, patients suffer from myopericarditis; if myocardial involvement is dominant, we are discussing permyocarditis. Interestingly, patients with pericarditis and elevated biomarkers of cardiomyocytolysis almost always have ST-segment elevation. A significant finding is that simultaneous myocardium involvement does not necessarily indicate a worse prognosis. These patients have recurrent pericarditis (RP) less often [22 , 23].

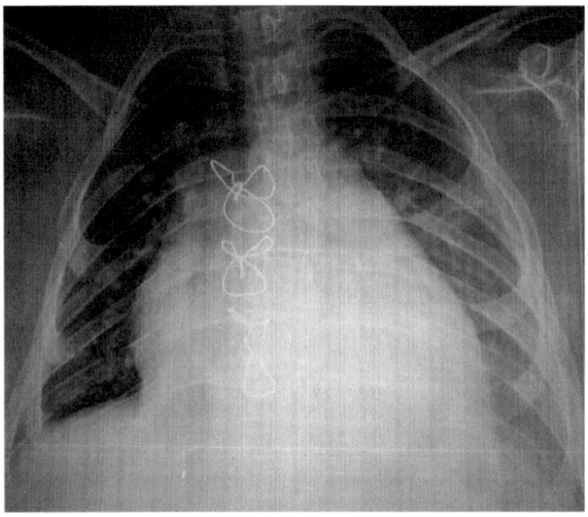

Figure 3.
CXR in a patient with postpericardiotomy syndrome after ASD operation (private collection).

2.4.5 Echocardiography

Echocardiography is widely available and provides valuable information about visualization of the thickened and hyperechoic pericardium, the presence or absence of pericardial effusion, its volume, and accompanying hemodynamic effects. Although echocardiography is normal in 40% of cases, it is essential to identify complications, such as tamponade or constrictive pericarditis. It could also be useful for monitoring the evolution of pericardial effusion over time and the response to medical therapy. Pericardial effusion is usually small and is evident in 60% of cases (**Figure 4**).

Pericardial effusion, based on size in diastole, is characterized as mild (<10 mm), moderate (10–20 mm), severe (21–25 mm), or very severe (> 25 mm). Trivial pericardial effusion is only seen in systole [4].

Echocardiographic signs of cardiac tamponade are 1) diastolic collapse of the right atrium (RA) (sensitivity 50–100%, specificity 33–100%); 2) duration of the diastolic RA collapse as a ratio of the cardiac cycle length > 0.34 (sensitivity >90%, specificity 100%); 3) diastolic collapse of the right ventricle (sensitivity 48–100%, specificity 72–100%); 4) respiratory changes of the mitral E velocity > 25%, and tricuspid E velocity > 40%; and 5) inferior vena cava (IVC) plethora (dilatation >20 mm and < 50% reduction in the inspiratory phase) (sensitivity 87%, specificity 40%) [24].

It may also aid in determining concomitant ventricular dysfunction, which may suggest a component of myocarditis. Patients with myocardial involvement might have lower ejection fraction and longitudinal and circumferential strain in all three myocardial layers and at the basal, midventricular, and apical levels [25].

2.4.6 Cardiac magnetic resonance

Cardiac magnetic resonance (CMR) is particularly useful in case of suspicion of myocardial involvement. CMR provides both morphological and hemodynamic information. The key CMR findings of pericarditis are the thickening of pericardial

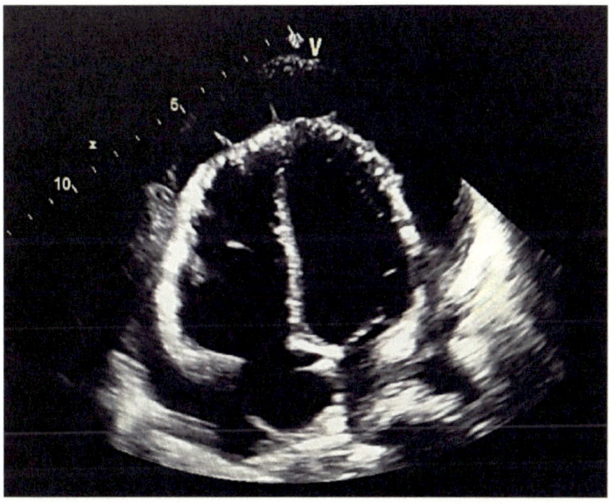

Figure 4.
The echocardiographic finding of a patient with idiopathic acute pericarditis (private collection).

layers and associated pericardial effusion on T1-weighted spin-echo CMR or cine CMR. In contrast, T2-weighted short tau inversion recovery (STIR) spin-echo CMR allows visualization of edema of the inflamed pericardial layers. Intense pericardial delayed hyperenhancement (DHE) in gadolinium-enhanced CMR studies represents objective evidence of pericardial inflammation. Additionally, higher quantitative pericardial DHE was independently associated with the ongoing recurrence of recurrent pericarditis [26]. Phase-sensitive inversion recovery (PSIR) sequence is central in diagnosing pericardial inflammation on magnetic resonance imaging (MRI) and surveillance, such as evaluating response to anti-inflammatory therapies. Adding a fat-suppression prepulse may enhance the visualization of pericardial inflammation [27]. The severity of pericardial late gadolinium enhancement (LGE) on initial MRI is significantly associated with recurrent pericarditis flares and escalation of therapy, and quantitative methods of pericardial LGE recently developed in the research setting have potential future clinical applications [28].

3. Therapy of acute pericarditis

Anti-inflammatory therapy is the cornerstone of pericarditis treatment. Understanding the inflammatory basis of pericarditis and the role of the inflammasome provides insight into the mechanisms of action of previously prescribed and new treatment options.

Nonsteroidal anti-inflammatory drugs (NSAIDs) are among the most commonly used agents in children with pericarditis. They act through the inhibition mechanism of cyclooxygenase inhibitors and decrease pericarditic pain associated with inflammation by inhibiting prostaglandin production. According to the ESC guidelines, high-dose NSAIDs should be used in pediatric pericarditis (class I, level C recommendation). Ibuprofen and indomethacin are the most frequently prescribed in the pediatric cohort. In contrast, naproxen and ketorolac were used in limited case reports and cohort studies. Acetylsalicylic acid (ASA) is not recommended in children <12 years due to the risk of Reye's syndrome and, therefore, is a class III level C recommendation for children in the 2015 ESC guidelines [4]. Failure to respond to an NSAID therapy within 7 days is associated with a relatively poorer prognosis in patients with pericarditis. On the other hand, we found that a CRP concentration $\geq$ 125 mg/L was determined to be an independent risk factor for recurrence in children with pericarditis [23].

Due to thrombocyte function inhibition, patients on NSAIDs are at risk for significant bleeding or bruising associated with the larger dose. Additionally, NSAID-treated children may be at increased risk of gastrointestinal (GI) bleeding due to diminished protective prostaglandin formation in the stomach. Consequently, they are at increased risk of GI bleeding, ulceration, and/or perforation, and the 2015 ESC guidelines recommend that patients treated should also receive a gastroprotective agent. Due to prostaglandin synthesis inhibition, NSAIDs could produce a prerenal injury, potentiating the possibility of an acute kidney injury (AKI), acute interstitial nephritis, and/or acute renal papillary necrosis, so the blood urea nitrogen (BUN) and creatinine should be monitored [4]. Indomethacin may be associated with the highest risk of neurologic manifestations, potentially exacerbating underlying psychiatric disturbances. At the same time, children with a history of asthma may develop an increased risk of asthma exacerbation due to an increase in leukotriene production [29].

According to the ESC recommendation, *colchicine* is recommended for treating acute pericarditis (class IIa, level C recommendation) in adults. The effectiveness of colchicine is related to the inhibitory effects on the activation of the NLRP3 inflammasome, which is involved in releasing the pro-inflammatory cytokine interleukin 1 (IL-1). Interleukin 1 is responsible for recruiting neutrophils and macrophages to the injury site. Colchicine also inhibits caspase-1 and the consequent release of tumor necrosis factor (TNF) and reactive oxygen species (ROS) [4]. Additionally, colchicine ameliorates the inflammatory cascade by inhibiting the assembly of the mitotic spindle, essentially stopping mitosis at metaphase [29].

By analyzing 72 of our patients with pericarditis who were treated from January 2011 to December 2019, we concluded that patients who are at higher risk for developing recurrent pericarditis (**Table 3**) should immediately start dual anti-inflammatory therapy (**Table 3**) [23, 30].

Relatively mild and common side effects of colchicine are gastrointestinal manifestations, such as abdominal pain, nausea, vomiting, and diarrhea, with diarrhea being the most common. Those symptoms are most frequently experienced within 24 hours of therapy and can be diminished by lowering the drug dose. On the other hand, patients with renal and liver failure may develop severe side effects such as blood dyscrasias, including myelosuppression, leukopenia, granulocytopenia, thrombocytopenia, pancytopenia, and aplastic anemia, which may develop within 24 to 72 hours. Great caution is especially needed in patients taking cytochrome P450 3A4 (CYP3A4) inhibitors simultaneously (like erythromycin and fluconazole), while colchicine is metabolized in the liver by this enzyme and eliminated via p-glycoprotein. So, the patients should avoid grapefruit juice. Neuromuscular toxicity

Drug	Dose	Treatment duration	Dose tapering
Ibuprofen	30–50 mg/kg in 3 divided doses	1–2 weeks	for 1–2 weeks after the normalization of inflammatory parameters
Colchicine	2015 ESC guideline dosing recommendations: • 0.5 mg/day in patients <5 yr. • 1.0–1.5 mg/day in 2 to 3 divided doses in patients >5 yr. Manufacturer package insert recommendations: • 4 to 6 yr.: 0.3–1.8 mg daily in 1–2 divided doses • 6 to 12 yr.: 0.9–1.8 mg daily in 1–2 divided doses • >12 yr.: Refer to adult dosing: 1 × 0.5 mg (BW <70 kg) 2 × 0.5 mg (BW > 70 kg)	3 months	Not often used in clinical practice / 0.5 mg on another day (BW < 70 kg) 0.5 mg once daily (BW > 70 kg) for a few weeks

Abbreviations: BW – body weight; ESC – European Society of Cardiology.

Table 3.
Recommendation for the treatment of acute pericarditis in children modified according to the recommendations of the European Association of Cardiologists.

may manifest as sensory neuropathy and/or rhabdomyolysis and occurs with chronic therapy. Chronic colchicine may also induce cyanocobalamin deficiency by disturbing intestinal absorption [29].

Historically, *corticosteroids* (CS) have been used in pericarditis treatment, leading to rapid resolution of symptoms and pericardial effusion. The mechanism of action of CS consists of blocking transcription factors, such as nuclear factor-kappa B (NF-kB) and activator protein-1 (AP-1), which are required for the transcription of pro-inflammatory mediators and the synthesis of many inflammatory cytokines [29]. However, CS increase the risk of pericarditis recurrence and prolong the disease course. At the same time, high doses of CS (1.0 mg/kg/day prednisone) are often associated with serious side effects and a higher rate of recurrence. Our series of patients showed that CS increase the recurrence frequency after acute pericarditis, especially in those treated with higher doses (0.5–1 mg/kg) [23]. The potential mechanism is that CS may potentiate DNA or RNA replication in pericardial tissue, leading to increased viral antigens, thus impairing the clearance of viral infections. Consequently, the 2015 ESC guidelines do not recommend corticosteroids as first-line therapy for pericarditis in children (class III, level C recommendation). On the other hand, in patients with recurrent pericarditis refractory to treatment with NSAID plus

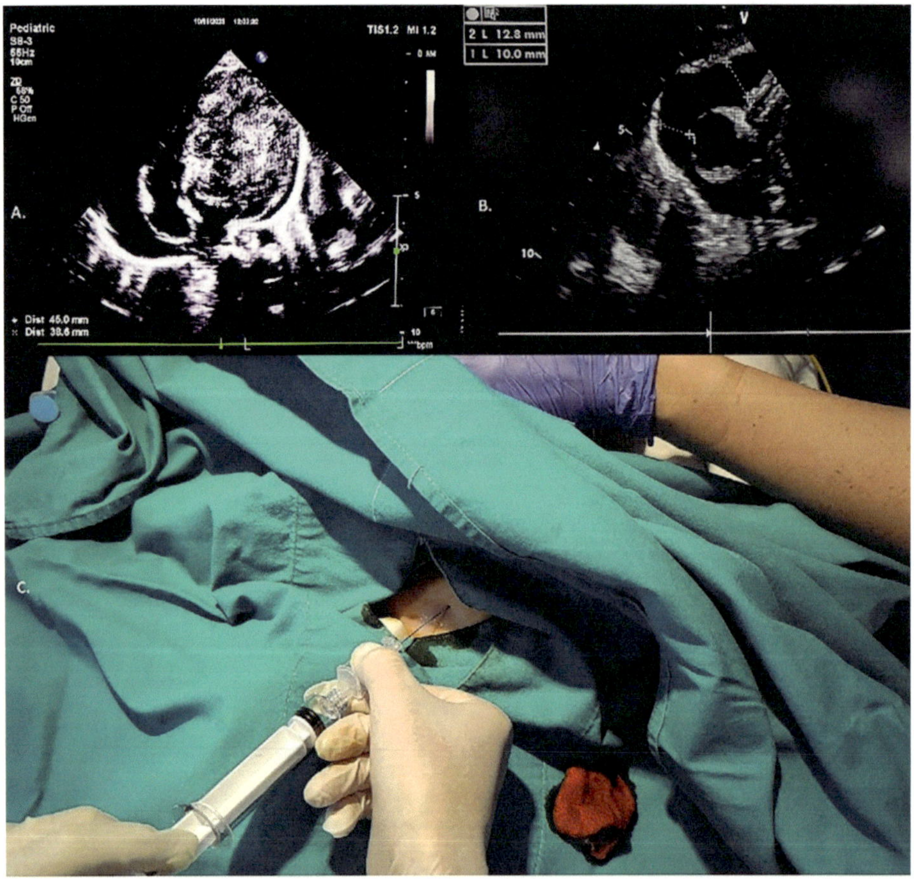

Figure 5.
Echo-guided pericardial puncture (C) in our 4-month-old infant with pericardial effusion (B) induced by huge left ventricle (LV) rhabdomyoma (45.0 × 38.6 mm) (C) treated with sirolimus within tuberous sclerosis.

colchicine, small CS doses are recommended (class IIa, level C recommendation) [4]. Patients with pericardial affection as a part of MIS-C were successfully treated with CS without any complications and episodes of recurrence [10, 11, 31].

Urgent *pericardiocentesis* or *drainage* of pericardial effusion is indicated for each patient with an established diagnosis of cardiac tamponade and hemodynamic shock. Pericardiocentesis is especially recommended when purulent, tuberculous, or neoplastic pericarditis is suspected or in patients who remain symptomatic despite medical treatment, and it could be urgent or elective, despite patients' signs and symptoms. According to the ESC's current opinion, a total score ≥ 6 warrants immediate pericardiocentesis in the absence of contraindications and rapidly deteriorating patients. The scoring system includes etiology, clinical presentation, and echocardiography findings [32].

In the last 12 years, our Institute has performed pericardial puncture in 3 patients (**Figure 5**), pericardial drainage in 12 patients, and simultaneous pleural drainage in 4 patients.

An inflammatory pseudotumor was extracted in one patient with bacterial pericarditis (**Figure 6**).

When bacterial pericarditis (purulent pericarditis—PP) is suspected, empiric broad-spectrum parenteral *antibiotics* should be administered immediately. The treatment duration varies (range: 2–8 weeks) and routes (oral/intravenous [IV]/ combination). For diagnosis and treatment, all of the reported cases of pediatric purulent required pericardial drainage (some with temporary pericardial drain left in place). Open surgical drainage through subxiphoid pericardiotomy is preferable,

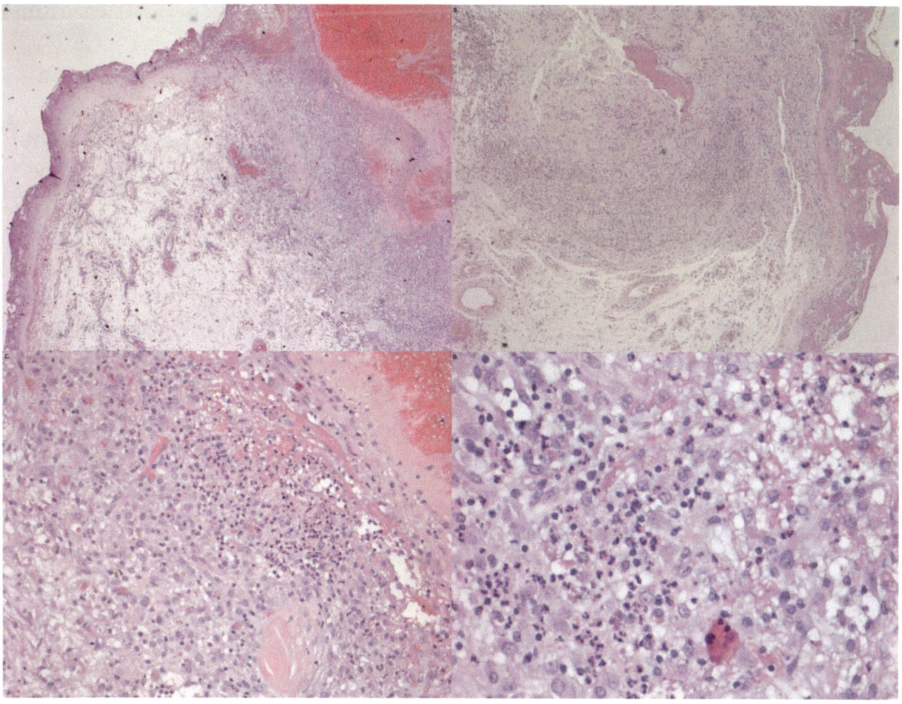

Figure 6.
Histological findings in a patient with pericardial inflammatory pseudotumor; A. hematoxylin–eosin × 25; B. hematoxylin–eosin × 50; C. hematoxylin–eosin × 200; D. hematoxylin–eosin × 400 (private collection). Courtesy of Dejana Bozic, MD.

but frequent irrigation of the pericardial cavity using large catheters may liquefy the purulent exudate. One study showed that early intervention for PP with pericardiectomy should be done if the patients have tamponade after initial pericardiocentesis or if the fever persists on appropriate antibiotics therapy [33]. *Intrapericardial fibrinolysis*, a less invasive procedure, has been proposed as an alternative to surgery for PP treatment (class IIa, level C recommendation). Two main options can be distinguished: primary fibrinolysis performed immediately after drain insertion and rescue fibrinolysis applied in cases of recurrence or incomplete evacuation of pus. Streptokinase, urokinase, and tissue plasminogen activators (tPAs) have all been used for pericardial fibrinolysis. Report a failure rate of 5% after using intrapericardial fibrinolysis to manage PP [15]. We treated a 4-month-old patient with *S. aureus* PP with intrapericardial tPA (2 mg in 10 ml of saline solution during 3 hours) installation due to incomplete evacuation of pus after surgical drainage.

4. Complications

The most common complications are recurrent or incessant pericarditis, which occurs in about 15 to 30% of cases. Recurrent pericarditis is the recurrence of symptoms after a minimum symptom-free interval of 4–6 weeks. If symptoms persist for more than 4–6 weeks after an acute episode, pericarditis is defined as incessant (**Table 1**) [4, 34, 35]. The study conducted by Imazio M et al. highlights that an incessant course of pericarditis is a possible new risk factor for complications and especially for developing constriction. Patients with incessant pericarditis more commonly had echocardiographic evidence of constriction and thickened pericardium on multimodality imaging [36].

Also, the development of chronic and constrictive pericarditis may occur in a smaller number of patients.

The incidence of *constrictive pericarditis (CP)* is very low in children, and it could be explained as a possible subdiagnosis and the insidious character of this disease and its complications. CP induces signs of heart failure due to loss of pericardial compliance (layers' adhesion) and restricting diastolic filling of both ventricles. It is a consequence of a chronic inflammatory process involving both pericardial layers, parietal and visceral, and/or scar. The main etiological factors in developed countries are idiopathic pericarditis, cardiac surgery, malignancy, and radiotherapy. Incomplete drainage of PP is a rare entity that should also be considered. However, tuberculosis remains the most prevalent cause in developing countries [37]. The increasing number of cardiac surgeries in the modern era leads to postpericardiotomy syndrome as the main cause of CP [38]. The ESC guidelines recommend using echocardiography to diagnose constrictive pericarditis. Two-dimensional (2D) echocardiography may show increased pericardial thickness with or without calcification, biatrial enlargement, reduced IVC collapsibility index, and septal bounce (a consequence of enhanced interventricular dependency). Pulsed-wave echocardiography Doppler indicates increased mitral E-wave velocity and shortened deceleration time (usually <160 ms), with a small or absent A-wave resembling a restrictive inflow pattern. With inspiration, there is a decrease in peak mitral E-wave velocity by >25% during the first beat of inspiration, while peak tricuspid E-wave velocity increases by >40%. An annulus reversus phenomenon means the lateral mitral tissue Doppler e' velocity is lower than the medial e' velocity due to the tethering of the adjacent fibrotic and

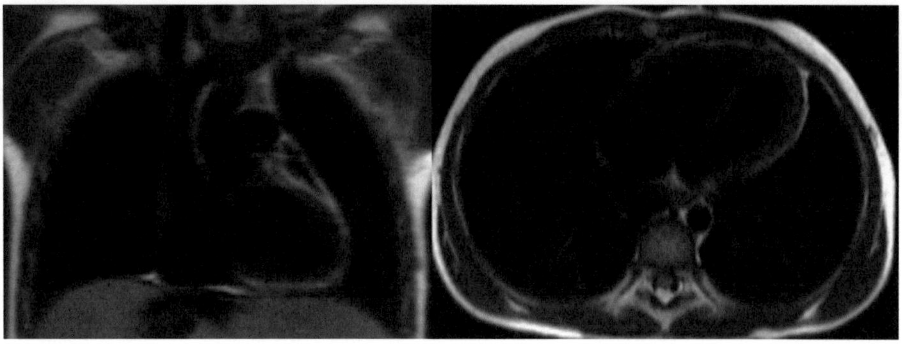

Figure 7.
Cardiac magnetic resonance in the patient with constrictive pericarditis (private collection).

scarred pericardium. Additionally, due to the same reasons, the 2D left ventricle (LV) speckle tracking technique points out the impairment of circumferential shortening and twist mechanics, while a longitudinal strain is well preserved [19]. CMR and computed tomography (CT) enable accurate measurements of pericardial thickness, while computed tomography scans can detect calcifications better. In patients with active inflammation, anti-inflammatory drugs are the first-line therapy. A pericardiectomy is the only definitive management of chronic refractory CP, with an operative mortality rate of 10–50%. Due to the possibility of transient constrictive pericarditis, patients with newly diagnosed CP who are hemodynamically stable and do not have stigmas of chronic constriction may be treated with anti-inflammatory agents for up to 3 months with close monitoring [39].

We treated one female patient with CP. She was examined due to hepatomegaly. Echocardiography and CMR findings pointed out CP (**Figure 7**). The patient underwent pericardiectomy at 12 years of age, and the ParvoB-19 virus was isolated from the pericardial tissue.

In one patient with bacterial pericarditis, partial anterior pericardiectomy was performed.

In some patients, during the pericardial healing process, after the inflammation, granulation tissue formation with subsequent fibrosis of the pericardium and obliteration of the pericardial cavity may lead to constrictive-effusive pericarditis [40].

5. Recurrent pericarditis

Recurrent pericarditis (RP) is an autoimmune reaction resulting from the exposure of previously hidden self-antigens and the production of cardiac autoantibodies after acute pericarditis [35]. On the other hand, in patients with RP, the inflammation is predominantly mediated by cytokines (mainly interleukin 1 (IL-1)), suggesting the effects of the innate immune system typical of auto-inflammatory diseases. In some genetically determined syndromes, such as familial Mediterranean fever and cryopyrin-associated periodic syndromes, recurrences of pericarditis occur more often, so genetic tests should be performed in patients with a high frequency of recurrences [29].

Risk factors for recurrent pericarditis in the adult patient population are clearly defined and are divided into factors associated with:

1. Treatment-related variables with increased risk in multivariable models:

    a. Corticosteroids' use.

    b. Lack of colchicine.

3. Patient-related variables with increased risk in multivariable models:

    a. Incomplete response to NSAIDs

    b. Elevated CRP.

1. Patient-related variables without increased risk in multivariable models:

    a. Younger patients.

    b. Males.

    c. Pericardial effusion [35].

Although the risk factors for RP are clearly defined in adults, we tried to define them in a group of pediatric patients. Through a detailed retrospective analysis and based on statistical processing, we defined that the independent risk factors for recurrent pericarditis are:

1. Non-idiopathic acute pericarditis.

2. Corticosteroids' use.

3. ESR > 50 mm/h.

4. CRP ≥ 125 mg/L.

5. Absence of myocardial inflammation [23].

Independent risk factors for recurrent pericarditis in children were classified into three groups (**Table 4**).

Patient-related variables with increased risk in multivariable models
• ESR > 50 mm/L
• CRP ≥ 125 mg/L
Disease-related variables with increased risk in multivariable models
• absence of myocardial inflammation
• non-idiopathic acute pericarditis
Treatment-related variables without increased risk in multivariable models
• corticosteroids' use
Abbreviations: ESR – erythrocyte sedimentation rate; CRP – C-reactive protein.

Table 4.
Risk factors for recurrence of pediatric pericarditis.

6. Therapy of recurrent pericarditis

The first line of therapy for patients with RP is similar to that for acute pericarditis, except that colchicine use lasts at least 6 months (**Table 4**), and more significant physical activity must be avoided.

Kumar et al. presented a stepwise treatment of pericarditis. They proposed further evaluation of inflammation for patients with ≥2 recurrences of pericarditis. Namely, in the case of elevated CRP and positive LGE, the use of IL-1 inhibitors is suggested. On the other hand, if CRP is normal and LGE is negative, corticosteroids should be considered. Additional drugs should be used in patients with colchicine-resistant and corticosteroid-dependent pericarditis [25].

The 2015 ESC guidelines gave a class IIb recommendation for using interleukin-1 (IL-1) inhibitor anakinra to treat recurrent pericarditis. Two recent randomized controlled trials, The Anakinra-Treatment of Recurrent Idiopathic Pericarditis (AIRTRIP) and Rilonacept inhibition of interleukin-1 alpha and beta for recurrent pericarditis: a pivotal symptomatology and outcomes study (RHAPSODY), strongly support the role of anakinra and Rilonacept in treating corticosteroid-dependent colchicine-resistant recurrent pericarditis [4].

Anakinra, a short-acting IL-1 receptor (IL-1α and IL-1β) antagonist that plays a crucial role in the auto-inflammatory pathway in the inflammatory cascade, is vital in treating refractory pericarditis—corticosteroid-dependent and colchicine-resistant. It is administered subcutaneously at 1–2 mg/kg (maximum dose 100 mg/kg) for several months with gradual tapering. The use of anakinra implies a gradual suspension of corticosteroids and colchicine. In the study of Finetti et al. [41], 10 pediatric patients (10/15) were included, and the average anakinra dose was 1.3 mg/kg, while the average therapy duration was 17.6 months (13–24 months). The disease control was established in all patients. Six had a new relapse after the dose decreased [42]. Caorsi et al. conducted a multicentric study that included 58 pediatric patients treated with IL-1 receptor blockers; 57 received anakinra and 1 received canakinumab as the first anti-IL-1 drug [42]. A complete response to treatment was achieved in 54 patients (95%) with complete control of clinical manifestations in a mean time of 2 ± 1.64 days. During daily treatment with anakinra, the cumulative number of relapses was two. On the other hand, during the tapering or withdrawal period, the cumulative number of relapses was 65. Consequently, daily treatment with anakinra was reintroduced in 17 of 21 patients with complete response. The mean treatment duration to achieve drug-free remission in their cohort was 1.82 years, much longer than those observed in the adults. They concluded that the early use of IL-1 blockers in patients resistant to adequate dosage of NSAIDs and colchicine, without a course of steroids, could lead to more rapid and effective control of the diseases, avoiding severe side effects [42]. Anakinra has been demonstrated as effective in patients with colchicine-resistant and steroid-dependent recurrent pericarditis.

Anakinra was used in three of our patients (one boy and two girls aged 14 and 15) who had colchicine-resistant and corticosteroid-dependent pericarditis (two idiopathic and one postpericardiotomy syndrome). After discontinuing corticosteroids and introducing anakinra, the resolution of iatrogenic Cushing syndrome was registered. No patient had a relapse during the anakinra administration. In two patients, anakinra was stopped after 6 and 12 months, but both had disease relapses after the treatment ended (after 5 days and 3 months). Anakira was started again in both patients, and no new relapses were registered. The second girl is still on the initial doses of the drug.

Anakinra's most common side effects include injection-site skin reactions (38–44%), myalgias and arthralgias (6%), elevated transaminases (3%), and neutropenia (1%), anaphylaxis, and soft tissue (3%) and respiratory infections (3%). It can lead to serious infections, including tuberculosis (TB) [43].

Rilonacept is a dimeric fusion protein that inhibits IL-1α and IL-1β by direct binding and is administered subcutaneously. The drug loading dose is 320 mg (4.4 mg/kg up to 320 mg in 12–17-year-olds), while the maintenance dose (weekly injections) is 160 mg weekly (2.2 mg/kg up to 160 mg in 12–17-year-olds). In adults with RP, Rilonacept led to a median normalization in symptoms of 5 days and C-reactive protein in 7 days, and significantly reduced pericarditis recurrence events (overall 6.7% (control group) versus 74.2% (placebo group), hazard ratio 0.04), along with having a persistent clinical response. The most frequent adverse events were injection-site reactions (34%) and upper respiratory tract infections (23%) [44].

Intravenous immunoglobulins (IVIGs) are potential immunomodulators that can be used in refractory pericarditis. IVIG's mechanism of action in autoimmune disorders involves blocking fragment crystallizable (Fc) receptors and Fc gamma-RIIB receptors on macrophages. The IVIG dose is 400–500 mg/kg/daily for 5 days.

Azathioprine, methotrexate, and mycophenolate mofetil (MMP) could also be used in RP [12].

In case of IL inhibitors' failure, pericardiectomy may be considered [35].

7. Conclusion

Acute pericarditis is the most common cardiogenic cause of chest pain, and the diagnosis can be established already in emergency pediatric services by careful auto- and hetero-anamnesis data, physical examination, ECG recording, and laboratory analyses. The use of anti-inflammatory therapy should be started immediately, i.e., ibuprofen, and in children who are at a higher risk for the development of recurrence (ESR > 50 mm/h, CRP ≥ 125 mg/L, absence of myocardial inflammation, non-infectious etiology), colchicine should also be given immediately. Corticosteroids should not be used in the treatment of acute pericarditis because they are an independent risk factor for the development of recurrent pericarditis. Patients with recurrent pericarditis should be treated with a combination of ibuprofen and colchicine (for 6 months). In the case of corticosteroid-dependent and colchicine-resistant pericarditis, anakinra can be safely and successfully administered in the pediatric population.

Author details

Stasa Krasic[1,2] and Vladislav Vukomanovic[1,2]*

1 Cardiology Department, Mother and Child Health Institute of Serbia, Belgrade, Serbia

2 Faculty of Medicine, University of Belgrade, Belgrade, Serbia

*Address all correspondence to: vvukomanovicdr@gmail.com

References

[1] Chen L, Duan H, Li X, Yang Z, Jiao M, Sun K, et al. The causes of chest pain in children and the criteria for targeted myocardial enzyme testing in identifying the causes of chest pain in children. Frontiers in Cardiovascular Medicine. 2021;**2**(8):582129. DOI: 10.3389/fcvm.2021.582129

[2] Pissarra R, Pereira M, Amorim R, Neto BP, Lourenço L, Santos LA. Chest pain in a pediatric emergency department: Clinical assessment and management reality in a third-level Portuguese hospital. Porto Biomedical Journal. 2022;**7**(3):e150. DOI: 10.1097/j.pbj.0000000000000150

[3] Hanson CL, Hokanson JS. Etiology of chest pain in children and adolescents referred to cardiology clinic. World Medical Journal. 2011;**110**(2):58-62

[4] Adler Y, Charron P, Imazio M, et al. ESC Scientific Document Group. 2015 ESC guidelines for the diagnosis and management of pericardial diseases: The Task Force for the Diagnosis and Management of Pericardial Diseases of the European Society of Cardiology (ESC) endorsed by: The European Association for Cardio-Thoracic Surgery (EACTS). European Heart Journal. 2015;**36**(42):2921-2964

[5] Shahid R, Jin J, Hope K, Tunuguntla H, Amdani S. Pediatric pericarditis: Update. Current Cardiology Reports. 2023;**25**(3):157-170

[6] Blank N, Lorenz HM. Idiopathic pericarditis-an autoinflammatory disease? Current Rheumatology Reports. 2019;**21**(5):18. DOI: 10.1007/s11926-019-0820-2

[7] Imazio M. Noninfectious pericarditis: Management challenges for cardiologists. Kardiologia Polska. 2020;**78**(5):396-403. DOI: 10.33963/KP.15353

[8] Gabaldo K, Sutlić Ž, Mišković D, Knežević Praveček M, Prvulović Đ, Vujeva B, et al. Postpericardiotomy syndrome incidence, diagnostic and treatment strategies: Experience AT two collaborative centers. Acta Clinica Croatica. 2019;**58**(1):57-62. DOI: 10.20471/acc.2019.58.01.08

[9] Heching HJ, Bacha EA, Liberman L. Post-pericardiotomy syndrome in pediatric patients following surgical closure of secundum atrial septal defects: Incidence and risk factors. Pediatric Cardiology. 2015;**36**(3):498-502. DOI: 10.1007/s00246-014-1039-7

[10] Krasic S, Ninic S, Prijic S, Popovic S, Pasic S, Petrovic G, et al. Analysis of cardiac manifestation and treatment of multisystem inflammatory syndrome in children related to SARS-CoV-2. Biomolecules and Biomedicine. 2023;**23**(2):335-343. DOI: 10.17305/bjbms.2022.7820

[11] Krasic S, Vukomanovic V, Ninic S, Pasic S, Samardzija G, Mitrovic N, et al. Mechanisms of redox balance and inflammatory response after the use of methylprednisolone in children with multisystem inflammatory syndrome associated with COVID-19. Frontiers in Immunology. 2023;**14**(14):1249582. DOI: 10.3389/fimmu.2023.1249582

[12] Chiabrando JG, Bonaventura A, Vecchié A, Wohlford GF, Mauro AG, Jordan JH, et al. Management of acute and recurrent pericarditis: JACC state-of-the-art review. Journal of the American College of Cardiology. 2020;**75**(1):76-92. DOI: 10.1016/j.jacc.2019.11.021

[13] Ozturk E, Tanidir IC, Saygi M, Ergul Y, Guzeltas A, Odemis E. Evaluation of non-surgical causes of cardiac tamponade in children at a cardiac surgery center. Pediatrics International. 2014;**56**(1):13-18. DOI: 10.1111/ped.12192

[14] Fowler NO. Cardiac tamponade. A clinical or an echocardiographic diagnosis? Circulation. 1993;**87**(5):1738-1741. DOI: 10.1161/01.cir.87.5.1738

[15] Augustin P, Desmard M, Mordant P, Lasocki S, Maury JM, Heming N, et al. Clinical review: Intrapericardial fibrinolysis in management of purulent pericarditis. Critical Care. 2011;**15**(2):220. DOI: 10.1186/cc10022

[16] Van Dam MN, Hashmi MF, Fitzgerald BM. Pulsus Paradoxus. Treasure Island, FL: StatPearls Publishing; 2024 https://www.ncbi.nlm.nih.gov/books/NBK482292/

[17] Roy CL, Minor MA, Brookhart MA, Choudhry NK. Does this patient with a pericardial effusion have Cardiac Tamponade? Journal of the American Medical Association. 2007;**297**(16):1810-1818. DOI: 10.1001/jama.297.16.1810

[18] Jensen JK, Poulsen SH, Mølgaard H. Cardiac tamponade: A clinical challenge. E-Journal of Cardiology Practice. 2017;**15**:17-27

[19] Brandt RR, Oh JK. Constrictive pericarditis: Role of echocardiography and magnetic resonance imaging. E-Journal of Cardiology Practice. 2017;**15**:22

[20] Saeed S, Mohamed Ali A, Wasim D, Saeed N, Lunde T, Solheim E, et al. Natural course of electrocardiogram changes and the value of multimodality imaging in acute pericarditis. Cardiology. 2023;**148**(3):219-227. DOI: 10.1159/000530207

[21] Ridley L. Chest radiograph signs suggestive of pericardial disease. Expert Analysis. 9 Sep 2019. Available from: https://www.acc.org/Latest-in-Cardiology/Articles/2019/09/09/10/46/Chest-Radiograph-Signs-Suggestive-of-Pericardial-Disease

[22] Imazio M, Brucato A, Barbieri A, Ferroni F, Maestroni S, Ligabue G, et al. Good prognosis for pericarditis with and without myocardial involvement: Results from a multicenter, prospective cohort study. Circulation. 2013;**128**(1):42-49

[23] Krasic S, Prijic S, Ninic S, Borovic R, Petrovic G, Stajevic M, et al. Predictive factors of recurrence after pediatric acute pericarditis. Jornal de Pediatria. 2021;**97**(3):335-341

[24] Pérez-Casares A, Cesar S, Brunet-Garcia L, Sanchez-de-Toledo J. Echocardiographic evaluation of pericardial effusion and Cardiac Tamponade. Frontiers in Pediatrics. 2017;**24**(5):79. DOI: 10.3389/fped.2017.00079

[25] Kumar S, Furqan M, Kafil T, Klein A. The paradigm shift in the management of recurrent pericarditis. Experts Analysis. 4 Jan 2023. Available from: https://www.acc.org/Latest-in-Cardiology/Articles/2022/12/19/14/52/The-Paradigm-Shift-in-the-Management-of-Recurrent-Pericarditis

[26] Kumar A, Sato K, Verma BR, Ala CK, Betancor J, Yzeiraj E, et al. Quantitative assessment of pericardial delayed hyperenhancement helps identify patients with ongoing recurrences of pericarditis. Open Heart. 2018;**5**(2):e000944. DOI: 10.1136/openhrt-2018-000944

[27] Bogaert J, Francone M. Cardiovascular magnetic resonance in pericardial diseases. Journal of Cardiovascular Magnetic

Resonance. 2009;**11**(1):14. DOI: 10.1186/1532-429X-11-14

[28] Wang TKM, Ayoub C, Chetrit M, Kwon DH, Jellis CL, Cremer PC, et al. Cardiac magnetic resonance imaging techniques and applications for pericardial diseases. Circulation Cardiovascular Imaging. 2022;**15**(7):e014283. DOI: 10.1161/CIRCIMAGING.122.014283

[29] Schwier NC, Stephens K, Johnson PN. Management of idiopathic viral pericarditis in the pediatric population. Journal of Pediatric Pharmacology and Therapeutics. 2022;**27**(7):595-608. DOI: 10.5863/1551-6776-27.7.595

[30] Vukomanovic V, Prijic S, Krasic S, Borovic R, Ninic S, Nesic D, et al. Does colchicine substitute corticosteroids in treatment of idiopathic and viral pediatric pericarditis? Medicina. 2019;**55**(10):609. DOI: 10.3390/medicina55100609

[31] Vukomanovic V, Krasic S, Prijic S, Ninic S, Popovic S, Petrovic G, et al. Recent experience: Corticosteroids as a first-line therapy in children with multisystem inflammatory syndrome and COVID-19-related myocardial damage. The Pediatric Infectious Disease Journal. 2021;**40**(11):e390-e394. DOI: 10.1097/INF.0000000000003260

[32] Ristić AD, Imazio M, Adler Y, Anastasakis A, Badano LP, Brucato A, et al. Triage strategy for urgent management of cardiac tamponade: A position statement of the European Society of Cardiology Working Group on myocardial and pericardial diseases. European Heart Journal. 2014;**35**(34):2279-2284. DOI: 10.1093/eurheartj/ehu217

[33] Tarun S, Makadia L, Demirhan S, Shah SS, Foca MD, Bacha EA, et al. Surgical and medical management of purulent bacterial pericarditis with pericardial mass in a young child. JACC: Case Reports. 2023;**5**(15):101834. DOI: 10.1016/j.jaccas.2023.101834

[34] Andreis A, Imazio M, Casula M, Avondo S, Brucato A. Recurrent pericarditis: An update on diagnosis and management. Internal and Emergency Medicine. 2021;**16**(3):551-558

[35] Cremer PC, Kumar A, Kontzias A, Tan CD, Rodriguez ER, Imazio M, et al. Complicated pericarditis: Understanding risk factors and pathophysiology to inform imaging and treatment. Journal of the American College of Cardiology. 2016;**68**(21):2311-2328. DOI: 10.1016/j.jacc.2016.07.785

[36] Imazio M, Pivetta E, Andreis A, Serra C, Carbone F, Masoero M, et al. Incessant pericarditis as a risk factor for complicated pericarditis and hospital admission. Circulation. 2021;**143**(4):401-402. DOI: 10.1161/CIRCULATIONAHA.120.051156

[37] Faustino M, Carmo Mendes I, Anjos R. Constrictive pericarditis: A challenging diagnosis in paediatrics. Case Reports in Cardiology. 2015;**2015**:402740. DOI: 10.1155/2015/402740

[38] Chang SA, Oh JK. Constrictive pericarditis: A medical or surgical disease? Journal of Cardiovascular Imaging. 2019;**27**(3):178-186. DOI: 10.4250/jcvi.2019.27.e28

[39] Yacoub M, Quintanilla Rodriguez BS, Mahajan K. Constrictive-effusive pericarditis. Treasure Island, FL: StatPearls Publishing; 2024 https://www.ncbi.nlm.nih.gov/books/NBK519579/

[40] Yadav NK, Siddique MS. Constrictive pericarditis. Treasure Island, FL:

StatPearls Publishing; 2024 https://www.ncbi.nlm.nih.gov/books/NBK459314

[41] Finetti M, Insalaco A, Cantarini L, Meini A, Breda L, Alessio M, et al. Long-term efficacy of interleukin-1 receptor antagonist (anakinra) in corticosteroid-dependent and colchicine-resistant recurrent pericarditis. The Journal of Pediatrics. 2014;**164**(6):1425-1431.e1. DOI: 10.1016/j.jpeds.2014.01.065

[42] Caorsi R, Insalaco A, Bovis F, Martini G, Cattalini M, Chinali M, et al. Pediatric recurrent pericarditis: Appropriateness of the standard of care and response to IL-1 blockade. The Journal of Pediatrics. 2023;**256**:18-26.e8. DOI: 10.1016/j.jpeds.2022.11.034

[43] Cheema AH, Chaludiya K, Khalid M, Nwosu M, Konka S, Agyeman WY, et al. Efficacy of Anakinra in pericarditis: A systematic review. Cureus. 2022;**14**(10):e29862. DOI: 10.7759/cureus.29862

[44] Wang TKM, Klein AL. Rilonacept (interleukin-1 inhibition) for the treatment of pericarditis. Current Cardiology Reports. Jan 2022;**24**(1):23-30. DOI: 10.1007/s11886-021-01621-0

Chapter 3

The Clinical Detection and Treatment of Myocarditis and Pericarditis

Effat Davoudi-Monfared, Kaveh Hedayati Emami and Kian Alipasandi

Abstract

Myocarditis is described as damage to the heart muscle, which causes inflammation of myocyte. The etiology consists of infectious and non-infectious diseases. The prevalence of myocarditis is estimated between 10.2 and 105.6 per 100,000 people worldwide. Although mortality decreased from 1990 to 2019, the incidence rate has risen. As part of treatment, the use of therapeutic strategies for the treatment of underlying cardiac presentations such as myocardial ischemia and heart failure should be considered. However, use of intravenous immunoglobulins and immunosuppressive medications will be discussed in this chapter. COVID-19 has been a prominent cause of myocarditis in recent years. Additionally, some new concepts like the effect of microbiota on the incidence of viral myocarditis and the influence of gut-heart axis will be discussed. Pericarditis is the presence of inflammation in the pericardial sac. Treatment strategies for pericarditis include the use of nonsteroidal anti-inflammatory drugs, colchicine, and glucocorticoids.

Keywords: myocarditis, cardiomyopathy, COVID-19, dilated cardiomyopathy, pericarditis

1. Introduction

Myocarditis is an inflammatory disease of cardiac muscles that can affect different age ranges [1]. The disease can be potentially life-threatening, although it can be self-limiting in non-severe forms. It is estimated that 1.8 million cases of myocarditis are happening annually [2]. The discrepancy in prevalence is high based on geographic location, age, and sex, and a 10.2–105.6 per 100,000 people has been reported [3]. This difference is related to challenges in diagnosis, clinicians' experience in each center, and epidemiologic considerations for viral disease. The prevalence rate decreased over time, but the global number of cases of myocarditis has increased by 49.8% [2]. The incidence and mortality rate of the disease seems to be higher in the male sex in comparison to females [4]. The disability adjusted life years (DALY) rate revealed a decreasing pattern, which may be related to advances in the treatment and medical interventions for myocarditis [4].

The most-known etiology of myocarditis is infectious disease, including viral, bacterial, helminthic, and autoimmune diseases, and other causes such as toxins, drugs, and hypersensitivity [5]. Classic symptoms include chest pain, fever, and dyspnea, which resemble many cardiac diseases [6]. Hence, additional invasive and non-invasive diagnostic tools should be applied to confirm the diagnosis. Endomyocardial biopsy (EBM) has stood as the gold standard for definite diagnosis of myocarditis. Histological evidence retrieved from the biopsy showed myocyte damage and necrosis with the nonischemic origin [7]. Infiltration of mononuclear cells or sometimes eosinophile or neutrophils results in histopathologic forms predominantly lymphocytic myocarditis (LM) and lymphohistiocytic myocarditis [8, 9]. Other forms such as eosinophilic, neutrophilic, giant cell myocarditis (GCM), cardiac sarcoidosis, and myocarditis with granulomata exist [8]. This histologic subtype can predict the patient's mortality, as GCM worsens prognosis of patients in comparison with LM [10]. However, non-invasive diagnostic tools such as cardiac magnetic resonance imaging have been proposed in recent years. The sooner the diagnosis is made, the better therapeutic strategies can be accomplished according to underlying reasons.

This chapter will review the etiology, diagnosis, prognosis, and treatment of acute myocarditis. It will also discuss invasive and noninvasive diagnostic tools. The presentation of findings will be in accordance with recent findings especially in the area of COVID-19 infection and vaccination.

2. Etiology and pathogenesis of myocarditis

The most common cause of myocarditis is infectious and autoimmune disease. Viral infections, such as parvovirus B19 (PVB19), influenza, adenovirus, enterovirus (including coxsackieviruses), human herpesvirus 6 (HHV-6), human immunodeficiency virus (HIV), and hepatitis C virus (HCV), are mostly responsible for virus-induced myocarditis [3]. After pandemic of COVID-19, which began in 2019, SARS-CoV-2 was inserted into the aforementioned list [11].

In the acute infectious phase (from day 1 to day 7 of viral disease) direct or indirect injury to myocardial cell may occur depending on the virus. Adenovirus and enterovirus enter the myocyte and cause a direct cytolytic effect, and PVB19 induces the release of inflammatory cytokines [12]. The innate immune system is critical in eradicating viruses, but excessive response causes damage to myocardial cells [13]. Between week 1 and week 4 after initial start of the viral symptoms, the signs of viral myocarditis will begin by T-cell mediated immune response [14]. In some patients, all viruses will be eliminated from cardiac cells and recovery will proceed. However, in genetically susceptible patients, persistent myocardial infection and subsequent dilated cardiomyopathy will happen [12].

Autoimmune diseases are the second most widespread cause of myocarditis. Diseases such as sarcoidosis, Behçet's disease, systemic lupus, and Eosinophilic granulomatosis with polyangiitis can induce myocarditis with almost the same mechanism [15–18]. Autoreactive T-cell that acts against α-MyHC (α isoform of myosin heavy chain) is the main cellular mechanism known for the induction of myocarditis [19]. Autoantibodies that are produced by B cells can also trigger myocarditis [20]. Macrophages have a critical role in the pathogenesis of giant cell myocarditis and sarcoidosis [21]. Other immune cells, such as dendritic cells and fibroblasts, can help the triggering and progression of myocarditis [22, 23]. This cascade of immune cells may lead to persistent inflammation of the myocardium and dilated cardiomyopathy. The details of infectious and non-infectious conditions that can cause myocarditis are presented in **Figure 1**.

Myocarditis induced by drugs is categorized as a direct toxicology effect (i.e., anthracyclines) or as a hypersensitivity response (like in case of cephalosporin or antibiotics). As a whole, five categories of drugs are defined to cause myocarditis: antipsychotics, salicylates, antineoplastic-immunotherapeutic agents, antineoplastic-cytotoxic agents, and vaccines [24]. One of the antipsychotics that have drawn attention as a prominent cause of myocarditis is clozapine. The occurrence of clozapine-induced myocarditis (CIM) was six times higher in males vs. females [25]. Although most of the investigations were case reports, some additional risk factors such as obesity, smoking, and inflammatory disease are related to CIM [25].

Immune checkpoint inhibitors (ICI) such as nivolumab and pembrolizumab also cause cardiomyopathy. The prevalence is 0.04–1.14%, yet the mortality is high (25–50%) compared to other immune-related adverse events of this pharmacologic category [26–28]. The exact mechanism is not defined, but the possible similarity between tumor and myocyte exists. Like other types of myocarditis, the role of T-cells is momentous [29]. Some studies revealed that the infiltration of CD8+ and CD4+ T cell in heart tissues was damaged due to ICIs [19, 29, 30].

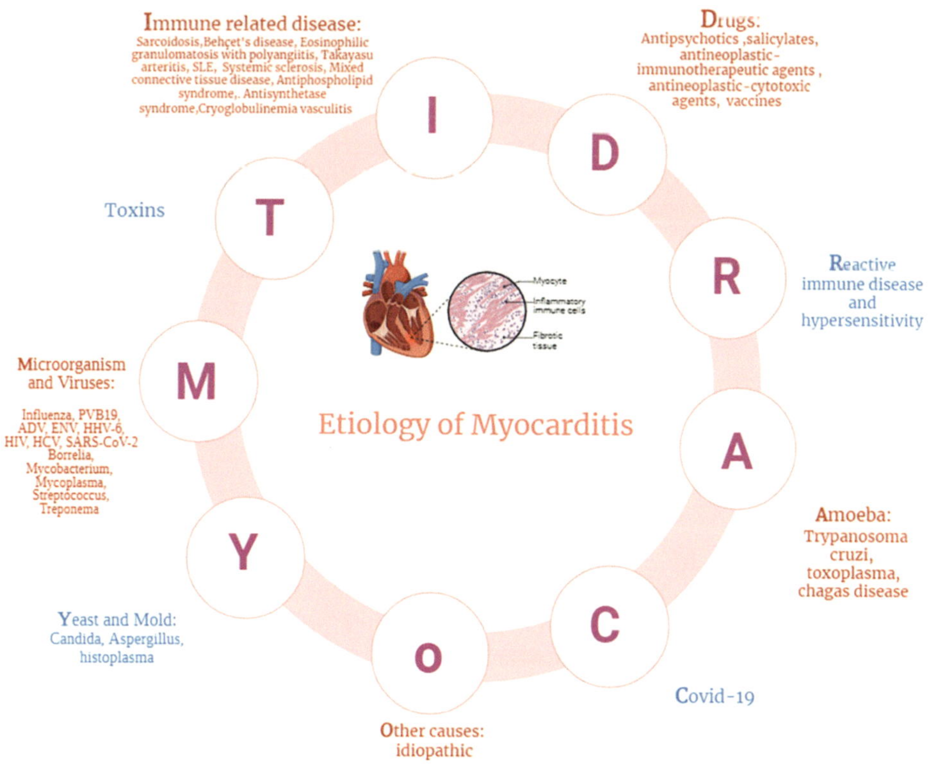

Figure 1.
Etiology of myocarditis with the abbreviation of "MYOCARDIT." Every alphabet is the representative of a category of etiology of disease.

3. Diagnosis of myocarditis

3.1 Clinical presentation

The clinical presentation of myocarditis is a wide range from symptomatic patients to patients with cardiogenic shock and sudden cardiac death [31]. The most common symptoms include chest pain, fever, and dyspnea, respectively [32]. However, most patients are asymptomatic. Other symptoms such as fatigue, palpitation, edema, and syncope may happen. In the case of fulminant myocarditis, severe hemodynamic compromise, fatal arrhythmia, and cardiogenic shock threaten patient's life [33].

The initial clinical presentation of myocarditis can be identical to myocardial infarction, new onset heart failure, chronic heart failure, or even a new onset severe arrhythmia [34]. As mentioned before, the symptoms are not specific and overlap with other cardiac crises. That's why, most of the time, the diagnosis is challenging and in favor of underdiagnosis of myocarditis.

In the cases when symptoms mimic acute coronary syndrome, electrocardiographic changes, and cardiac enzyme elevation may happen. If the cardiac angiography rules out dysfunction of coronary arteries, vasospasm or embolism may be assumed as the reason for infarction [35]. However, in most of such cases myocarditis is underdiagnosed [35]. When the symptoms are identical to heart failure, the chance of accurate diagnosis is enhanced, especially in the absence of ischemic heart disease, hypertension, or valvular disease. In the case of arrhythmia, ventricular tachycardia and atrial fibrillation are common [36]. However, atrioventricular (AV) block, sustained ventricular tachycardia, ventricular fibrillation, and ventricular flutter may happen [37]. In fact, one of the main reasons for sudden cardiac death in the young population is myocarditis and secondary fatal arrhythmia [38]. Finally, if the patient is presenting symptoms in accordance with chronic heart failure and myocarditis is a possible diagnosis, and if the acute phase has been passed, resulting in dilated cardiomyopathy (DCM), sustained inflammation is the main cause leading to such conditions [39]. Otherwise, DCM may results from other conditions, and many differentials may exist.

Some patients (18–80% according to different investigations) with suspected viral myocarditis may present with prodromal symptoms within the past 2–4 weeks, such as flu-like symptoms or gastrointestinal disturbance, indicative of a viral disease [32]. However, most patients may not report such symptoms. Acute myocarditis is proposed, if the time interval is less than 1 month. However, it may be within 3 months, so the definition is according to "subacute myocarditis."

3.2 Laboratory tests

Routine cardiac markers such as the N-terminal of B-type natriuretic peptide (Nt-Pro BNP), troponin I, and troponin T are the current markers for diagnosis of acute myocarditis. High-sensitivity cardiac troponin T (hs-cTnT) is both diagnostic and prognostic markers in acute myocarditis [40, 41]. Some studies suggest elevated cTnT/cTnI shows cell necrosis [5]. A persistently high level of troponin is associated with a bad prognosis, and a fast decline indicates a good outcome for the patient, even if the early levels are high [10].

BNP is elevated in acute and chronic heart failure and also in myocarditis [42]. However, one study disclosed that elevated cardiac troponin and simultaneous normal levels of BNP are related to the worse prognosis in patients with fulminant myocarditis [43]. The hypothesis behind this is the protective role of BNP in maintaining neurohormonal hemostasis. In other words, high cTnT level and lack of high production of BNP result from massive myocyte injury and surrendering of hemodynamic compromise. However, BNP is neither a specific marker nor a sensitive one for acute myocarditis. Other tests such as C-reactive protein (CRP), erythrocyte sedimentation rate (ESR), and leukocyte count may be used, yet they are not specific [5].

3.3 Echocardiography

Transthoracic echocardiography (TTE) is one of the first diagnostic steps for acute myocarditis. Common findings in TTE consist of diastolic dysfunction, reduction in left ventricular ejection fraction (LVEF), segmental or global wall motion abnormalities, disturbance in the echogenicity of the myocardium, change in wall thickness, and accumulation of fluid in pericardium (in case of concomitant pericarditis) [6]. Such presentation may be observed in other cardiac disease such as heart failure or different kind of cardiomyopathies.

Although the findings of TTE are non-specific, it is the first widely available diagnostic strategy that can illicit the clinical and hemodynamic status of the patient and has no limitation regarding arrhythmia or cardiac function. Other important points about TTE are as follows:

- TTE helps diagnose other causes for related clinical presentations such as valvular disease and the detection of intracardiac thrombi.

- The degree of left ventricular (LV) dysfunction should be determined to specify the therapeutic strategy for the patient [44].

- In emergency conditions, particularly when fulminant myocarditis is suspected, and the patient is hemodynamically unstable, other specific modalities such as cardiac magnetic resonance imaging (C-MRI) and endomyocardial biopsy (EMB) are not easily accessible. Hence, echocardiography is the best non-invasive informative diagnostic method.

- Some specific findings may raise the possibility of myocarditis like focal wall motion abnormalities and simultaneous pericardial edema.

- Echocardiography is essential in the assessment of response to the therapy, and it will be repeated during follow-up course.

3.4 Electrocardiography

Electrocardiographic (ECG) exploration may show ST-segment elevation or abnormalities in T-wave [45]. Patients with specific form of myocarditis, like sarcoidosis, may manifest third-degree AV block [46]. About 51% of patients presented with premature ventricular contraction (PVC) have some degree of cardiac inflammation [47]. Hence, PVC records in electrocardiograms should be taken into particular account. ECG exploration can help in the determination of prognosis. For instance, wide QRS and Q-wave, QRS-T angle $\geq$100°, and QT_c interval prolongation are associated with poor prognosis [5]. Normal ECG is hardly seen in patients with myocarditis but is associated with better prognosis [48].

3.5 Cardiovascular magnetic resonance imaging

The most non-invasive diagnostic modality for myocarditis is cardiac/cardiovascular magnetic resonance imaging (CMRI). CMRI gives a complete view of the heart's function, structure, and tissue, so abundant valuable data can be obtained. The first official inclusion of CMRI in the diagnosis of myocarditis was in Lake Louise Criteria (LLC) in 2009 [49]. Suggested criteria were defined according to classic CMRI. Abnormality in two sequencing out of the following three could establish the diagnosis of myocarditis: abnormality in T2-weighted imaging that is suggestive of edema, abnormality in early gadolinium enhancement (EGE); a marker for capillary leak, disturbance in late gadolinium enhancement (LGE); and indicative of scarring or necrosis. The data showed acceptable accuracy and good positive predictive value for such criteria.

Next to the LLC 2009, an assessment of the components of the criteria was performed by different investigations to determine the accuracy and positive predictive value in practice [50]. Simultaneously, new techniques in CMRI, like parametric mapping, were proposed, and the CMRI was evolving in diagnosis of myocarditis [51, 52]. The update of LLC in 2018 confirms the diagnosis of myocarditis if at least one abnormality in each T1-based technique and T2-based technique exists [53]. Segmental or global left ventricular hypokinesia and pericardial effusion were supportive criteria for diagnosis of myocarditis in updated LLC [53]. However, one technique may be used in patients with more evidences in favor of myocarditis.

CMRI has some limitations like any other diagnostic tool. For example, CMRI cannot be easily used in case of sustained arrhythmia. Recent investigations suggest ^{18}F-fluorodeoxyglucose positron emission tomography (FDG-PET) scan instead of CMRI in such conditions [54]. Another issue is that CMRI will not discriminate chronic cardiomyopathy from acute type. Also, subendocardial lesions may not be easily recognized by CMRI [55]. It should be noted that CMRI should be performed within week 1 or 2 of the onset of symptoms. If not, the sensitivity and specificity of CMRI will decrease substantially [56].

3.6 Endomyocardial biopsy

Endomyocardial biopsy (EMB) is the gold standard for diagnosis of myocarditis. Although the procedure is invasive, it brings essential data regarding tissue and immunohistochemistry. However, due to risks and adverse effects, EMB is performed if only the results of non-invasive strategies are inconclusive or the biopsy findings will modify the therapeutic plan. The general indication of EMB is unexplained ventricular tachy- or bradyarrhythmia, unexplained new-onset heart failure, discriminating different kinds of cardiomyopathy (that the diagnosis affects the whole treatment plan), and in cases like heart mass or heart transplant [57].

The method involves the safe insertion of the bioptome into the cardiac muscle by the direction of fluoroscopy or ultrasound imaging. The samples can be taken from the right ventricle (through various veins) or the left ventricle (through the brachial or femoral artery or direct septal puncture) [58]. Other imaging techniques, such as echocardiography, can be applied to guide an optimum sampling [59]. Generally, three or four samples are retrieved and some technical considerations should be taken into account in accordance with the most probable diagnosis [57].

The samples will be assessed histologically and interpreted according to Dallas criteria [7]. The criteria require evidence of infiltration of immune cells into myocytes, showing degeneration of myocardial cells and necrosis due to non-ischemic causes. Immunohistochemistry assessment should contain at least 14 leukocytes per mm^3 and a minimum of 7 CD^{3+}/mm^3 [7]. In the case of viral myocarditis, tissue polymerase chain reaction (PCR) may be considered to guide immunosuppressant therapy.

Like any other procedure, EMB carries a certain risk of complication. However, the overall risk is less than 1%. The most common complication is hematoma. Other adverse events, such as arteriovenous fistula, pneumothorax, post-procedural infection, valvular complication, arrhythmia or block, chamber perforation, and subsequent cardiac tamponade, are possible [57].

4. Treatment approach of myocarditis

The initial steps in the treatment of myocarditis are supportive and in accordance with underlying clinical presentation. Patients with uncomplicated myocarditis may present with chest pain and non-steroidal anti-inflammatory drugs (NSAIDs) and aspirin can help to suppress the pain [60, 61]. When fulminant myocarditis with cardiogenic shock is the diagnosis, inotrope and vasopressor should be used according to the clinical conditions of the patient [62]. The use of pharmacologic treatment for heart failure, acute coronary syndrome, or ventricular arrhythmia in the context of myocarditis corresponds to related guidelines [63–65].

4.1 Mechanical circulatory support

Patients whose initial clinical presentation is cardiogenic shock need hemodynamic support, including vasopressors and inotropes to maintain perfusion of the heart and other major organs. Anyway, the use of vasoactive drugs in patients with marked systolic dysfunction will increase cardiac workload and predispose patients to succedent ischemic events. That's why the use of a temporary mechanical circulatory support (MCS) device was proposed in the treatment of fulminant myocarditis. The primary objectives for the use of temporary MCS were maintaining systemic and coronary perfusion, decreasing the workload on ventricles, and venous decongestion. The most popular methods for temporary MCS are intra-aortic balloon pump (IABP), percutaneous LV assist device (i.e., Impella), and venous-arterial extracorporeal membrane oxygenation (VA-ECMO). Such devices can improve prognosis, postpone heart transplants, decrease the need for durable devices, and finally decrease the risk of mortality [66].

4.2 Pharmacologic treatment for myocarditis

Immunosuppressive agents are frequently used for the treatment of myocarditis, both autoimmune disease-related forms and isolated forms of myocarditis. Corticosteroids have the largest evidence and are prescribed as initial pulse doses and maintenance therapy. Other immunomodulators such as tocilizumab, tofacitinib, antithymocyte globulin, interferon-α, and lots of other medications may be used, but the generally prescribed ones are brought in **Table 1**, with relevant precautions and warnings [67, 85]. The great challenge with such therapies is immunosuppression and increasing risk of various infections. It should be noted that some of these medications are accused of inducing myocarditis, that is, cyclophosphamide.

Pharmacologic intervention	Dose	Type of myocarditis	Precaution and warnings	References
First-line treatment				
Corticosteroids	IV methylprednisolone pulse (500–1000 mg for 3 days) and maintenance of 1 mg/kg	Almost all types of myocarditis	Hyperglycemia, hypertension, increased risk of infection, gastrointestinal side effect including bleeding, malaise, insomnia, irritability, acne, adrenal insufficiency, osteopenia and osteoporosis, glaucoma, cataracts	[67]
IVIG	1–2 g/kg for 1 day 1 g/kg for 2 days 400 mg/kg for 5 days	Mostly viral myocarditis, autoimmune disease-related myocarditis (mostly systemic lupus erythematosus)	Anaphylaxis, hypersensitivity reactions, infusion-related reaction, antibody development, pulmonary edema, thromboembolic events, hemolysis and positive Coombs test, hematoma, aseptic meningitis, nephrotoxicity	[68–70]
Azathioprine	2 mg/kg for 6 months as maintenance treatment	Virus-negative myocarditis	Bone marrow suppression, immunosuppression and increase in risk of infection, nausea/vomiting, hepatotoxicity	[71, 72]
Cyclophosphamide	600 mg/m^2 (BSA) on day 1, 15, 30	Autoimmune disease related myocarditis (SLE, vasculitis), eosinophilic myocarditis	Bone marrow suppression, impaired wound healing, immunosuppression and increasing risk of infection, hemorrhagic cystitis, cardiotoxicity*	[72, 73]
Mycophenolate mofetil	2 g/d for 6 months as maintenance treatment	Lymphocytic myocarditis, virus-negative myocarditis	Bone marrow suppression, immunosuppression and increasing risk of infection, difference in pharmacokinetic of delayed-release and oral dosage form	[74–76]
Second line or less frequently used pharmacologic interventions				
Rituximab	375 mg/m^2 weekly for 4 weeks	Myocarditis induced by eosinophilic granulomatosis with polyangiitis	Hypersensitivity reactions, infusion-related reaction, immunosuppression and increase in risk of infection, late-onset neutropenia, hepatitis B virus reactivation, reactivation of tuberculosis, PML	[77, 78]

Pharmacologic intervention	Dose	Type of myocarditis	Precaution and warnings	References
Methotrexate	20 mg weekly for 3–12 months	Virus-negative myocarditis, sarcoidosis	Bone marrow suppression, gastrointestinal adverse effects, hepatotoxicity, errors in dosing schedule (by patient) and risk of drug toxicity	[79, 80]
Infliximab	5 mg/kg single dose	ICI-mediated myocarditis	Increase risk of infection, hypersensitivity reactions, infusion-related reaction, antibody formation, reactivation of hepatitis B virus, reactivation of tuberculosis	[81]
Abatacept	500 mg every 2 weeks for 5 doses	ICI-mediated myocarditis	Increase risk of infection, hypersensitivity reactions, infusion-related reaction	[82, 83]
Alemtuzumab	30 mg single dose	ICI-mediated myocarditis	Bone marrow suppression, immunosuppression and increase in risk of infection, hypersensitivity reactions, infusion-related reaction, thrombocytopenia, stroke and cervicocephalic arterial dissection, PML, fatal autoimmune conditions	[84]

Abbreviation: ICI: immune checkpoint inhibitor, IV: intravenous, IVIG: intravenous immunoglobulin, PML: progressive multifocal leukoencephalopathy.
**Please consider that cyclophosphamide is one of the medications that causes cardiomyopathy. Besides, it has immunomodulating effect for treatment of cardiomyopathy.*

Table 1.
Summary of pharmacological immunosuppressive interventions for the treatment of myocarditis.

5. Myocarditis and COVID-19

COVID-19 was the first pandemic of the twenty-first century that presented various immune-related complications [86]. Cardiovascular complications were among the most common complications, and myocarditis was the one that was detected not only in severe COVID-19, but also in mild cases [11, 87, 88]. The initial pathogenesis was assumed to be related to Angiotensin Receptor Enzyme 2 (ACE2) receptor. The spike protein of the virus binds ACE2 receptor and adherence to the human type 2 TMPRSS2 (transmembrane serine protease 2) causes entry of the virus into cell [89]. The expression of ACE2 is observed in many organs and tissue, like lungs, kidneys, brain, gastrointestinal tract, and heart [90]. While ACE2 receptor and TMPRSS2 are expressed in myocyte, pericyte, and other immune cells, penetration of the virus to such cells can happen [91]. The entry of the SARS-CoV-2 can elucidate a complex of immune reactions, leading to myocarditis.

The prevalence of COVID-19-related myocarditis is not clear, but is estimated at 150 COVID-19-related myocarditis per 100,000 people versus 9 non-COVID-19 myocarditis per 100,000 people at the same time [92]. The typical presentation of the COVID-19-related myocarditis is the same as other phenotypes of myocarditis that mentioned earlier in this chapter, that is, fever, chest pain, palpitation, and syncope. Although some studies suggest that some variants of SARS-CoV-2, like Delta, may cause more damage to cardiomyocytes in comparison with Alpha, it seems that expression of ACE2 in endothelial cells of coronary arteries is much more prominent [93, 94]. Increased biomarkers such as troponin and Nt-pro-BNP were the risk factors for mortality despite of the severity of COVID-19 illness [95–97].

Another important issue is COVID-19 vaccination-related myocarditis. Early after the start of vaccination, case reports of myocarditis and pericarditis following vaccination were released, especially after the second dose. Old reports of vaccination-related myocarditis indicate the importance of mRNA vaccines [98]. The same was true for COVID-19 vaccination. The mRNA-base COVID-19 vaccine (Moderna and Pfizer) had the highest risk of myocarditis [99]. These mRNA vaccines encode the spike glycoprotein of the virus. The age below 30 was another independent risk factor [99]. Fortunately, most cases of COVID-19 vaccination-related myocarditis were mild with a good prognosis [100].

6. Pericarditis

Pericarditis is an inflammatory disease involving the pericardium that can range from a minimal pericardial effusion to infective pericarditis [101]. Most of the time, pericarditis goes along with myocarditis or endocarditis. In rare cases, it can present as an isolated form. The disease is frequently mild and self-limiting. In some cases, the disease has a recurrent identity, causing irritating signs and symptoms and multiple admissions to the hospital and emergency department. The second recurrence is observed in 25–50% of patients and the third recurrence is observed in 20–40% [102]. However, it can be complicated in rare cases, in which the disease causes cardiac tamponade that endangers the patient's life.

The etiology of the disease is viral infections in more than 80% of cases [102]. Finding the etiology will not change the diagnostic and therapeutic plan. Taking a complete medical history, heart auscultation, electrocardiography, echocardiography, and blood tests (especially CRP and troponin) are necessary for diagnostic work-up. If two of the following criteria exist, the diagnosis can be confirmed: chest pain, pericardial effusion, pericardial rubbing, and ST elevation or PR depression on electrocardiogram [103]. Invasive procedures are rarely required.

The first-line treatment of pericarditis consists of aspirin or NSAID, colchicine, and proton pump inhibitors. Sometimes, exercise restriction is proposed to be performed by patient [101]. Corticosteroids are not recommended as the first line, due to increasing risk of relapse [104]. But they are prescribed in the second line or third line. Other immunosuppressive agents may be used in the non responsive form, and pericardiectomy is that last treatment option for those resistant to pharmacotherapy [105].

7. Future of myocarditis

One of the greatest challenges in myocarditis is the early diagnosis (tools, time, and differential diagnosis). Some new non-invasive diagnostic tools are required to detect patients with myocarditis so the proper treatment can be started. Biomarkers may help in this field. Such markers can have diagnostic and prognostic value and should be specific enough to differentiate myocarditis from another cardiac disease with similar presentations [106].

Genetic biomarkers such as microRNA (miRNA) have drawn attention in recent years. Animal models have shown that one miRNA named mmu-miR-721 produced by Th17 cells can be used in diagnosis of myocarditis. Such biomarker is observed in animal models of autoimmune myocarditis and coxsackievirus and is not present in ischemic cardiac disease [106]. The humanized analog of this biomarker, Hsa-miR-Chr8:96/mmumiR-721, was elevated in four distinct human investigations and could produce a ROC curve with area under curve (AUC) of 0.972, meaning a good distinguishing ability between myocarditis and ischemic events [107]. Another investigation found high levels of miR-4763-3p in patients with fulminant myocarditis [108]. In addition, this study revealed that miRNA enrichment can be associated with the severity of the disease. It seems miRNA will have a more prominent role in determining the diagnosis and prognosis of myocarditis in the near future.

Another potential treatment of myocarditis may be the regulation of microbiota. The human gut microbiome is considered a "distinct organ" that contains beneficial microorganisms and is a treasure of genomes, a 100 times more than the human genome and involved in various human related hemostasis especially nutrition and immunity [109, 110]. Recent investigations have shown the effect of gut-heart axis on incidence of cardiovascular disease and the underlying mechanism is systemic inflammation and endothelial dysfunction. Hu et al. performed fecal microbial transplantation in mouse models and showed that increase in diversity and richness of microbiota, especially higher firmicutes/bacteroidetes was accompanied by less myocardial injury [111]. This was a result of less IFN-γ gene expression in cardiomyocyte and decreased CD4 + IFN-γ + cells in the spleen.

8. Conclusions

Myocarditis is the inflammation of cardiomyocyte that can have symptoms resembling other cardiovascular disease. Many infectious and non-infectious disease can cause myocarditis. The early and accurate diagnostic strategy should be reached, so the therapeutic strategy can be placed in right direction. However, diagnosis is still challenging. EMB is the gold standard, but is not possible in every cases. That's why non-invasive tools, that is, CMRI are recommended as first line. Stabilizing hemodynamic is the first goal in patients presenting with fulminant myocarditis. Use of temporary MCDs and immunosuppressive agents should be considered in accordance with probable etiology. New biomarkers and non-invasive diagnostic and prognostic tools may help in future.

Acknowledgements

We appreciate all the nursing staff of Intensive Care Unit of Yas Hospital Complex for their cooperation and kind support throughout the current research. Words cannot express our gratitude to our colleague Dr. Mahgol Hedayati for her invaluable support in writing this chapter.

Conflict of interest

All authors state that they have no conflict of interest to declare.

Author details

Effat Davoudi-Monfared[1*], Kaveh Hedayati Emami[2] and Kian Alipasandi[3]

1 Yas Hospital Complex, Department of Clinical Pharmacy, Faculty of Pharmacy, Tehran University of Medical Sciences, Tehran, Iran

2 Imam Khomeini Hospital Complex, Department of Anesthesiology and Critical Care, Faculty of Medicine, Tehran University of Medical Sciences, Tehran, Iran

3 Tehran Heart Center, Faculty of Medicine, Tehran University of Medical Sciences, Tehran, Iran

*Address all correspondence to: edavudimonfared@gmail.com

References

[1] Ammirati E, Moslehi JJ. Diagnosis and treatment of acute myocarditis: A review. JAMA. 2023;**329**(13):1098-1113

[2] Dai H et al. Global, regional, and National Burden of myocarditis and cardiomyopathy, 1990-2017. Frontiers in Cardiovascular Medicine. 2021;**8**:610989, 1-12

[3] Pollack A et al. Viral myocarditis—Diagnosis, treatment options, and current controversies. Nature Reviews Cardiology. 2015;**12**(11):670-680

[4] Roth GA et al. Global burden of cardiovascular diseases and risk factors, 1990-2019: Update from the GBD 2019 study. Journal of the American College of Cardiology. 2020;**76**(25):2982-3021

[5] Piccirillo F, Watanabe M, Di Sciascio G. Diagnosis, treatment and predictors of prognosis of myocarditis. A narrative review. Cardiovascular Pathology. 2021;**54**:107362

[6] Lampejo T et al. Acute myocarditis: Aetiology, diagnosis and management. Clinical Medicine (London, England). 2021;**21**(5):e505-e510

[7] Aretz HT. Myocarditis: The Dallas criteria. Human Pathology. 1987;**18**(6):619-624

[8] Leone O et al. The spectrum of myocarditis: From pathology to the clinics. Virchows Archiv. 2019;**475**(3):279-301

[9] Baughman KL. Diagnosis of myocarditis. Circulation. 2006;**113**(4):593-595

[10] Ammirati E et al. Update on acute myocarditis. Trends in Cardiovascular Medicine. 2021;**31**(6):370-379

[11] Irabien-Ortiz A et al. Fulminant myocarditis due to COVID-19. Revista Española de Cardiología (English Edition). 2020;**73**(6):503

[12] Baldeviano GC et al. Interleukin-17A is dispensable for myocarditis but essential for the progression to dilated cardiomyopathy. Circulation Research. 2010;**106**(10):1646-1655

[13] Khawaja A, Bromage DI. The innate immune response in myocarditis. The International Journal of Biochemistry & Cell Biology. 2021;**134**:105973

[14] Sozzi FB et al. Viral myocarditis: Classification, diagnosis, and clinical implications. Frontiers in Cardiovascular Medicine. 2022;**9**:908663

[15] Demirelli S et al. Cardiac manifestations in Behcet's disease. Intractable & Rare Diseases Research. 2015;**4**(2):70-75

[16] Blauwet LA, Cooper LT. Idiopathic giant cell myocarditis and cardiac sarcoidosis. Heart Failure Reviews. 2013;**18**:733-746

[17] Du Toit R et al. Lupus myocarditis: Review of current diagnostic modalities and their application in clinical practice. Rheumatology. 2023;**62**(2):523-534

[18] Colantuono S et al. Early benralizumab for eosinophilic myocarditis in eosinophilic granulomatosis with polyangiitis. Allergology International. 2020;**69**(3):483-484

[19] Won T et al. Cardiac myosin-specific autoimmune T cells contribute to immune-checkpoint-inhibitor-associated myocarditis. Cell Reports. 2022;**41**(6):111611, 1-13

[20] Won T et al. Autoimmune myocarditis, old dogs and new tricks. Circulation Research. 2024;**134**(12):1767-1790

[21] Gilotra NA et al. Sarcoidosis-related cardiomyopathy: Current knowledge, challenges, and future perspectives state-of-the-art review. Journal of Cardiac Failure. 2022;**28**(1):113-132

[22] Pistulli R et al. Characterization of dendritic cells in human and experimental myocarditis. ESC Heart Failure. 2020;**7**(5):2305-2317

[23] Amoah BP et al. Immunopathogenesis of myocarditis: The interplay between cardiac fibroblast cells, dendritic cells, macrophages and CD4+T cells. Scandinavian Journal of Immunology. 2015;**82**(1):1-9

[24] Nguyen LS et al. Systematic analysis of drug-associated myocarditis reported in the World Health Organization pharmacovigilance database. Nature Communications. 2022;**13**(1):25

[25] Richardson N, Greenway SC, Bousman CA. Clozapine-induced myocarditis and patient outcomes after drug rechallenge following myocarditis: A systematic case review. Psychiatry Research. 2021;**305**:114247

[26] Johnson DB et al. Fulminant myocarditis with combination immune checkpoint blockade. New England Journal of Medicine. 2016;**375**(18):1749-1755

[27] Moslehi JJ et al. Increased reporting of fatal immune checkpoint inhibitor-associated myocarditis. The Lancet. 2018;**391**(10124):933

[28] Salem J-E et al. Cardiovascular toxicities associated with immune checkpoint inhibitors: An observational, retrospective, pharmacovigilance study. The Lancet Oncology. 2018;**19**(12):1579-1589

[29] Palaskas N et al. Immune checkpoint inhibitor myocarditis: Pathophysiological characteristics, diagnosis, and treatment. Journal of the American Heart Association. 2020;**9**(2):e013757

[30] Wei SC et al. A genetic mouse model recapitulates immune checkpoint inhibitor–associated myocarditis and supports a mechanism-based therapeutic intervention. Cancer Discovery. 2021;**11**(3):614-625

[31] Guglin M, Smith C, Rao R. The spectrum of lupus myocarditis: From asymptomatic forms to cardiogenic shock. Heart Failure Reviews. 2021;**26**:553-560

[32] Ammirati E et al. Management of acute myocarditis and chronic inflammatory cardiomyopathy: An expert consensus document. Circulation: Heart Failure. 2020;**13**(11):e007405

[33] Veronese G et al. Fulminant myocarditis: Characteristics, treatment, and outcomes. Anatolian Journal of Cardiology/Anadolu Kardiyoloji Dergisi. 2018;**19**(4):279-286

[34] Biesbroek PS et al. Diagnosis of myocarditis: Current state and future perspectives. International Journal of Cardiology. 2015;**191**:211-219

[35] Gallagher S et al. Diagnosis and management of patients with acute cardiac symptoms, troponin elevation and culprit-free angiograms. Heart. 2012;**98**(13):974-981

[36] Adegbala O et al. Predictors, burden, and the impact of arrhythmia on patients admitted for acute myocarditis. The American Journal of Cardiology. 2019;**123**(1):139-144

[37] Baksi AJ, Kanaganayagam GS, Prasad SK. Arrhythmias in viral myocarditis and pericarditis. Cardiac Electrophysiology Clinics. 2015;7(2):269-281

[38] Doolan A, Semsarian C, Langlois N. Causes of sudden cardiac death in young Australians. Medical Journal of Australia. 2004;**180**(3):110-112

[39] Jefferies JL, Towbin JA. Dilated cardiomyopathy. The Lancet. 2010;**375**(9716):752-762

[40] Ukena C et al. Diagnostic and prognostic validity of different biomarkers in patients with suspected myocarditis. Clinical Research in Cardiology. 2014;**103**(9):743-751

[41] Liu C et al. The absolute and relative changes in high-sensitivity cardiac troponin I are associated with the in-hospital mortality of patients with fulminant myocarditis. BMC Cardiovascular Disorders. 2021;**21**(1):571

[42] Mahmood SS et al. Myocarditis in patients treated with immune checkpoint inhibitors. Journal of the American College of Cardiology. 2018;**71**(16):1755-1764

[43] Yu S-R et al. An hypothesis: Disproportion between cardiac troponin and B-type natriuretic peptide levels—A high risk and poor prognostic biomarker in patients with fulminant myocarditis? Heart, Lung & Circulation. 2021;**30**(6):837-842

[44] Rroku A, Kottwitz J, Heidecker B. Update on myocarditis—What we know so far and where we may be heading. European Heart Journal - Acute Cardiovascular Care. 2020;**10**(4):455-467

[45] Cooper LT Jr. Myocarditis. New England Journal of Medicine. 2009;**360**(15):1526-1538

[46] Gilotra N et al. Management of cardiac sarcoidosis in 2020. Arrhythmia & Electrophysiology Review. 2020;**9**(4):182-188

[47] Lakkireddy D et al. Myocarditis causing premature ventricular contractions. Circulation: Arrhythmia and Electrophysiology. 2019;**12**(12):e007520

[48] Sinagra G et al. Myocarditis in clinical practice. Mayo Clinic Proceedings. 2016;**91**(9):1256-1266

[49] Friedrich MG et al. Cardiovascular magnetic resonance in myocarditis: A JACC white paper. Journal of the American College of Cardiology. 2009;**53**(17):1475-1487

[50] Wei S et al. Performance of cardiac magnetic resonance imaging for diagnosis of myocarditis compared with endomyocardial biopsy: A meta-analysis. Medical Science Monitor. 2017;**23**:3687-3696

[51] Luetkens JA et al. Incremental value of quantitative CMR including parametric mapping for the diagnosis of acute myocarditis. European Heart Journal - Cardiovascular Imaging. 2016;**17**(2):154-161

[52] Bohnen S et al. Performance of t1 and t2 mapping cardiovascular magnetic resonance to detect active myocarditis in patients with recent-onset heart failure. Circulation: Cardiovascular Imaging. 2015;**8**(6):e003073

[53] Ferreira VM et al. Cardiovascular magnetic resonance in nonischemic myocardial inflammation: Expert recommendations. Journal of the American College of Cardiology. 2018;**72**(24):3158-3176

[54] Peretto G et al. Clinical applications of FDG-PET scan in arrhythmic

myocarditis. JACC: Cardiovascular Imaging. 2022;**15**(10):1771-1780

[55] Li J-H et al. Subendocardial involvement as an underrecognized cardiac MRI phenotype in myocarditis. Radiology. 2022;**302**(1):61-69

[56] Popa A et al. The role of magnetic resonance imaging in risk stratification of patients with acute myocarditis. Diagnostics. 2024;**14**(13):1426, 1-13

[57] Leone O et al. 2011 consensus statement on endomyocardial biopsy from the Association for European Cardiovascular Pathology and the Society for Cardiovascular Pathology. Cardiovascular Pathology. 2012;**21**(4):245-274

[58] Bermpeis K et al. Safety of right and left ventricular endomyocardial biopsy in heart transplantation and cardiomyopathy patients. Heart Failure. 2022;**10**(12):963-973

[59] Pearman JL et al. Intracardiac echocardiographic-guided right-sided cardiac biopsy: Case series and literature review. Catheterization and Cardiovascular Interventions. 2021;**98**(5):1000-1005

[60] Ammirati E et al. Clinical presentation and outcome in a contemporary cohort of patients with acute myocarditis: Multicenter Lombardy registry. Circulation. 2018;**138**(11):1088-1099

[61] Younis A et al. Epidemiology characteristics and outcome of patients with clinically diagnosed acute myocarditis. The American Journal of Medicine. 2020;**133**(4):492-499

[62] Hang W et al. Fulminant myocarditis: A comprehensive review from etiology to treatments and outcomes. Signal Transduction and Targeted Therapy. 2020;**5**(1):287

[63] Byrne RA et al. 2023 ESC guidelines for the management of acute coronary syndromes: Developed by the task force on the management of acute coronary syndromes of the European Society of Cardiology (ESC). European Heart Journal - Acute Cardiovascular Care. 2024;**13**(1):55-161

[64] Authors/Task Force Members et al. 2021 ESC Guidelines for the diagnosis and treatment of acute and chronic heart failure: Developed by the Task Force for the diagnosis and treatment of acute and chronic heart failure of the European Society of Cardiology (ESC). With the special contribution of the Heart Failure Association (HFA) of the ESC. European Journal of Heart Failure. 2022;**24**(1):4-131

[65] Brugada J et al. 2019 ESC guidelines for the management of patients with supraventricular tachycardia the task force for the management of patients with supraventricular tachycardia of the European society of Cardiology (ESC) developed in collaboration with the association for European paediatric and congenital Cardiology (AEPC). European Heart Journal. 2020;**41**(5):655-720

[66] Kondo T et al. Differences in prognosis and cardiac function according to required percutaneous mechanical circulatory support and histological findings in patients with fulminant myocarditis: Insights from the CHANGE PUMP 2 study. Journal of the American Heart Association. 2022;**11**(4):e023719

[67] Winter M-P et al. Immunomodulatory treatment for lymphocytic myocarditis—A systematic review and meta-analysis. Heart Failure Reviews. 2018;**23**(4):573-581

[68] Robinson J et al. Intravenous immunoglobulin for presumed viral myocarditis in children and adults. Cochrane Database of Systematic Reviews. 2020;**8**(8):CD004370, 1-34

[69] Yen C-Y et al. Role of intravenous immunoglobulin therapy in the survival rate of pediatric patients with acute myocarditis: A systematic review and meta-analysis. Scientific Reports. 2019;**9**(1):10459

[70] Thomas G et al. Lupus myocarditis: Initial presentation and longterm outcomes in a multicentric series of 29 patients. The Journal of Rheumatology. 2017;**44**(1):24-32

[71] Grzechocińska J et al. Immunosuppressive therapy of biopsy-proven, virus-negative, autoimmune/immune-mediated myocarditis—Focus on azathioprine: A review of existing evidence and future perspectives. Biology. 2023;**12**(3):356

[72] Cheng C-y et al. Efficacy of immunosuppressive therapy in myocarditis: A 30-year systematic review and meta analysis. Autoimmunity Reviews. 2021;**20**(1):102710

[73] Guerra M et al. Treatment options in lupus myocarditis—A systematic review. Acta Reumatológica Portuguesa. 2019

[74] Vennier A et al. Clinical features and outcomes of patients admitted to the ICU for cyclophosphamide-associated cardiac toxicity: A retrospective cohort. Supportive Care in Cancer. 2023;**31**(8):474

[75] De Luca G et al. Efficacy and safety of mycophenolate mofetil in patients with virus-negative lymphocytic myocarditis: A prospective cohort study. Journal of Autoimmunity. 2020;**106**:102330

[76] Allaoui A et al. Mycophenolate mofetil use in severe myocarditis complicating systemic lupus. Cureus. 2022;**14**(6):e25789, 1-6

[77] Higashitani K et al. Rituximab and mepolizumab combination therapy for glucocorticoid-resistant myocarditis related to eosinophilic granulomatosis with polyangiitis. Modern Rheumatology Case Reports. 2021;**6**(1):87-92

[78] Wang C-R, Tsai Y-s, Tsai H-W. Acute myocarditis in patients with antineutrophil cytoplasmic antibody–positive microscopic polyangiitis and receiving rituximab therapy. The Journal of Rheumatology. 2019;**46**(12):1645-1646

[79] Campochiaro C et al. Efficacy and safety of methotrexate for the treatment of autoimmune virus-negative myocarditis: A case series. JCR: Journal of Clinical Rheumatology. 2021;**27**(4):e143-e146

[80] Ballul T et al. Treatment of cardiac sarcoidosis: A comparative study of steroids and steroids plus immunosuppressive drugs. International Journal of Cardiology. 2019;**276**:208-211

[81] Zhang RS et al. Treatment of corticosteroid refractory immune checkpoint inhibitor myocarditis with infliximab: A case series. Cardio-Oncology. 2021;**7**(1):13

[82] Salem J-E et al. Abatacept for severe immune checkpoint inhibitor–associated myocarditis. New England Journal of Medicine. 2019;**380**(24):2377-2379

[83] Nguyen LS et al. Reversal of immune-checkpoint inhibitor fulminant myocarditis using personalized-dose-adjusted abatacept and ruxolitinib: Proof of concept. Journal for Immunotherapy of Cancer. 2022;**10**(4):e004699corr1, 1-5

[84] Esfahani K et al. Alemtuzumab for immune-related myocarditis due to PD-1 therapy. New England Journal of Medicine. 2019;**380**(24):2375-2376

[85] Ammirati E et al. Immunomodulating therapies in acute myocarditis and recurrent/acute pericarditis. Frontiers in Medicine. 2022;**9**:838564, 1-27

[86] Yazdanpanah N, Rezaei N. Autoimmune complications of COVID-19. Journal of Medical Virology. 2022;**94**(1):54-62

[87] Nedeljkovic IP et al. Focal myocarditis after mild COVID-19 infection in athletes. Diagnostics. 2021;**11**(8):1519

[88] Shahrami B et al. Management of a critically ill patient with COVID-19-related fulminant myocarditis: A case report. Respiratory Medicine Case Reports. 2022;**36**:101611

[89] Hoffmann M et al. SARS-CoV-2 cell entry depends on ACE2 and TMPRSS2 and is blocked by a clinically proven protease inhibitor. Cell. 2020;**181**(2):271-280.e8

[90] Zou X et al. Single-cell RNA-seq data analysis on the receptor ACE2 expression reveals the potential risk of different human organs vulnerable to 2019-nCoV infection. Frontiers in Medicine. 2020;**14**:185-192

[91] Hikmet F et al. The protein expression profile of ACE2 in human tissues. Molecular Systems Biology. 2020;**16**(7):e9610

[92] Boehmer TK. Association between COVID-19 and myocarditis using hospital-based administrative data—United States, March 2020–January 2021. MMWR. Morbidity and Mortality Weekly Report. 2021;**70**:1228-1232

[93] Nchioua R et al. Strong attenuation of SARS-CoV-2 omicron BA.1 and increased replication of the BA.5 subvariant in human cardiomyocytes. Signal Transduction and Targeted Therapy. 2022;**7**(1):395

[94] Wagner JU et al. Increased susceptibility of human endothelial cells to infections by SARS-CoV-2 variants. Basic Research in Cardiology. 2021;**116**:1-12

[95] Nie S-F et al. Cardiac troponin I is an independent predictor for mortality in hospitalized patients with COVID-19. Circulation. 2020;**142**(6):608-610

[96] Selçuk M et al. Prognostic significance of N-terminal pro-BNP in patients with COVID-19 pneumonia without previous history of heart failure. Journal of Cardiovascular and Thoracic Research. 2021;**13**(2):141

[97] Gaze DC. Clinical utility of cardiac troponin measurement in COVID-19 infection. Annals of Clinical Biochemistry. 2020;**57**(3):202-205

[98] Arness MK et al. Myopericarditis following smallpox vaccination. American Journal of Epidemiology. 2004;**160**(7):642-651

[99] Diaz GA et al. Myocarditis and pericarditis after vaccination for COVID-19. JAMA. 2021;**326**(12):1210-1212

[100] Montgomery J et al. Myocarditis following immunization with mRNA COVID-19 vaccines in members of the US military. JAMA Cardiology. 2021;**6**(10):1202-1206

[101] Lazarou E et al. Acute pericarditis: Update. Current Cardiology Reports. 2022;**24**(8):905-913

[102] Cremer PC et al. Complicated pericarditis: Understanding risk factors and pathophysiology to inform

imaging and treatment. Journal of the American College of Cardiology. 2016;**68**(21):2311-2328

[103] Adler Y et al. 2015 ESC guidelines for the diagnosis and management of pericardial diseases: The task force for the diagnosis and management of pericardial diseases of the European Society of Cardiology (ESC) endorsed by: The European Association for Cardio-Thoracic Surgery (EACTS). European Heart Journal. 2015;**36**(42):2921-2964

[104] Andreis A et al. Recurrent pericarditis: An update on diagnosis and management. Internal and Emergency Medicine. 2021;**16**:551-558

[105] Tzani A et al. Meta-analysis of population characteristics and outcomes of patients undergoing pericardiectomy for constrictive pericarditis. The American Journal of Cardiology. 2021;**146**:120-127

[106] Suresh A, Martens P, Tang WW. Biomarkers for myocarditis and inflammatory cardiomyopathy. Current Heart Failure Reports. 2022;**19**(5):346-355

[107] Blanco-Domínguez R et al. A novel circulating microRNA for the detection of acute myocarditis. The New England Journal of Medicine. 2021;**384**(21):2014-2027

[108] Nie X et al. Circulating miR-4763-3p is a novel potential biomarker candidate for human adult fulminant myocarditis. Molecular Therapy - Methods & Clinical Development. 2020;**17**:1079-1087

[109] Zheng D, Liwinski T, Elinav E. Interaction between microbiota and immunity in health and disease. Cell Research. 2020;**30**(6):492-506

[110] Riccio P, Rossano R. The human gut microbiota is neither an organ nor a commensal. FEBS Letters. 2020;**594**(20):3262-3271

[111] Hu X-F et al. Fecal microbiota transplantation alleviates myocardial damage in myocarditis by restoring the microbiota composition. Pharmacological Research. 2019;**139**:412-421

Section 2

Imaging for Inflammatory Myocardial Diseases

Chapter 4

The Role of Advanced Multimodality Cardiovascular Imaging in the Diagnosis and Management of Myocarditis and Pericarditis

Nana Osei, Abena Agyekum, Kai Shiang Lin and Inna Bukharovich

Abstract

This chapter provides a comprehensive review of the pivotal role advanced multimodality cardiovascular imaging plays in the diagnosis and management of myocarditis and pericarditis. It highlights the unique strengths and limitations of key imaging modalities, including echocardiography, cardiac magnetic resonance imaging (CMR), cardiac computed tomography (CCT), and nuclear imaging, demonstrating their contributions to informed clinical decision-making. Additionally, the chapter explores emerging imaging techniques and highlights future research directions, offering valuable insights into their potential to enhance the understanding and man-agement of these inflammatory conditions. By adopting an evidence-based approach, this chapter seeks to equip clinicians and researchers with the knowledge and tools necessary to optimize patient outcomes.

Keywords: pericarditis, myocarditis, cardiovascular diseases, cardiac imaging, inflammation

1. Introduction

Myocarditis and pericarditis are inflammatory diseases of the myocardium and pericardium, respectively. They present with a broad spectrum of clinical manifestations that can range from mild, self-limiting symptoms to life-threatening complications such as heart failure, obstructive shock, arrhythmias, and sudden cardiac death [1, 2]. Timely and accurate diagnosis is paramount to improving patient outcomes, particularly given the considerable overlap in clinical presentations with other cardiovascular and systemic diseases.

Advancements in cardiovascular imaging have transformed the diagnostic landscape for myocarditis and pericarditis. Multimodality imaging now facilitates noninvasive assessment of the structural, functional, and tissue characteristics of the myocardium and pericardium. While echocardiography remains the cornerstone of initial evaluation, advanced imaging techniques such as cardiac magnetic resonance imaging (CMR), cardiac computed tomography (CCT), and nuclear cardiac imaging—particularly positron emission tomography (PET)—offer deeper insights into disease pathophysiology and play a pivotal role in guiding therapeutic strategies.

This chapter explores the evolving role of advanced multimodality cardiovascular imaging in the diagnosis and management of myocarditis and pericarditis. It examines the unique capabilities and limitations of each imaging modality, emphasizing their integration into clinical practice. Additionally, the chapter highlights emerging imaging techniques and future directions, underscoring their potential to deepen our understanding of these complex conditions. Through a comprehensive review, this chapter aims to equip clinicians and researchers with practical insights to optimize the care of patients with myocarditis and pericarditis.

2. Phenotypes and genotypes

The study of myocarditis and pericarditis encompasses a wide range of clinical manifestations (phenotypes) and underlying genetic factors (genotypes). This dual perspective is crucial for accurate diagnosis, effective management, and potential future therapies for these inflammatory heart conditions.

2.1 Phenotypes of myocarditis

The clinical manifestations of myocarditis vary widely, influenced by the histological severity, stage at presentation, and etiology of the disease. Myocarditis can present as acute, subacute, chronic, or fulminant [3]. Mild symptoms include sharp, angina-like chest pain, fatigue, generalized weakness, and reduced exercise tolerance, and severe presentations may include heart failure and arrhythmias, with complications such as dilated cardiomyopathy, cardiogenic shock, and sudden cardiac death [4, 5].

2.2 Genotypes of myocarditis

Genetic predisposition plays a significant role in the susceptibility and clinical course of myocarditis.

2.2.1 Genetic variations

Structural protein mutations: Mutations in structural proteins, such as Titin (TTN) and Dystrophin, result in a defective myocardium that is more susceptible to inflammation and damage, especially following insults like viral infections. These mutations are significant because in one study, 22% of patients with suspected myocarditis possessed pathogenic variants of cardiac related genes [6].

Immune response gene variants: Specific single nucleotide polymorphisms (SNPs) in immune-related genes, such as Toll-like receptor 3 (TLR3), have been linked to increased susceptibility to viral myocarditis [7].

Pathogenic mutations: Variants in the HLA-DR4 gene have been associated with heightened inflammatory responses in myocarditis [8].

2.3 Phenotype of pericarditis

Pericarditis, characterized by inflammation of the pericardial sac, displays diverse phenotypes depending on its etiology, symptom severity, and clinical features. The most common symptoms include sharp, pleuritic chest pain alleviated by sitting up or leaning forward, and may be accompanied by a pericardial friction rub on auscultation [2, 9]. Systemic symptoms such as low-grade fever, general malaise, and chills may also be present, and further complications include cardiac tamponade and constrictive pericarditis, which can result in hemodynamic compromise and heart failure from fibrotic pericardial changes, respectively [2, 10].

2.4 Genotypes of pericarditis

While the genetic underpinnings of pericarditis are less understood than those of myocarditis, emerging evidence highlights potential genetic contributors.

Genetic variants

Interleukin-1 cytokine variants: Variants within the IL-1 gene locus may modulate inflammatory responses, with some conferring protection against pericarditis [11].

Mutations in immune response genes: Genetic alterations, such as those affecting the NLRP12 gene, have been implicated in recurrent pericarditis, pointing to a role for innate and adaptive immune dysregulation [12].

3. Clinical pathophysiology

The pathophysiology of myocarditis and pericarditis is diverse, with overlapping features, and the conditions often co-occur as myopericarditis. While myocarditis primarily affects the myocardium, pericarditis involves inflammation of the protective pericardial sac. Both conditions share common triggers and pathophysiologic mechanisms.

Myocarditis is most often caused by viral infections, including coxsackievirus, human immunodeficiency virus (HIV), Epstein-Barr virus (EBV), and hepatitis C virus (HCV), which directly injure cardiomyocytes. The progression of viral myocarditis typically occurs in three phases: acute, autoimmune, and chronic. The acute phase begins with an insult to myocardial tissue, activating the innate immune system and leading to the release of pro-inflammatory cytokines and the recruitment of immune cells like neutrophils, macrophages, and natural killer cells. It is followed by the autoimmune phase, which is driven by molecular mimicry between viral antigens and myocardial proteins, triggering an amplified humoral and cellular immune response, ultimately resulting in fibrosis [4, 13, 14]. In the setting of a regulated immune response, the infection resolves, and the inflammation subsides, limiting further myocardial damage. If the immune response is dysregulated, however, prolonged autoimmune inflammation may lead to fulminant myocarditis [15]. In the chronic phase, patients achieve either full recovery or progression to chronic dilated cardiomyopathy from irreversible myocardial remodeling [14].

Pericarditis involves inflammation of the pericardium due to infectious, autoimmune, or traumatic etiologies. The inflammatory response leads to a cascade of pathological events, including the release of pro-inflammatory cytokines, particularly IL-1, and activation of the innate immune system, which results in increased vascular permeability and extravasation of inflammatory cells and fluid into the pericardial sac. IL-1 plays a pivotal role in pathogenesis, supported by the efficacy of IL-1 inhibitors in treatment, and severe effusion can result in cardiac tamponade or constrictive pericarditis [2, 16].

Both myocarditis and pericarditis highlight the delicate balance between protective immune responses and pathological tissue injury. While the immune response is essential for eliminating infectious agents and initiating repair, excessive or dysregulated inflammation can cause significant damage, leading to severe complications. This underscores the importance of timely diagnosis and targeted interventions to mitigate immune-mediated injury and optimize patient outcomes.

4. Biomarkers and electrocardiographic (ECG) features in myocarditis and pericarditis

The diagnostic evaluation of myocarditis and pericarditis relies on a combination of clinical, biochemical, and ECG findings to identify myocardial or pericardial involvement and distinguish these conditions from other cardiac etiologies.

In myocarditis, cardiac biomarkers such as troponin T and troponin I are elevated in at least 50% of patients, reflecting myocardial injury or necrosis. Erythrocyte sedimentation rate (ESR) and C-reactive protein (CRP) levels are typically elevated as well, indicating an active inflammatory process. Leukocytosis is often present, and eosinophilia may also be noted, particularly in eosinophilic myocarditis. While not essential for diagnosing myocarditis, ECG aids in ruling out other cardiac etiologies and detecting arrhythmias such as atrioventricular (AV) blocks and ventricular ectopy. Certain ECG findings, such as ST-segment elevations, can mimic acute coronary syndromes [3, 17].

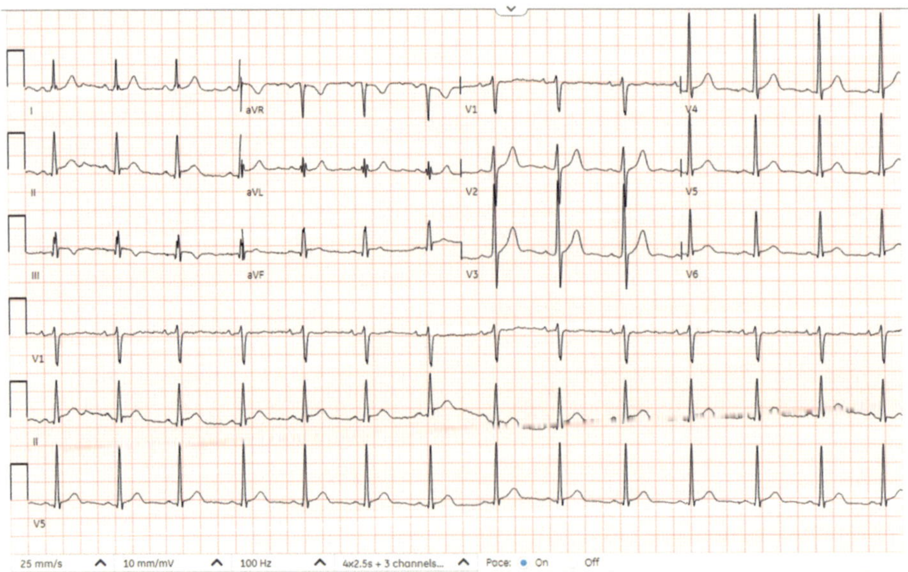

Figure 1.
An ECG showing normal sinus rhythm, diffuse PR-segment depressions, and diffuse ST-segment elevations consistent with both myocarditis and pericarditis.

Similarly to that seen in myocarditis, inflammatory markers such as ESR and CRP are typically elevated in pericarditis, reflecting systemic inflammation. ECG findings often include diffuse concave ST-segment elevations and PR-segment depressions, and reciprocal ST-segment depressions are also commonly observed in lead aVR (**Figure 1**) [18].

5. Imaging modalities

5.1 Echocardiography

Echocardiography is a cornerstone diagnostic and management tool for myocarditis and pericarditis, offering detailed, real-time insights into cardiac structure and function in these inflammatory conditions.

In myocarditis, echocardiography is the initial imaging modality of choice as it provides critical information on cardiac function, wall motion, and the presence of effusions. A key finding is global or regional left ventricular (LV) dysfunction, as evidenced by reduced ejection fraction (EF) and wall motion abnormalities such as hypokinesis, akinesis, or dyskinesis [3, 19]. Echocardiography also helps in identifying complications such as intracardiac thrombi in the setting of regional wall motion abnormalities and pericardial effusion, as well as excluding alternative causes of presenting symptoms, guiding management decisions [19]. However, while invaluable for assessing functional and structural changes, echocardiography lacks the sensitivity and specificity required to characterize myocardial inflammation definitively.

Similarly, in pericarditis, echocardiography is the primary tool for assessing pericardial thickening, which is indicative of chronic inflammatory changes. It is widely available, cost-effective, and can be performed urgently. Echocardiography can also detect the presence and quantify the magnitude of a pericardial effusion and, therefore, help its hemodynamic effects (**Figures 2** and **3**) [18, 21].

5.2 Cardiac magnetic resonance imaging

Cardiac MRI (CMR) has emerged as an indispensable tool for diagnosing and managing myocarditis and pericarditis, offering unmatched tissue characterization and diagnostic precision through advanced imaging techniques.

Guided by the updated Lake Louise Criteria, which utilizes T1/T2 mapping and late gadolinium enhancement (LGE), CMR is considered the gold standard non-invasive modality for diagnosing myocarditis, even in patients with biopsy-proven pathology [19]. T1 mapping quantifies longitudinal relaxation times, reflecting myocardial inflammation and fibrosis, and elevated native T1 values are indicative of acute myocardial injury, whereas post-contrast T1 mapping assesses extracellular volume (ECV), a marker of diffuse fibrosis.

In pericarditis, T1 mapping can detect concurrent pericardial inflammation, while T2 mapping quantifies myocardial water content, directly measuring edema. Elevated T2 values are highly sensitive to myocardial inflammation in myocarditis and pericardial edema in pericarditis, and excel in detecting diffuse changes, which are often missed by conventional T2-weighted imaging. Notably, the diagnostic accuracy of CMR in myocarditis is highest when performed within the first 2–3 weeks of symptom onset, as myocardial edema diminishes over time.

LGE identifies areas of myocardial damage through gadolinium accumulation in regions of necrosis, inflammation, or fibrosis. In myocarditis, LGE typically presents

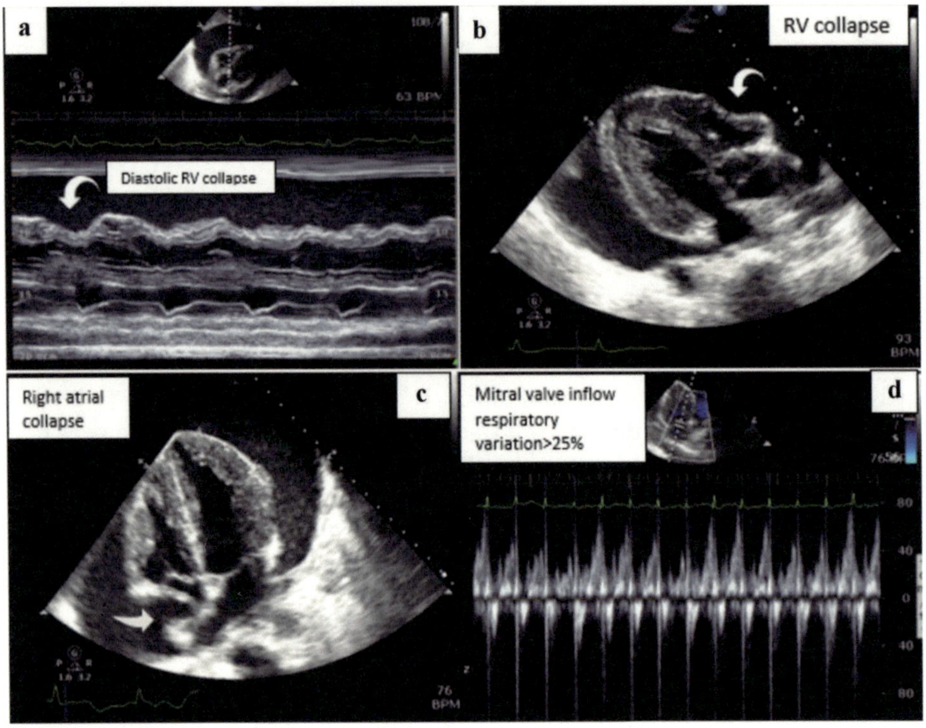

Figure 2.
Transthoracic echocardiography showing the following findings: (a) M-mode with large pericardial effusion and right ventricular (RV) diastolic collapse. (b) The parasternal long-axis view is consistent with RV diastolic collapse. (c) The collapse of the right atrium (d) Mitral valve inflow velocity with respiratory variation greater than 25% [20].

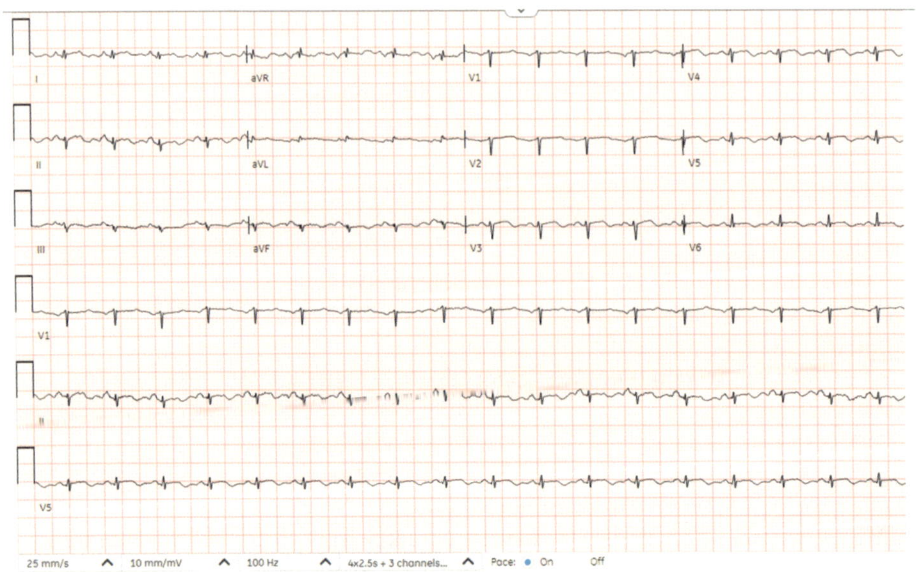

Figure 3.
ECG showing normal sinus rhythm and low-voltage QRS in the setting of a pericardial effusion post-myocarditis.

as a nonischemic, patchy distribution in the sub epicardium or mid-wall layers [14]. In pericarditis, LGE highlights inflamed pericardial tissue and helps differentiate acute pericarditis from chronic constrictive forms [22].

The combined use of T1/T2 mapping and LGE offers complementary insights, with T1/T2 mapping excelling in detecting diffuse disease and LGE providing superior spatial resolution for focal injury. Together, these techniques enhance diagnostic accuracy, facilitate risk stratification, and guide therapeutic decisions, transforming the management of myocarditis and pericarditis [1, 18]. Limitations include practical constraints, including high cost, limited accessibility, contraindications in patients with renal impairment or implanted devices, and reduced sensitivity in chronic myocarditis (**Figures 4–6**) [24, 25].

CMR also is helpful in solidifying the diagnosis of restrictive versus constrictive pericarditis as a complication after myocarditis and pericarditis (**Figure** 7).

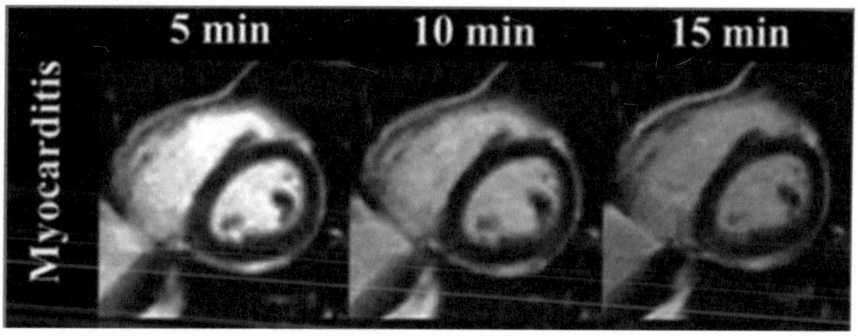

Figure 4.
Diffuse inflammation is seen in myocarditis.

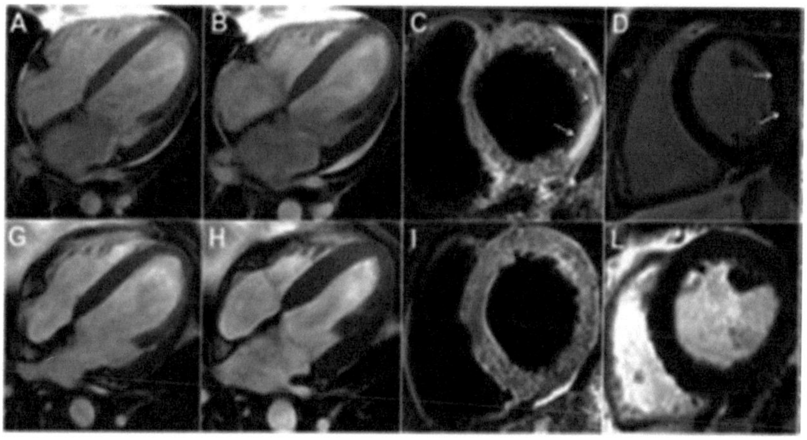

Figure 5.
CMR of a biopsy-proven autoimmune myocarditis in HIV-associated dilated cardiomyopathy showing long-axis images (panel A = diastole, panel B = systole) with a severely dilated and dysfunctional LV recovering from an EF of 20% to an EF of 45% after 4 months of steroid therapy (panel G = diastole, panel H = systole), T2 short-tau inversion recovery images (T2-STIR) in the midventricular short-axis showing subepicardial edematous imbibition of the inferolateral segment of the LV myocardium (panel C, arrows) and thickening of pericardial layers with a minimal amount of effusion (panel C, arrowheads) that correspond to LGE with the same distribution (panel D, arrows), and T2w-STIR LGE images (panel I and L) that show complete regression of tissue edema and late enhancement at a 4-month follow-up [23].

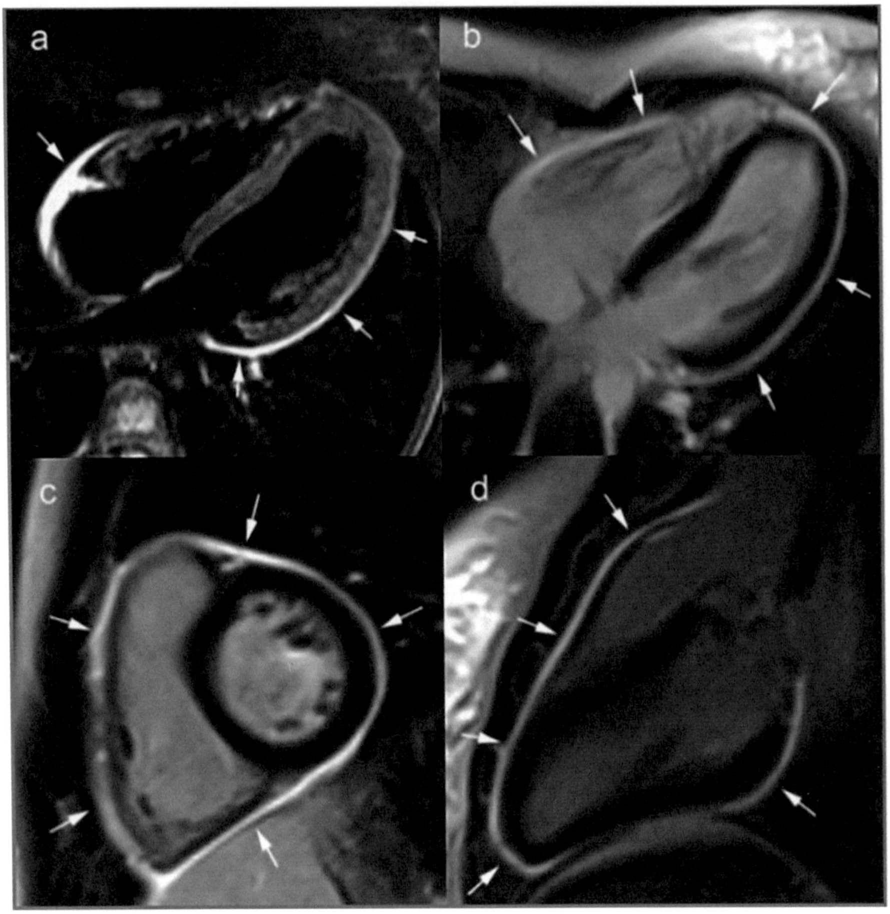

Figure 6.
CMR showing acute viral inflammatory pericarditis in a 15-year-old girl, with T2-weighted short-tau inversion recovery spin-echo CMR (a), LGE CMR in horizontal long-axis (b), short-axis (c), and vertical long-axis plane (d). There is diffuse hyperintense appearance of the pericardium on T2-weighted short-tau inversion recovery spin-echo CMR (panel a, arrows) and strong, homogeneous enhancement of the entire pericardium following gadolinium administration (panels b, c, d, arrows) [23].

5.3 Computed tomography (CT)

CT is often used in ruling out other conditions and for diagnosing pericarditis rather than myocarditis. It helps visualize pericardial thickening, calcification, and effusion and is particularly useful in cases of suspected constrictive pericarditis (**Figure 8**) [18, 21].

5.4 Nuclear imaging

18F-Fluorodeoxyglucose Positron Emission Tomography (PET) provides robust information on myocardial inflammation and pericarditis. Increased glucose uptake, suggestive of inflammatory activity, helps differentiate active inflammation from scarring secondary to prior viral infections (**Figure 9**) [1].

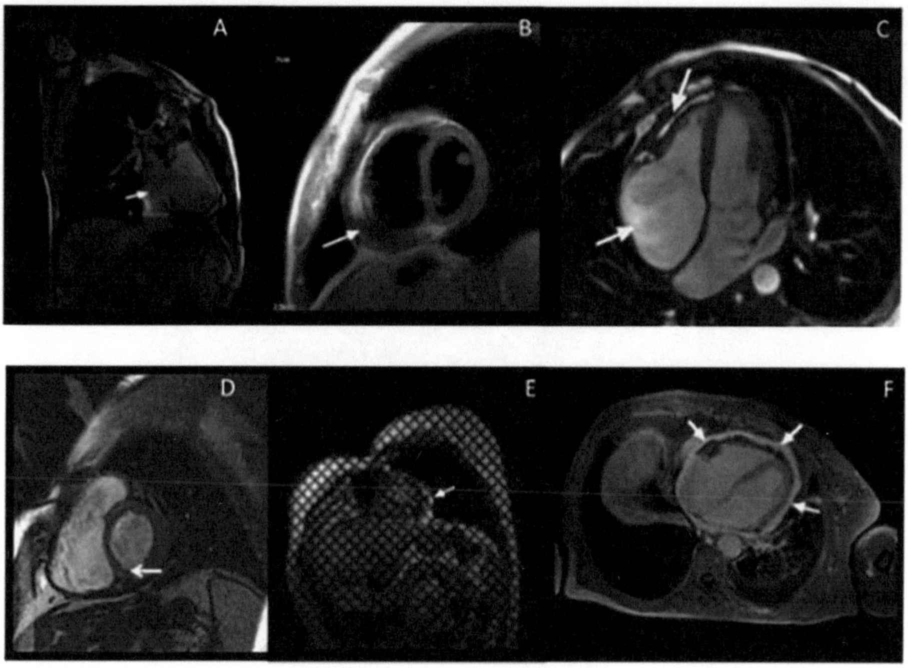

Figure 7.
CMR of constrictive pericarditis. A: Right ventricular vertical long-axis image showing circumferential pericardial thickening and an enlarged inferior vena cava; B: short-axis image showing circumferential pericardial thickening, encysted pericardial effusion; C: four-chamber image showing focal pericardial thickening in front of the right ventricle lateral wall, an encysted pericardial effusion, an enlarged right atrium; D: short-axis image showing focal pericardial thickening in front of the left ventricular inferior and lateral walls; E: short-axis tagging image showing focal pericardial thickening and adherence in front of the left ventricular lateral wall; F: four-chamber late gadolinium enhancement image showing enhancing pericardium [23].

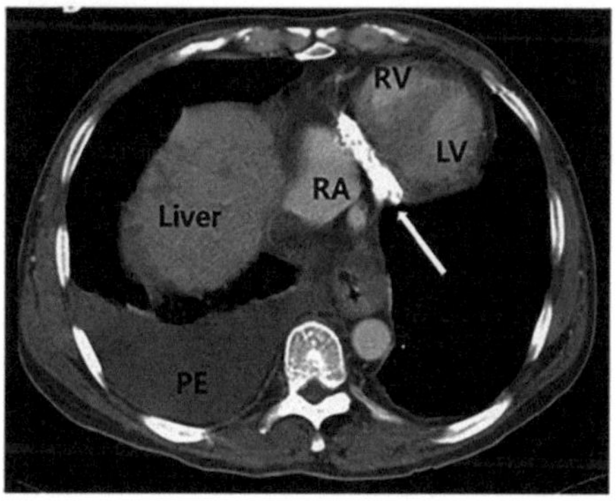

Figure 8.
A chest CT revealing dense calcifications (arrow) along the atrioventricular groove, and pleural effusion [26].

5.5 Hybrid techniques

The combination of CT, PET, CMR with traditional echocardiography has emerged as valuable tools in the diagnosis and management of both pericarditis and

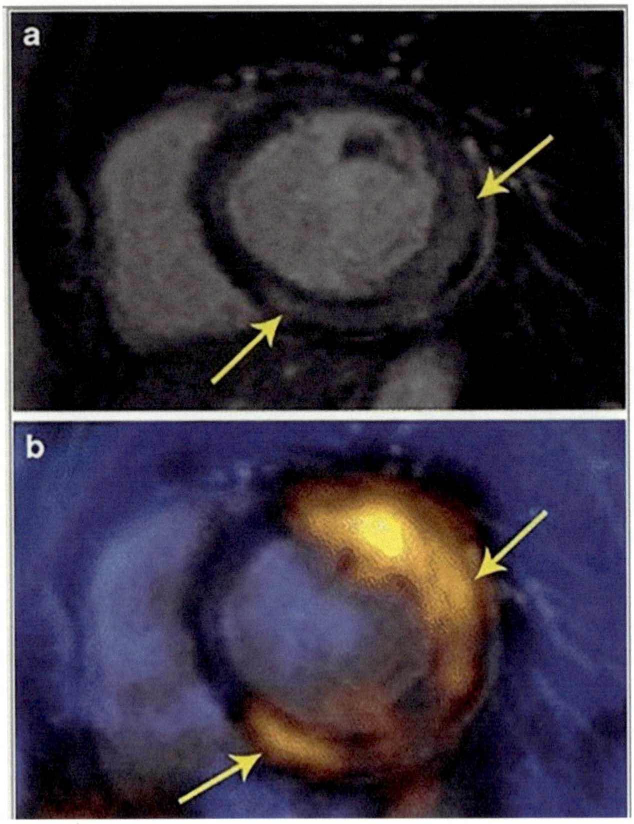

Figure 9.
Myocarditis. A: short-axis delayed enhancement MRI in a patient with acute onset chest pain and elevated enzymes shows mid-myocardial enhancement in the mid-lateral and inferior segments (arrow). B: Fused PET/MR image obtained after glucose diet shows patchy areas of intense uptake in the lateral and inferior wall, indicative of active inflammation [27].

myocarditis. They enhance precision in diagnosing active inflammation and assessing the extent of myocardial involvement, enabling improved risk stratification and therapeutic strategies [28].

6. General considerations and guidelines

For myocarditis, the American College of Radiology (ACR) recommends echocardiography as the initial imaging modality for assessing ventricular function, regional wall abnormalities, and pericardial effusion, and recommends CMR as the next imaging modality should echocardiography findings remain equivocal, as it is the gold standard for noninvasive imaging due to its superior ability to characterize tissue and assess cardiac function [29]. The updated Lake Louise Criteria in CMR is particularly effective for distinguishing myocarditis from other cardiomyopathies and ischemic heart disease, while also providing prognostic information [30]. The presence of cardiac biomarkers such as troponins, along with LV dysfunction, should be incorporated into management decisions, including the potential need for endomyocardial biopsy. Serial imaging can be used to monitor disease progression and assess response to treatment.

For pericarditis, echocardiography and CMR retain the same roles. CMR or cardiac CT are indicated in complex cases where additional anatomic detail is required, such as when there is suspicion of constrictive pericarditis or significant pericardial effusion potentially requiring intervention [18, 31]. Accurate diagnosis of pericarditis involves combining imaging findings with clinical history, physical examination, and laboratory results. Imaging findings often guide treatment strategies, such as pericardiocentesis or surgical intervention in cases of significant effusion or constriction.

Overall, a multimodality approach to imaging is recommended for both myocarditis and pericarditis.

7. Conclusion

Echocardiography, along with advanced imaging modalities such as CMR and cardiac CT, is cornerstones in the diagnosis and management of myocarditis and pericarditis. These imaging techniques are integral for evaluating cardiac function, guiding therapeutic decisions, and enabling the early detection of complications. As advancements in imaging technology progress, their contribution to refining treatment strategies and improving patient outcomes will continue to expand, reinforcing their pivotal role in modern cardiovascular care.

Author details

Nana Osei[1], Abena Agyekum[1], Kai Shiang Lin[1] and

Inna Bukharovich[2]* 1 SUNY Downstate Medical Center,

Brooklyn, New York, USA 2 Kings County Hospital Center,

Brooklyn, New York, USA

*Address all correspondence to: inna.bukharovich@nychhc.org

References

[1] Urzua Fresno C, Sanchez Tijmes F, Shaw KE, Huang F, Thavendiranathan P, Khullar S, et al. Cardiac imaging in myocarditis: Current evidence and future directions. Canadian Association of Radiologists Journal. 2023;**74**(1):147-159

[2] Dababneh E, Siddique MS. Pericarditis. [Updated 2023 Aug 8]. In: StatPearls [Internet]. Treasure Island (FL): StatPearls Publishing; Jan 2025. Available from: https://www.ncbi.nlm.nih.gov/books/NBK431080/

[3] Lampejo T, Durkin SM, Bhatt N, Guttmann O. Acute myocarditis: Aetiology, diagnosis and management. Clinical Medicine (London, England). 2021;**21**(5):e505-ee10

[4] Al-Akchar M, Shams P, Kiel J. Acute Myocarditis. Treasure Island (FL): StatPearls; 2024

[5] Heymans S, Van Linthout S, Kraus SM, Cooper LT, Ntusi NAB. Clinical characteristics and mechanisms of acute myocarditis. Circulation Research. 2024;**135**(2):397-411

[6] Bueno, Marinas M, De Gaspari M, Baritussio A, Cason M, Celeghin R, et al. Genetic testing in inflammatory cardiomyopathy/myocarditis: A red flag for cardiomyopathy-like histologic findings. European Heart Journal. November 2023;**44**(Suppl. 2):ehad655.1828. DOI: 10.1093/eurheartj/ehad655.1828

[7] Favere K, Bosman M, Klingel K, Heymans S, Van Linthout S, Delputte PL, et al. Toll-like receptors: Are they taking a toll on the heart in viral myocarditis? Viruses. 2021;**13**(6):1003. DOI: 10.3390/v13061003

[8] Baggio C, Gagno G, Porcari A, Paldino A, Artico J, Castrichini M, et al. Myocarditis: Which role for genetics? Current Cardiology Reports. 2021;**23**(6):58

[9] Lazarou E, Tsioufis P, Vlachopoulos C, Tsioufis C, Lazaros G. Acute pericarditis: Update. Current Cardiology Reports. 2022;**24**(8):905-913

[10] Andreis A, Imazio M, Casula M, Avondo S, Brucato A. Recurrent pericarditis: An update on diagnosis and management. Internal and Emergency Medicine. 2021;**16**(3):551-558

[11] Thorolfsdottir RB, Jonsdottir AB, Sveinbjornsson G, Aegisdottir HM, Oddsson A, Stefansson OA, et al. Variants at the interleukin 1 gene locus and pericarditis. JAMA Cardiology. 2024;**9**(2):165-172

[12] Cinteza E, Stefan D, Iancu MA, Ioan A, Vasile CM, Vatasescu R, et al. Autoinflammatory recurrent pericarditis associated with a new NLRP12 mutation in a male adolescent. Life (Basel, Switzerland). 2023;**13**(11):2131. DOI: 10.3390/life13112131

[13] Uccello G, Bonacchi G, Rossi VA, Montrasio G, Beltrami M. Myocarditis and chronic inflammatory cardiomyopathy, from acute inflammation to chronic inflammatory damage: An update on pathophysiology and diagnosis. Journal of Clinical Medicine. 2024;**13**(1):150

[14] Bozkurt B, Colvin M, Cook J, Cooper LT, Deswal A, Fonarow GC, et al. Current diagnostic and treatment strategies for specific dilated cardiomyopathies: A scientific statement from the American Heart

Association. Circulation. 2016;**134**(23):e579-e646

[15] He W, Zhou L, Xu K, Li H, Wang JJ, Chen C, et al. Immunopathogenesis and immunomodulatory therapy for myocarditis. Science China. Life Sciences. 2023;**66**(9):2112-2137

[16] Vecchié A, Bonaventura A, Golino M, Thomas G, Abbate A. Novel therapeutic insights into the treatment of pericarditis: Targeting the innate immune system. Journal of Cardiovascular Pharmacology. 2024;**83**(5):377-383. DOI: 10.1097/FJC.0000000000001553

[17] Crisci G, Bobbio E, Gentile P, Bromage DI, Bollano E, Ferone E, et al. Biomarkers in acute myocarditis and chronic inflammatory cardiomyopathy: An updated review of the literature. Journal of Clinical Medicine. 2023;**12**(23)

[18] Malik AA, Lloyd JW, Anavekar NS, Luis SA. Acute and complicated inflammatory pericarditis: A guide to contemporary practice. Mayo Clinic Proceedings. 2024;**99**(5):795-811

[19] Martens P, Cooper LT, Tang WHW. Diagnostic approach for suspected acute myocarditis: Considerations for standardization and broadening clinical Spectrum. Journal of the American Heart Association. 2023;**12**(17):e031454

[20] Khatun N, Akivis Y, Ji B, Chandrakumar HP, Bukharovich I, John S. Tuberculous pericarditis presenting as cardiac tamponade: Role of echocardiography. Journal of Medical Cases. 2023;**14**(8):271-276

[21] Khandaker MH, Espinosa RE, Nishimura RA, Sinak LJ, Hayes SN, Melduni RM, et al. Pericardial disease: Diagnosis and management. Mayo Clinic Proceedings. 2010;**85**(6):572-593

[22] Imazio M, Pivetta E, Palacio Restrepo S, Sormani P, Pedrotti P, Quarta G, et al. Usefulness of cardiac magnetic resonance for recurrent pericarditis. The American Journal of Cardiology. 2020;**125**(1):146-151

[23] Lachhab A, Doghmi N, Zouhairi A, Seghrouchni A, Wahid FA, Boulahya A, et al. Use of magnetic resonance imaging in assessment of constrictive pericarditis: A Moroccan center experience. International Archives of Medicine. 2011;**4**:36

[24] O'Halloran CP, Robinson JD, Watanabe K, Zumpf KB, Petito LC, Marino BS, et al. Magnetic resonance imaging in Pediatric myocarditis: Trends and associations with cost and outcome. JACC: Cardiovascular Imaging. 2022;**15**(7):1230-1238

[25] Bhatt AB, Foster E, Kuehl K, Alpert J, Brabeck S, Crumb S, et al. Congenital heart disease in the older adult: A scientific statement from the American Heart Association. Circulation. 2015;**131**(21):1884-1931

[26] Lee MS, Choi JH, Kim YU, Kim SW. Ring-shaped calcific constrictive pericarditis strangling the heart: A case report. International Journal of Emergency Medicine. 2014;7:40

[27] Chalian H, O'Donnell JK, Bolen M, Rajiah P. Incremental value of PET and MRI in the evaluation of cardiovascular abnormalities. Insights Into Imaging. 2016;**7**(4):485-503

[28] Hutt E, Kaur S, Jaber WA. Modern tools in cardiac imaging to assess myocardial inflammation and infection. European Heart Journal Open. 2023;**3**(2):oead019

[29] Rajiah P, Kirsch J, Bolen MA, Batlle JC, Brown RKJ, Francois CJ, et al.

ACR appropriateness criteria® nonischemic myocardial disease with clinical manifestations (ischemic cardiomyopathy already excluded). Journal of the American College of Radiology. 2021;**18**(5s):S83-s105

[30] Gannon MP, Schaub E, Grines CL, Saba SG. State of the art: Evaluation and prognostication of myocarditis using cardiac MRI. Journal of Magnetic Resonance Imaging. 2019;**49**(7):e122-ee31

[31] Antonopoulos AS, Vrettos A, Androulakis E, Kamperou C, Vlachopoulos C, Tsioufis K, et al. Cardiac magnetic resonance imaging of pericardial diseases: A comprehensive guide. European Heart Journal Cardiovascular Imaging. 2023;**24**(8):983-998

Chapter 5

Imaging in Myocarditis and Pericarditis

Mayuresh Chaudhari, Aiswarya Pillai and Mahi L. Ashwath

Abstract

Myocarditis and pericarditis represent inflammatory conditions of cardiac tissue. A variety of etiologies can result in myocarditis and pericarditis, including inflammatory and infectious causes. This chapter aims to provide a detailed overview of the various diagnostic methods for these conditions, focusing on the utility of imaging tests—echocardiography, cardiac CT, 18F FDG-PET, and CMR in the diagnostic work-up, utility, diagnostic features, and limitations of the various modalities. The role of imaging in the diagnosis of recurrent pericarditis and chronic constrictive pericarditis is discussed in this chapter. A brief overview of the management of myocarditis and pericarditis is also presented.

Keywords: echocardiogram, cardiovascular imaging, cardiac computed tomography (CT), cardiac magnetic resonance imaging (CMR), T1 and T2 mapping, myocarditis, pericarditis

1. Introduction

The myocardium and surrounding pericardium are both vulnerable to inflammatory pathologies that present along a common spectrum. Pericarditis, or inflammation of the pericardium, often presents with sharp, pleuritic chest pain that is typically worsened upon inspiration or when lying down and improved upon leaning forward. Patients may report a history of viral prodrome, and the physical exam typically reveals a friction rub. The evolution of acute pericarditis over time can be tracked using electrocardiogram (EKG) and typically follows four stages: Stage 1 changes involve diffuse ST elevations with PR depression, Stage 2 sees the return of EKG- ST and PR segments to baseline with T wave flattening, Stage 3 the inversion of T waves, and Stage 4 the normalization of the EKG with or without persistent T wave inversion.

Myocarditis, or inflammation of the myocardium, can present with a range of symptoms, ranging from progressive LV dysfunction to arrhythmias to acute myocardial infarction, except without any coronary involvement (ruled out by coronary angiography). Milder forms of the disease may, however, present similarly to acute pericarditis, including a viral prodrome, fatigue, and pleuritic chest pain. Myocardial injury may be suspected when diagnostic workups reveal elevated troponins and creatine kinase (CK-MB) levels. Elevated nonspecific inflammatory markers, such as elevated white blood cell counts, are, however, nonspecific and may be encountered in either disease.

Thus, myocardial and pericardial diseases exist upon a spectrum that occasionally shares overlapping clinical features and even common etiologies (**Tables 1** and **2**). The term myopericarditis refers to cases of confirmed acute pericarditis with elevated troponin but without left ventricular (LV) systolic dysfunction. Perimyocarditis on the other hand refers to cases presenting as confirmed acute pericarditis with elevated biomarkers and a depressed LV function.

Pericarditis

- Idiopathic
- *Viral*: influenza, coxsackievirus
- *Less commonly associated*: cardiac surgery damaging pericardium, infection (e.g., tuberculosis, histoplasmosis), pulmonary embolism, malignancy, radiation, rheumatic fever, trauma, connective tissue disease, etc.

Myocarditis

- *Viral*: coxsackievirus, adenovirus, hepatitis C virus, parvovirus B19, HIV, HHV6, CMV, EBV
- *Non-viral infections*: bacterial (*Corynebacterium diphtheriae*), protozoal (*Trypanosoma cruzi* i.e., Chagas disease), spirochetal (*Borrelia burgdorferi* i.e., Lyme disease), fungal, parasitic, etc.
- *Inflammatory disease*: sarcoidosis, systemic lupus erythematosus, scleroderma, giant cell myocarditis, hypersensitivity reactions, etc.
- *Myocardial toxins*: cocaine

**This list is not exhaustive, and there exist other etiologies causing myocarditis or pericarditis not listed above.*

Table 1.
Select etiologies of pericarditis and myocarditis.*

History	Upper respiratory tract infection, + fever, chest pain, sudden onset breathlessness
Physical examination	Pericardial friction rub (35–85%) + evidence of pericardial knock, gallop sounds [1]
EKG findings	ST concave elevation, PR depression except for avR Sensitivity 47–77%, specificity unknown [1]
Lab investigations	Raised WBC (neutrophilia in bacterial inf., neutropenia & Lymphocytosis in viral inf. and TB, monocytosis in parasitic, TB and viral inf., Eosinophilia in parasitic, collagen vascular disorders, hypereosinophilic syndrome.) ESR, CRP, cardiac Troponin I elevation - (Sensitivity 34%, specificity 89%, PPV 82%, NPV 47%) [1–3]
Coronary angiography	Normal
Echocardiography	Refer to **Table 3**
Cardiac MRI	
Endomyocardial biopsy	
CT/FDG-PET	

Table 2.
Summary of presentation, clinical features, and lab findings in myopericarditis.

Echocardiography

- Useful in detecting LV wall thickness, changes in LV geometry, changes in LV wall contractility and function, any focal echocardiogram (ECHO) bright spots, as well as any posterior pericardial effusions.
- Acute myocarditis is characterized by normal or increased LV diastolic dimensions, normal or increased septal thickness, and a spherical chamber on echocardiography.
- Two-dimensional strain echocardiography can additionally be used to map and quantify the regional contractile function of the myocardium when evaluating for myocarditis.

Cardiac magnetic resonance

- Can characterize using parametric mapping any myocardial inflammation, hyperemia, capillary leak, edema, necrosis, and/or fibrosis.
- Enables global or regional myocardial T1 and T2 relaxation times to be estimated and correlated back to edema, fibrosis, etc.
- Unique CMR patterns can also be used to distinguish between cardiac sarcoidosis, viral myocarditis, giant cell myocarditis, and eosinophilic myocarditis.
- Temporally distinguishes acute vs. chronic vs. healed myocarditis based on fibrosis, edema, necrosis, and hyperemia values.
- Temporally distinguishes acute vs. subacute vs. healed vs. burned-out pericarditis based on dark blood characterization of pericardial thickness, T2 STIR, and late Gadolinium enhancement data.
- Useful to evaluate pericardial fluid and/or pericardial layers edema in those with inflammatory pericarditis.

Computed tomography

- CT is the best imaging modality for morphological observation of the pericardium and pericardial space.
- CT has a higher spatial resolution than CMR (0.4 to 2 mm and is much better at showing pericardial calcifications and constriction.
- CT however is less adept at tissue characterization and temporal resolution than CMR.

Fluorodeoxyglucose positron emission technology

- Increased standardized uptake of 18F-FDG in the pericardium can be useful in identifying sources of inflammation, as well as detecting the metabolic activity of the pericardium due to underlying malignancy or systemic auto-immune disease.
- Tuberculomas have a characteristic pattern on PET, with high max 18F-FDG uptake values greater than those seen in idiopathic pericarditis.
- PET scans are useful in evaluating the pericardium of patients with contraindications to CMR (advanced kidney disease, recently placed pacemakers, severe claustrophobia, etc.)

Endomyocardial biopsy

- Gold standard for diagnosis of myocarditis.
- Useful in the diagnosis of cardiac sarcoidosis, eosinophilic, giant cell, and lymphocytic myocarditis.
- May be subject to differences in histologic interpretation between clinicians, random sampling of unaffected areas causing to inability to either rule out nor confirm the disease, as well as procedural risks of biopsy itself.

Table 3.
Overview of useful modalities in the diagnostic evaluation of myocarditis.

Due to overlap in clinical features and presentation, the diagnostic approach to both diseases is more or less the same, with various imaging modalities, including the conventional 2-dimensional echocardiography, Cardiac Magnetic Resonance Imaging (CMR), and in complex undiagnosed cases, cardiac Fluorine-18 Fluorodeoxyglucose Positron Emission Tomography/Computed Tomography (PET-CT) with or without endomyocardial biopsy (EMB). This chapter aims to provide a brief overview of commonly used imaging tests in the diagnostic work-up of patients with clinically suspected myopericarditis.

2. Diagnostic evaluation

2.1 General approach

Any patient with chest discomfort with or without palpitations, dyspnea, or syncope should undergo a prompt 12-lead EKG within 10 minutes to look for ST–T changes suggestive of the acute coronary syndrome (ACS)/pericarditis and to rule out life-threatening AV block or arrhythmias necessitating emergency care. If the initial laboratory evaluation reveals a troponin level above the upper normal reference limit, a bedside screening echocardiogram can often be useful to look for regional or global LV dysfunction, LV chamber dilatation, pericardial effusion, or valvular pathologies. There are many methods for Troponin I (cTnI) and high sensitivity Troponin I (hs-cTnI) quantification and these all carry their own assay-specific cut-off values. It is thereby recommended that clinicians refer to the local assay in use and adopt the appropriate 99th percentile upper limit of normal.

EKG changes (mainly generalized or localized ST-segment elevation) are more common in patients with myopericarditis than in patients with simple pericarditis. Patients with suspected myopericarditis require hospitalization for evaluation and treatment. It is mandatory to rule out life-threatening causes of troponin elevation (e.g., acute coronary syndromes [ACS], acute aortic syndromes, pulmonary embolism) by conventional coronary angiography or noninvasive CT angiography. A prospective observational study by Pasupathy et al. showed that up to 33% of patients initially diagnosed with myocardial infarction without coronary artery occlusion (MINOCA) had myocarditis [2, 4]. Another study on 107 patients of MINOCA with CMR at a mean delay of 6.9 days by Leurent et al. showed that myocarditis was diagnosed in 60%, AMI in 16%, takotsubo cardiomyopathy in 14%, and normal findings in 10% cases [5]. A high index of suspicion for myocarditis includes younger age, recent viral prodrome, dynamic EKG changes involving more than one vascular territory, absence of reciprocal ST changes, and global LV hypokinesia on echocardiography. Also, ST elevation in myocarditis is temporary and may subside within 24 (49%) or 48 hours (74%) [2]. Coronary angiography can be circumvented in young patients with a cardiac history with no/minimal cardiovascular risk factors and low pre-test probability for coronary artery disease (CAD), and in whom clinical suspicion for myopericarditis is high, prompt cardiac MRI should be performed [1].

Transthoracic 2-dimensional echocardiography is a noninvasive, rapidly accessible bedside imaging tool that helps the clinician during the initial bedside evaluation of the patient with suspected acute myopericarditis. Certain echocardiographic parameters which if present, have a high index of suspicion for myopericarditis are discussed later.

CMR can identify alterations induced by myocardial inflammation, regardless of the underlying cause, and has consequently changed the clinical decision-making approach for patients suspected of having myopericarditis once CAD has been excluded [6]. The multiparametric tissue characterization capability of CMR in exploiting changes in extracellular volume to visualize myocardial inflammation includes tissue edema, hyperemia, capillary leak, necrosis, as well as fibrosis. CMR has the potential to highlight these changes at varying stages and times of the disease process as it progresses from an acute to subacute and later a chronic stage. Thus, it is favorable to perform CMR at any stage of the disease.

In complex, yet undiagnosed cases with nonspecific and diffuse myocardial involvement on CMR, further evaluation with PET/CT may be useful in diagnosing conditions like cardiac sarcoidosis.

In suspected cases of immune-mediated myopericarditis, endomyocardial biopsy (EMB), considered a gold standard in the diagnosis of myocarditis based on established histological, immunological, and immunohistochemical criteria can be useful in the diagnosis of cardiac sarcoidosis, eosinophilic, giant cell, and lymphocytic myocarditis.

3. Echocardiography findings in myopericarditis

The most important parameters to look for in 2D echocardiography include assessment of LV wall thickness, changes in LV geometry, LV wall contractility and function, any focal ECHO bright spot (especially in the posterolateral wall), and the presence of posterior pericardial effusion (**Figure 1**). Patients with increased LV wall thickness and preserved LV diastolic dimensions suggest fulminant disease, whereas those with mildly increased LV diastolic dimensions and normal septal thickness suggest the acute, early stage of myocarditis. A thinned-out LV wall with massive LV enlargement usually suggests scarred myocardium or long-standing involvement and helps in considering other etiologies, such as idiopathic dilated cardiomyopathy [3].

LV dysfunction is usually reversible over several months in patients with fulminant myocarditis, whereas it is less common in patients with acute myocarditis [3], with a gradual change in LV chamber geometry to its original elliptical shape. In doubtful cases, an abnormal tissue Doppler (TDI) signal may be helpful in supplementing the diagnosis [7]. It is important to note that in the acute myopericarditis group,

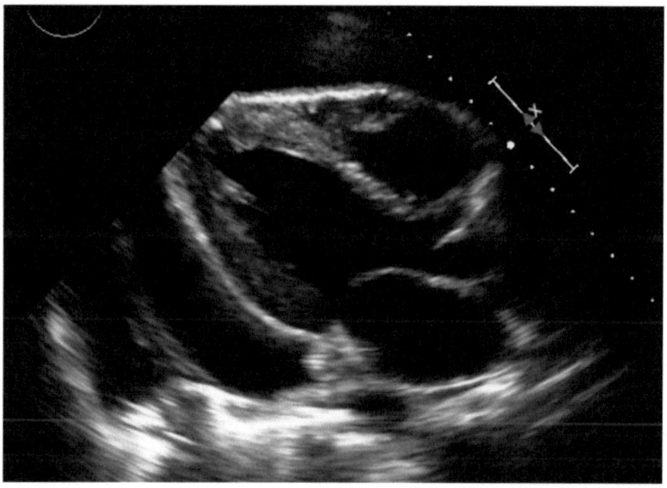

Figure 1.
Parasternal long axis view 2D ECHO image in a patient with pericardial effusion.

segmental wall motion abnormalities do not correspond to electrocardiographic and echocardiographic segments. For instance, EKG changes of ST-segment elevation in anterior leads may show as regional wall hypokinesia on echocardiography affecting postero-lateral walls. However, in a study by Saricam et al. late gadolinium enhancement in the subepicardial region on CMR coincided with echocardiographic focal echobright spot seen in the LV posterolateral wall showing the correlation between CMR and ECHO findings [3].

The earliest evidence of focal myopericarditis is usually some edema in the subepicardial layer of the LV wall on CMR imaging before any evident wall motion abnormality is visualized on routine 2-dimensional echocardiography.

Global longitudinal strain on speckle imaging was found to be more sensitive than ejection fraction estimation especially in patients with preserved LV function. This is due to the ability to differentiate between subtle myocardial movements in the form of speckles, favorable signal-to-noise ratio and angle independence useful to map and quantify regional contractile dysfunction despite normal LV function [6].

4. Cardiac magnetic resonance imaging for detection of myopericarditis

The strength of CMR lies in its unique ability for tissue characterization to differentiate myocardial inflammation, hyperemia, capillary leak, edema, necrosis, as well as fibrosis using parametric mapping.

Initial CMR sequences with blood and fat suppression algorithms are used to delineate the anatomy of the myocardium and pericardium. Volumetric quantification and ventricular function can be assessed by cine MRI which uses a balanced steady-state free precision (bSSFP) technique. Native T1 mapping utilizing saturation recovery methods (saturation recovery single-shot acquisition- SASHA) and inversion recovery techniques (like modified Look-Locker inversion recovery - MOLLI) or abbreviated modified Look-Locker inversion recovery (ShMOLLI), or hybrid sequences provides a "baseline" T1 value for comparison with post-contrast T1 relaxation time to calculate extracellular volume (ECV) and identify focal fibrosis and scarring. Myocardial tissue characterization is done using the injection of gadolinium-based contrast agents and estimating the late gadolinium enhancement (LGE) using a T1-weighted rapid gradient echo MRI (GRE) sequence combined with an inversion recovery pre-pulse to null the signal of normal myocardium. Focal myocardial fibrosis and scarring are better visualized with LGE; however, the signal intensity of the affected myocardium is not vividly enhanced to decipher diffuse and interstitial fibrosis [8]. Hence, quantification of pre-contrast T1 relaxation time is done prior to contrast injection. However, native T1 mapping lacks the ability to differentiate acute from chronic disease. This pitfall can be mitigated by native T2 mapping techniques using gradient or spin-echo sequences which have the advantages of better signal-to-noise ratio, fewer motion artifacts, and better image resolution in comparison to classic T2-weighted imaging, using a black-blood short-tau inversion recovery sequence. Parametric mapping techniques allow not only spatial visualization but also objective quantification of T1 and T2 relaxation times of regional or global myocardial tissue. From pre- and post-contrast T1 imaging, including adjustment for the current hematocrit value, extracellular volume can be calculated, which can be useful for detecting edema, hyperemia, capillary leakage, and fibrosis. Essentially, T1 is better for visualizing structure, while T2 is better for detecting pathology. Fat appears bright on T1 images, whereas fluid appears bright on T2 images. In assessing myocardial fibrosis, a T1-weighted image is typically better for visualizing normal anatomy and detecting potential areas of fibrosis. A normal T1 map of healthy left ventricular myocardium is between 990 ± 31 ms. The prolongation of T1 relaxation times (**Figure 2**) is mainly due to two biological factors, namely the increase of interstitial space due to edema (increased water volume due to acute inflammation) and fibrosis (later stages of myocardial inflammation or a healed condition). T2 imaging techniques may be more specific than T1 imaging for detecting fluid accumulation in acute inflammation, and more sensitive than T1 imaging for detecting edema in chronic fibrotic tissue [9]. Thus, T1 and T2 imaging techniques appear to be of complementary diagnostic value and hence are recommended as part of a comprehensive CMR examination in patients with clinically suspected myocarditis [9–11].

In acute stages of myocarditis, there is capillary leakage, hyperemia, and interstitial space expansion, resulting in increased uptake and volume of distribution of gadolinium-based contrast agents. Increased contrast uptake, described early after the use of gadolinium-based contrast agents, showed decreased sensitivity, specificity, and diagnostic accuracy in the detection of myocarditis, as reported by Lagan et al. and later in a meta-analysis by Kotanidis et al. [12] and thus early gadolinium enhancement was replaced with parametric mapping (elevated T1, T2 relaxation times or nonischemic LGE pattern) as one of the criteria in the revised Lake Louise criteria (LLC) in 2018 to diagnose patients with clinically apparent myocarditis (**Figure 3**) [13, 14].

The late gadolinium enhancement on inversion recovery gradient echo sequences depicted improved detection of myocardial necrosis, and later fibrosis and scar formation showing characteristic nonischemic patterns (a typically patchy appearance with most often subendocardial, mid-wall or subepicardial localization peculiar to different etiologies) (**Tables 4** and **5**) [9, 10].

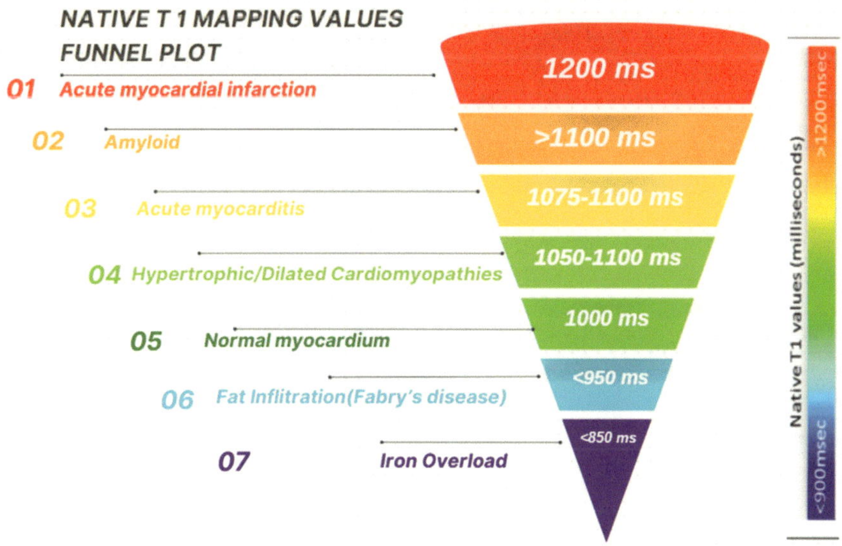

Figure 2.
Native T1 mapping values and ECV in different cardiac diseases. Figure adopted and modified from Martin Ugander (SCMR 2014) and Phillip Haff [8].

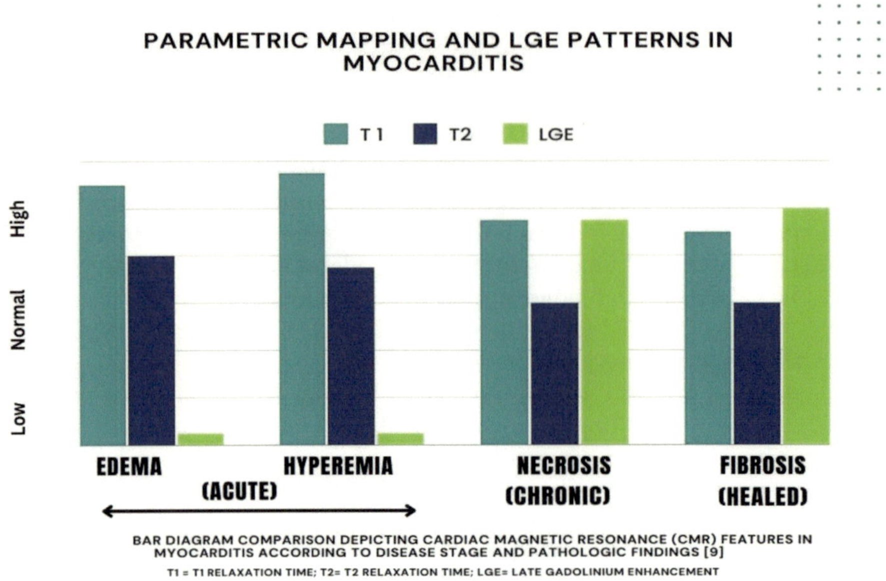

Figure 3.
Cardiac magnetic resonance (CMR) features in myocarditis according to disease stage and pathologic findings [9].

Viral Myocarditis	**Basal, mid-infero-lateral walls predominantly subepicardial and/or midmyocardial segments may be involved.**
Cardiac Sarcoidosis	Patchy, multifocal pattern, typically located in the mid-wall and subepicardial regions of the basal septum and inferolateral wall. LGE can be present in the right ventricular insertion points – "hook sign."
Giant Cell Myocarditis	Widespread late gadolinium enhancement (LGE) across multiple myocardial layers in both ventricles, mimics sarcoid, however overall LGE mass smaller than in cardiac sarcoidosis.
Eosinophilic Myocarditis	Patchy or multifocal subendocardial LGE not confined to a single region.

Table 4.
Cardiac magnetic resonance imaging patterns in different forms of myocarditis [9].

Midmyocardial	Epicardial	Subendocardial global	Subendocardial/transmural focal
• Idiopathic dilated cardiomyopathy • Myocarditis • Hypertrophic cardiomyopathy • Sarcoidosis, Chagas, Anderson - Fabry's disease	• Myocarditis • Sarcoidosis • Chagas disease • Anderson-Fabry's disease	• Amyloidosis • Systemic sclerosis • Post cardiac transplant • Eosinophilic myocarditis	• Ischemic cardiomyopathy

Table 5.
Late gadolinium enhancement patterns in cardiomyopathies [15].

5. Cardiac magnetic resonance in pericardial inflammation

Although computed tomography (CT) is the best imaging method for morphological assessment of pericardium and pericardial space, CMR gains an advantage over CT due to its dynamic and functional assessment properties in clarifying the complex relationship between pericardial constriction and cardiac filling.

Black blood T1-weighted spin-echo CMR using fast, segmental sequences is helpful in visualizing the heart, pericardium, and mediastinum [16, 17]. T2-weighted spin-echo CMR may also be utilized with the short-tau inversion recovery (STIR sequence, also referred to as "triple" spin-echo), which is highly effective at displaying myocardial edema [18] and assessing pericardial fluid and/or pericardial layer edema in individuals with inflammatory pericarditis (**Figure 4**). LGE sequences are

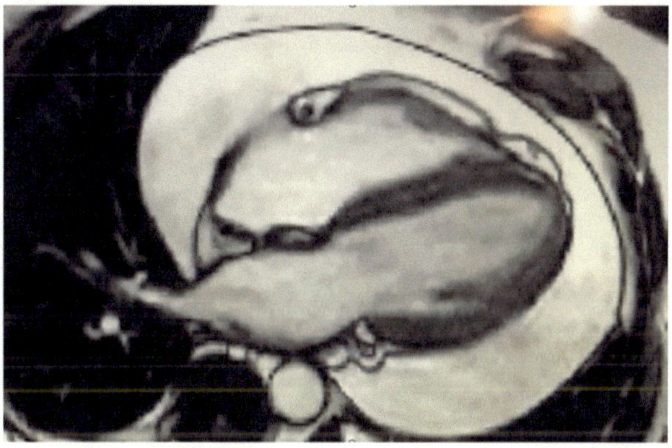

Figure 4.
Cardiac cine MRI sequence showing evidence of pericardial effusion.

2D-Echocardiography:

- Thickened pericardium
- Abnormal ventricular septal motion
- Flattening of LV posterior wall in diastole
- Dilated inferior vena cava

Doppler echocardiography:

- Dissociation of intracardiac and intrathoracic pressures
- Diastolic septal bounce and respiratory phase septal shift
- Hepatic diastolic forward-flow velocity increase in inspiration
- Hepatic vein diastolic reversal wave upon expiration
- Diastolic forward flow greater than systolic forward flow
- Normal or increased velocity of early diastolic transmitral flow (color M-mode)
- Mitral medial e' velocity greater than mitral lateral e' velocity (anulus reversus)
- Higher mitral annular e' velocity
- Reduced longitudinal strain in free wall of both ventricles

Table 6.
Echocardiographic findings in constrictive pericarditis [19–21].

useful in distinguishing between inflammatory and constrictive pericarditis, and to rule out any pericardial mass and concomitant myocardial involvement (**Table 6**).

Presence of pericardial effusion in addition to increased pericardial thickness can be fully demonstrated on T1-weighted spin-echo CMR or cine CMR, but inflammatory pericardial layer edema can be seen on T2-weighted STIR spin-echo CMR. Pericardial enhancement on gadolinium-enhanced CMR studies is an accurate method for detecting pericardial inflammation (**Figures 5** and **6**) [22]. Both LGE CMR and spin-echo CMR are complimentary. Pericardial inflammation can be further highlighted using the addition of fat suppression sequences. Another interesting aspect is the association of the pericardial signal with the adjacent layers, which can show enhancement of the surrounding fat and irregularity in chronic pericarditis or enhancement of the adjacent myocardial tissue in myocarditis (**Figure 7**) [22].

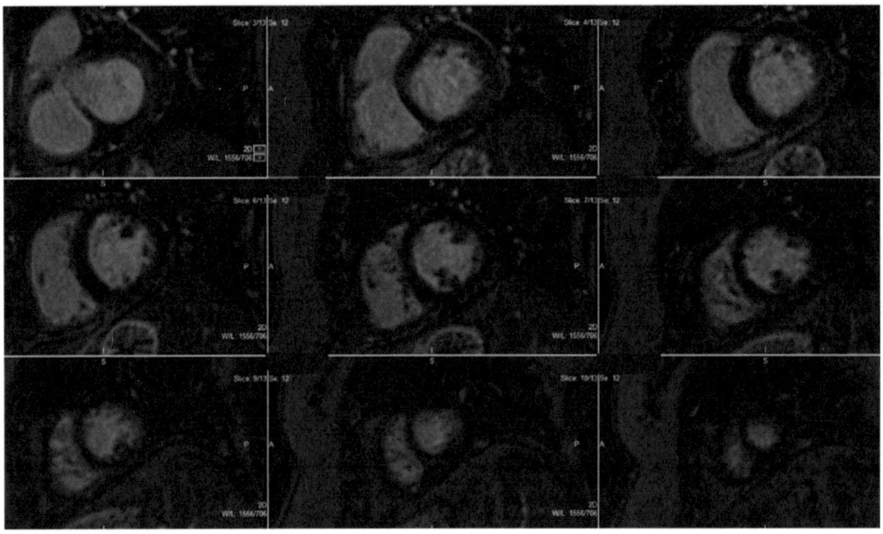

Figure 5.
Cardiac MRI LGE sequence with no pericardial enhancement.

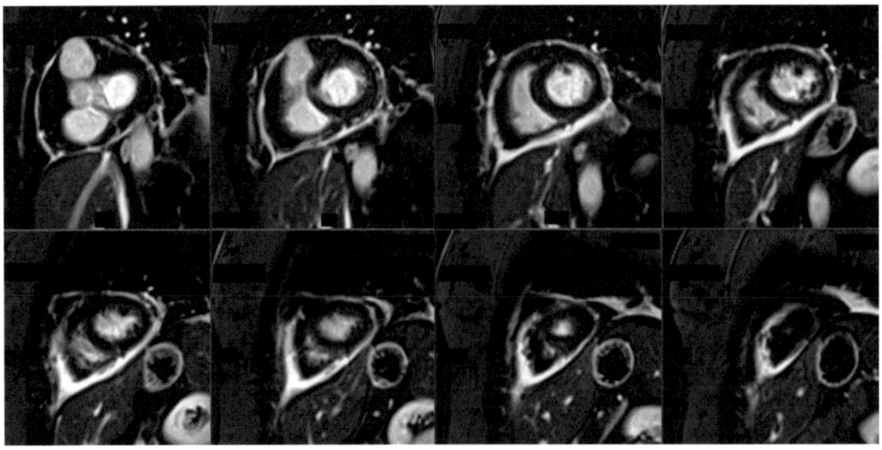

Figure 6.
Cardiac MRI LGE sequence with pericardial enhancement.

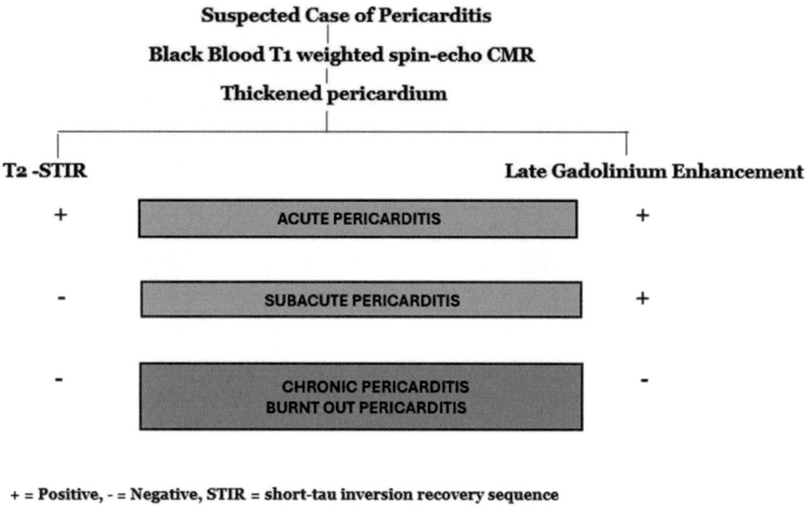

Figure 7.
Pericardial characterization findings in the various stages of pericarditis [16–18, 22].

The disadvantage of CMR is that it is time-consuming and impractical, especially in critically ill, hemodynamically unstable patients unable to hold their breath for a long time, and contraindicated in those who have metallic implantable electronic devices.

6. Computed tomography in the diagnosis of myopericarditis

In the diagnosis of myopericarditis, CT has a higher spatial resolution than MR (0.4 to 1 to 2 mm) and is much better at showing pericardial calcification and constriction. In acute pericarditis, pericardial thickness is minimal and, if present, pericardial effusion is also minimal.

Various case reports have highlighted the importance of detecting coincidental myopericarditis, especially in young individuals undergoing TRO (triple rule out) protocol for chest pain evaluation with a low index of suspicion for CAD. These reports reiterate the fact that CT imaging has the potential to diagnose and detect cases of early myopericarditis. Also, due to faster acquisition times in a single breath hold, it is more practical to acquire the images in critically ill, orthopneic, and hemodynamically unstable patients. However, with the advent of CMR's additional capability of better tissue characterization and better temporal resolution than CT (30–50 vs. 80–160 ms), CMR imaging is preferred over CT scan in the evaluation of suspected cases of myopericarditis whenever feasible [23].

7. Fluorodeoxyglucose positron emission technology scan in myocarditis and pericarditis

18F-fluorodeoxyglucose (18F-FDG-PET) works by injecting a radioactive tracer into a patient's body, which is taken up by active inflammatory cells. The use of PET/CT in various etiologies of myocarditis is well documented [24–26]. 18F-FDG-PET has been shown to be especially useful in establishing diagnosis and monitoring the response to treatment in patients with cardiac sarcoidosis [27].

A novel PET radiopharmaceutical with an affinity for the somatostatin receptor at the 68Ga labeled peptides has been shown to be more diagnostically accurate than 18F- FDG for cardiac sarcoidosis [28].

18F-FDG-PET is also useful in suspected cases of malignancy associated with pericarditis and pericardial effusions. Up to 5% of pericarditis cases are attributed to an underlying cancer, with the most common malignancies being breast cancer, lung cancer, and Hodgkin's lymphoma [29, 30]. In suspected cases of tuberculous pericarditis, 18F-FDG-PET has a definite role in the diagnosis, especially in tuberculomas which have a characteristic high standardized uptake value (SUVmax) [31]. If the pericardial SUVmax is very high (>9) and the 18FDG uptake pattern does not suggest a typical malignancy, the possibility of tuberculous pericarditis should be presumed. Additionally, it can also be useful in selecting an optimum site for tissue biopsy. Many PET protocols require a prolonged fast with a preceding high-fat/low-carbohydrate diet, limiting its ability in rapid diagnosis, albeit useful in situations with contraindications to CMR [32].

In summary, PET may have utility in evaluating myopericarditis due to granulomatous conditions, underlying malignancy, or systemic inflammatory conditions.

8. Recurrent pericarditis

8.1 Introduction

Recurrent pericarditis is defined as a new episode of pericarditis detected on evaluation with chest pain after an asymptomatic period, arbitrarily defined as at least 4–6 weeks according to the European Society of Cardiology 2015 guidelines, despite adequate anti-inflammatory therapy [33, 34]. It is often due to inappropriate treatment of pericarditis (e.g., early discontinuation of anti-inflammatory therapy, low drug dosage, lack of specific recommendations on exercise restriction) rather than a true relapse [33]. It is important to distinguish from incessant pericarditis in which there is no symptom-free period between the two episodes, as it can progress directly to constriction [34]. The term "chronic pericarditis" instead is used to describe any pericardial involvement lasting >3 months.

Acute pericarditis can recur in about 20–30% of cases, and the frequency increases up to 50% in cases receiving inadequate treatment regimens [35]. According to an Italian study, recurrent episodes were more common in patients with isolated pericarditis (31.8%) than in patients with myopericarditis (10.5%) [36].

8.2 Epidemiology

The etiology of recurrent pericarditis is thought to be immune-related. This is supported by evidence of non-organ-specific antibodies and a good response to corticosteroid therapy. Factors associated with an increased risk of recurrence include female gender, inadequate dose and duration of corticosteroid and colchicine use.

8.3 Clinical features and diagnosis

Evidence of symptoms of pericarditis after a symptom-free interval of 4–6 weeks, documented by recurrent chest pain compatible with pericarditis and one or more of the following: a pericardial friction rub, EKG changes, or echocardiographic evidence of new or worsening pericardial effusion, elevation in blood-based inflammatory markers like white-cell count, erythrocyte sedimentation rate, or C-reactive protein (CRP) level with confirmation on CMR study, if feasible [37].

8.4 Imaging in recurrent pericarditis

Diagnosis is primarily based on baseline echocardiographic findings of moderate to large pericardial effusion or worsening pericardial effusion, cardiac tamponade, and exclusion of other etiologies (e.g., tuberculosis, systemic inflammatory disease, neoplastic disease) that may have been missed in previous evaluations.

The normal pericardial thickness is less than 2 mm and appears as a thin hypo-intense (dark) lining surrounded by hyper-intense (bright) lining suggestive of mediastinal and epicardial fat on T1-weighted CMR images [16, 17]. Recurrent pericarditis is suspected when there is increased pericardial thickness with increased signal intensity (bright) of the pericardium on short-tau inversion recovery (STIR)-T2 weighted sequences with hyper-intense (bright) signals on T1-weighted late gadolinium enhancement sequences.

The latter may suggest residual fibrosis and a potential therapeutic target with appropriate anti-inflammatory therapy. Recently, a CMR-guided treatment strategy has been shown not only to reduce new relapses but also to minimize the duration of corticosteroid therapy [22].

CT is a complementary imaging modality to detect thickened pericardium, calcifications, and pericardial effusion based on varying attenuation values of the pericardial fluid. Low attenuation values of pericardial fluid (e.g. 0–20 HU) suggest a transudate, intermediate values (e.g., 20–60 HU) are indicative of exudative effusions, while high attenuation values (>60 HU) mostly suggest hemorrhage [23].

In fact, in a recent study in patients with acute pericarditis and pericardial effusion, an increased 18F-FDG- PET uptake of the pericardium suggestive of ongoing inflammation was considered a risk factor for further recurrences [29].

9. Constrictive pericarditis

9.1 Introduction

Constrictive pericarditis (CP) is a chronic process, a sequela to long-standing pericardial inflammation involving the fibrous pericardium that impairs normal diastolic filling of the ventricles. Symptoms are related to decreased cardiac output and increased pulmonary venous congestion and include fatigue, exercise intolerance, dyspnea, anorexia, and symptoms of right heart failure, such as abdominal distension and pedal edema. Clinical examination reveals raised jugular venous pressure with rapid x- and y-descent waves and paradoxically increased waveform during inspiration (Kussmaul's sign) [38]. On auscultation, a pericardial knock may be observed in up to 47% of patients. Pulsus paradoxus (inspiratory drop of >10 mmHg in systolic blood pressure) has also been reported. There is no pathognomonic EKG pattern [38].

9.2 Epidemiology

CP can occur irrespective of the presence of pericardial effusion. With a slight male predominance, tuberculosis is the most common etiology in developing countries in contrast to the developed world where idiopathic or viral etiology is the most common, followed by cardiac injury, post-radiotherapy, rheumatic diseases, malignancies, and trauma. The incidence of CP is 20–30% after tuberculous pericarditis. This risk is lower with other bacteria or viral etiological agents [39].

9.3 Role of imaging in diagnosis

In patients with strong clinical suspicion for CP, chest radiography may show pericardial calcification in 25–30% of cases, mostly associated with tuberculous pericarditis. Two-dimensional echocardiography may show a concomitant pericardial effusion in 30–40% of patients. In addition to a dilated inferior vena cava, diastolic septal bounce and respiratory phase septal shift due to interventricular dependence can be seen in four-chamber view. Doppler mitral flow velocities usually show a restrictive filling pattern (E/A > 1 and deceleration time < 150 ms). Mitral lateral e′ velocity might be lower than medial e′ velocity due to tissue tethering (anulus reversus). Higher mitral annular e′ velocities in patients with symptoms and signs of right heart failure are highly suggestive of constrictive pericarditis (i.e., >8 cm/s). Normal or increased propagation velocity of early diastolic transmitral flow on color M-mode may also be observed, while expiratory hepatic vein diastolic flow reversal is the most specific echocardiographic sign [19]. On strain imaging, global longitudinal strain and early diastolic tissue velocities are generally preserved in early stages, whereas circumferential strain, torsion, and early diastolic untwisting are reduced (**Table 6**) [20, 21].

The role of CMR in CP is to look for underlying active inflammation in addition to constriction, which can predict reversibility with the complete course of anti-inflammatory therapy. Therefore, assessment of LGE on CMR can be very useful in identifying the stage of disease and predicting response to treatment [40].

CT is more sensitive than chest X-ray for detecting pericardial thickening, calcification, and preoperative planning of pericardiectomy. Failure to visualize the posterolateral LV wall on dynamic CT may indicate myocardial fibrosis or atrophy, which is associated with poor surgical outcomes. Interestingly, positron emission tomography/CT using 18F-fluorodeoxyglucose can also serve the same diagnostic information as CMR in detecting active inflammation and predicting response to anti-inflammatory therapy [41].

Cardiac catheterization is currently reserved in complex cases with effusive-constrictive overlap where there is a dilemma in treatment plans. The main findings on invasive hemodynamics are elevation and equalization of cardiac diastolic pressures in both ventricles (<5 mm Hg difference), prominent rapid diastolic LV filling waveform (≥5 mm Hg, referred to as a square root sign), reduced cardiac output and an exaggerated inspiratory decrease in systolic blood pressure (>10 mm Hg) [42]. These findings may be masked due to aggressive prior diuretic therapy and hence an intravenous fluid challenge may be reasonable in selected cases for unmasking the invasive hemodynamic patterns.

10. Treatment/management

Medical therapy in myopericarditis depends on the predominant presentation. In pericarditis predominant presentation with chest pain, mild pericardial effusion, and preserved LV function, Nonsteroidal anti-inflammatory drugs (NSAIDs) are the first line of drugs used. Colchicine is used routinely in patients with recurrent pericarditis, but its role in myopericarditis is not well established. However, a combination regime of aspirin (650–1000 mg three times daily) or ibuprofen (600–800 mg three times daily) with colchicine (0.5–0.6 mg twice daily for patients weighing ≥70 kg. and once daily in ≤70 kg) [43].

A meta-analysis of five controlled clinical trials in patients with recurrent pericarditis showed a significant reduction in recurrences with colchicine. Similarly, low-dose corticosteroids (0.2–0.5 mg/kg) are commonly used and are associated with high treatment outcomes [43]. Colchicine is usually continued for 3 months, then stopped without reducing the dose. Pericardiocentesis or surgical drainage is recommended for hemodynamic stabilization in patients with massive pericardial effusion often with cardiac tamponade.

In patients with predominant myocarditis with depressed LV function and signs and symptoms of left heart failure, standard heart failure therapy with diuretics, beta-blockers, and angiotensin-converting enzyme inhibitors/angiotensin receptor blockers (ARBs) are recommended. Ventilatory support, inotropes, and extracorporeal membrane oxygenation (ECMO) may be considered in refractory heart failure patients with cardiogenic shock. Corticosteroids are usually used in specific conditions like giant cell myocarditis or recurrent pericarditis refractory to first-line therapy [1].

Medical management of CP includes diuretics and salt restriction. Sinus tachycardia being a compensatory response in CP due to poor ventricular filling and reduced cardiac output, beta blockers and calcium channel antagonists that slow the heart rate should be avoided. In patients with atrial fibrillation and a rapid ventricular response, digoxin is the drug of choice for rate control. Surgical pericardiectomy is the definitive treatment in CP provided there are no comorbidities or radiation induced disease.

Exercise restriction — limitation of fitness activity to walking and/or lightweight training is recommended for at least 3 months or until complete clinical remission. For competitive sports activities, a longer restriction time of up to 6 months may be considered on an individual basis and therapeutic response [44, 45].

11. Prognosis

The condition has an overall good prognosis even at a relatively long-term follow-up of above 2.5 years with no significant long-term sequelae. A meta-analysis showed a recurrence rate of 13%, 3.5% for residual left-ventricular dysfunction, and 0.9% for cardiac tamponade and/or constriction [44]. In a study by Imazio et al., 114 patients with myopericarditis were followed for a mean duration of 36 months. Recurrence was seen in 10.5%, 0.9% developed constriction and LV dysfunction persisted in 7.9% of patients [45]. Prognosis is generally poor in symptomatic patients refractory to medical therapy.

Patient education, reassurance, and the importance of salt and fluid optimization in addition to compliance with medical therapy should be reinforced [46].

Although the prognosis is generally good, patient triage is of utmost importance and therapy should focus on the severity and stage of the disease to prevent morbidity and mortality. In the absence of data from randomized trials, treatment recommendations for myopericarditis are largely based on expert opinion [35].

12. Conclusion

Myopericarditis is not an uncommon problem and is usually viral in etiology. With the current Covid-19 pandemic leading to cardiac manifestations and case reports of

Covid m-RNA vaccine-associated myopericarditis, one needs to have a low threshold in suspecting myopericarditis, especially in individuals with cardiac symptoms following a viral prodrome and febrile illness. There are currently different modalities to detect myopericarditis, which is best managed with an interdisciplinary approach that includes an intensivist, cardiologist, radiologist, infectious disease specialist, physical therapist, and internist. Although the overall prognosis is good, these patients often need aggressive medical therapies and supportive care in an intensive care setting to mitigate the long-term sequelae thereby reducing mortality and morbidity. Prompt treatment before constriction develops is of utmost importance as the prognosis later is generally dismal.

Conflicts of interest

The authors declare that there is no conflict of interest.

Appendix and nomenclature

18F-FDG	18F-fluorodeoxyglucose
ACS	acute coronary syndrome
CCTA	coronary computed tomography angiography
CMR	cardiac magnetic resonance
COVID-19	coronavirus disease 2019
CT	computed tomography
CP	constrictive pericarditis
EKG	electrocardiogram
ECV	extracellular volume
EGE	early gadolinium enhancement
GBCA	gadolinium-based contrast agent
LGE	late gadolinium enhancement
LLC	lake Louise criteria
LVEF	left ventricular ejection fraction
PE	pulmonary embolism
PET	positron emission tomography
SPECT	single-photon emission computed tomography
STE	speckle tracking echocardiography
STIR	short-tau inversion recovery
TDI	tissue Doppler imaging
TTE	transthoracic echocardiography

Author details

Mayuresh Chaudhari[1*], Aiswarya Pillai[2] and Mahi L. Ashwath[3]

1 UT Health Sciences Centre, Glen Biggs Institute, San Antonio, Texas, USA

2 Joe R. and Teresa Lozano Long School of Medicine, UT Health San Antonio, Texas, USA

3 Inaugural Reuben Jacobs Chair in Internal Medicine, UHS/UT Heart and Vascular Institute, San Antonio, Texas, USA

*Address all correspondence to: chaudharim@uthscsa.edu

References

[1] Imizio M. Myopericarditis In - UpToDate, Gesh Bernard, editor. Wolter Kluwer. Waltham, USA; 2024

[2] Lasica R, Djukanovic L, Savic L, Krljanac G, Zdravkovic M, Ristic M, et al. Update on myocarditis: From etiology and clinical picture to modern diagnostics and methods of treatment. Diagnostics. 2023;**13**(19):3073

[3] Saricam E, Saglam Y, Hazirolan T. Clinical evaluation of myocardial involvement in acute myopericarditis in young adults. BMC Cardiovascular Disorders. 2017;**17**:129

[4] Pasupathy S, Tavella R, McRae S, Beltrame JF. Myocardial infarction with non-obstructive coronary arteries – Diagnosis and management. European Cardiology Review. 2015;**10**(2):79-82

[5] Leurent G, Langella B, Fougerou C, Lentz PA, Larralde A, Bedossa M, et al. Diagnostic contributions of cardiac magnetic resonance imaging in patients presenting with elevated troponin, acute chest pain syndrome and unobstructed coronary arteries. Archives of Cardiovascular Diseases. 2011;**104**(3):161-170

[6] Adeboye A, Alkhatib D, Butt A, Yedlapati N, Garg N. A review of the role of imaging modalities in the evaluation of viral myocarditis with a special focus on COVID-19-related myocarditis. Diagnostics. 2022;**12**(2):549

[7] Bobbio E, Amundsen J, Oldfors A, Bollano E, Bergh N, Björkenstam M, et al. Echocardiography in inflammatory heart disease: A comparison of giant cell myocarditis, cardiac sarcoidosis, and acute non-fulminant myocarditis. IJC Heart & Vasculature. 2023;**46**:101202

[8] Haaf P, Garg P, Messroghli DR, et al. Cardiac T1 mapping and extracellular volume (ECV) in clinical practice: A comprehensive review. Journal of Cardiovascular Magnetic Resonance. 2017;**18**:89. DOI: 10.1186/s12968-016-0308-4

[9] Polte CL, Bobbio E, Bollano E, Bergh N, Polte C, Himmelman J, et al. Cardiovascular magnetic resonance in myocarditis. Diagnostics. 2022;**12**(2):399

[10] Abdel-Aty H, Simonetti O, Friedrich M. T2-weighted cardiovascular magnetic resonance imaging. Journal of Magnetic Resonance Imaging JMRI. 2007;**26**:452-459

[11] Joudar I, Aichouni N, Nasri S, Kamaoui I, Skiker I. Diagnostic criteria for myocarditis on cardiac magnetic resonance imaging: An educational review. Annals of Medicine and Surgery. 2023;**85**(8):3960-3964

[12] Kotanidis CP, Bazmpani MA, Haidich AB, Karvounis C, Antoniades C, Karamitsos TD. Diagnostic accuracy of cardiovascular magnetic resonance in acute myocarditis: A systematic review and meta-analysis. JACC: Cardiovascular Imaging. 2018;**11**(11):1583-1590

[13] Lagan J, Schmitt M, Miller CA. Clinical applications of multi-parametric CMR in myocarditis and systemic inflammatory diseases. The International Journal of Cardiovascular Imaging. 2018;**34**(1):35-54

[14] Ferreira VM, Schulz-Menger J, Holmvang G, Kramer CM, Carbone I, Sechtem U, et al. Cardiovascular magnetic resonance in nonischemic myocardial inflammation: Expert recommendations. Journal of the

American College of Cardiology. 2018;**72**(24):3158-3176

[15] Adam RD, Shambrook J, Flett AS. The prognostic role of tissue characterisation using cardiovascular magnetic resonance in heart failure. Cardiac Failure Review. 2017, 2017. Available from: https://www.cfrjournal.com/articles/prognostic-role-tissue-characterisation-using-cardiovascular-magnetic-resonance-heart;**3**(2):86-96 [Accessed: May 28, 2024]

[16] Bogaert J, Francone M. Cardiovascular magnetic resonance in pericardial diseases. Journal of Cardiovascular Magnetic Resonance. 2009;**11**(1):14

[17] Misselt AJ, Harris SR, Glockner J, Feng D, Syed IS, Araoz PA. MR imaging of the pericardium. Magnetic Resonance Imaging Clinics of North America. 2008;**16**(2):185-199, vii

[18] Aletras AH, Tilak GS, Natanzon A, Hsu LY, Gonzalez FM, Hoyt RF, et al. Retrospective determination of the area at risk for reperfused acute myocardial infarction with T2-weighted cardiac magnetic resonance imaging: Histopathological and displacement encoding with stimulated echoes (DENSE) functional validations. Circulation. 2006;**113**(15):1865-1870

[19] Welch TD, Ling LH, Espinosa RE, et al. Echocardiographic diagnosis of constrictive pericarditis: Mayo Clinic criteria. Circulation. Cardiovascular Imaging. 2014;**7**:526-534

[20] Kusunose K, Dahiya A, Popovic ZB, et al. Biventricular mechanics in constrictive pericarditis comparison with restrictive cardiomyopathy and impact of pericardiectomy. Circulation. Cardiovascular Imaging. 2013;**6**:399-406

[21] Sengupta PP, Khandheria BK, Korinek J, et al. Apex-to-base dispersion in regional timing of left ventricular shortening and lengthening. Journal of the American College of Cardiology. 2006;**47**:163-172

[22] Taylor AM, Dymarkowski S, Verbeken EK, Bogaert J. Detection of pericardial inflammation with late-enhancement cardiac magnetic resonance imaging: Initial results. European Radiology. 2006;**16**(3):569-574

[23] Hoey ETD, Shahid M, Watkin RW. Computed tomography and magnetic resonance imaging evaluation of pericardial disease. Quantitative Imaging in Medicine and Surgery. 2016;**6**(3):274-284

[24] Schneider S, Batrice A, Rischpler C, Eiber M, Ibrahim T, Nekolla SG. Utility of multimodal cardiac imaging with PET/MRI in cardiac sarcoidosis: Implications for diagnosis, monitoring and treatment. European Heart Journal. 2014;**35**(5):312

[25] von Olshausen G, Hyafil F, Langwieser N, Laugwitz KL, Schwaiger M, Ibrahim T. Detection of acute inflammatory myocarditis in Epstein Barr virus infection using hybrid 18F-fluoro-deoxyglucose-positron emission tomography/magnetic resonance imaging. Circulation. 2014;**130**(11):925-926

[26] Lamacie MM, Almufleh A, Nair V, Stadnick E, Birnie D, Beanlands RSB, et al. Serial 18F-Fluorodeoxyglucose positron emission tomography imaging in a patient with Giant cell myocarditis. Circulation. Cardiovascular Imaging. 2020;**13**(2):e009940

[27] Mathijssen H, Tjoeng TWH, Keijsers RGM, Bakker ALM, Akdim F, van Es HW, et al. The usefulness of

repeated CMR and FDG PET/CT in the diagnosis of patients with initial possible cardiac sarcoidosis. EJNMMI Research. 2021;**11**:129

[28] Castiglione V, Aimo A, Todiere G, Barison A, Fabiani I, Panichella G, et al. Role of imaging in cardiomyopathies. Cardiac Failure Review. 2023;**9**:e08

[29] Kim MS, Kim EK, Choi JY, Oh JK, Chang SA. Clinical utility of [18F]FDG-PET/CT in pericardial disease. Current Cardiology Reports. 2019;**21**(9):107

[30] Xu B, Huang SSL, Jellis C, Flamm SD. Diagnosis of active pericarditis by positron emission tomography (PET)/cardiac magnetic resonance (CMR) imaging. European Heart Journal. 2018;**39**(2):179

[31] Hyeon CW, Yi HK, Kim EK, Park SJ, Lee SC, Park SW, et al. The role of 18F-fluorodeoxyglucose-positron emission tomography/computed tomography in the differential diagnosis of pericardial disease. Scientific Reports. 2020;**10**:21524

[32] Klein AL, Abbara S, Agler DA, Appleton CP, Asher CR, Hoit B, et al. American Society of Echocardiography clinical recommendations for multimodality cardiovascular imaging of patients with pericardial disease: Endorsed by the Society for Cardiovascular Magnetic Resonance and Society of cardiovascular computed tomography. Journal of the American Society of Echocardiography. 2013;**26**(9):965-1012.e15

[33] Soler-Soler J, Sagristà-Sauleda J, Permanyer-Miralda G. Relapsing pericarditis. Heart. 2004;**90**(11):1364-1368

[34] Adler Y, Charron P, Imazio M, et al. ESC Scientific Document Group. 2015 ESC Guidelines for the diagnosis and management of pericardial diseases: The Task Force for the Diagnosis and Management of Pericardial Diseases of the European Society of Cardiology (ESC)Endorsed by: The European Association for Cardio-Thoracic Surgery (EACTS). European Heart Journal. 7 Nov 2015;**36**(42):2921-2964. DOI: 10.1093/eurheartj/ehv318. Epub 2015 Aug 29

[35] McNamara N, Ibrahim A, Satti Z, Ibrahim M, Kiernan TJ. Acute pericarditis: A review of current diagnostic and management guidelines. Future Cardiology. Mar 2019;**15**(2):119-126. DOI: 10.2217/fca-2017-0102. Epub 2019 Mar 8

[36] Imazio M, Brucato A, Barbieri A, et al. Good prognosis for pericarditis with and without myocardial involvement results from a multicenter. Prospective Cohort Study Circulation. 2013;**128**:42-49

[37] Imazio M, Gribaudo E, Gaita F. Recurrent pericarditis. Progress in Cardiovascular Diseases. 2017;**59**(4):360-368

[38] Ling LH, Oh JK, Schaff HV, et al. Constrictive pericarditis in the modern era: Evolving clinical spectrum and impact on outcome after pericardiectomy. Circulation. 1999;**100**:1380-1386

[39] Chiabrando J, Bonaventura A, Vecchié A, et al. Management of acute and recurrent pericarditis: JACC state-of-the-art review. Journal of the American College of Cardiology. 2020;**75**(1):76-92

[40] Cremer PC, Tariq MU, Karwa A, et al. Quantitative assessment of pericardial delayed hyper enhancement predicts clinical improvement in patients with constrictive pericarditis treated with anti-inflammatory therapy.

Circulation. Cardiovascular Imaging. 2015;**8**:e003125

[41] Chang SA, Choi JY, Kim EK, et al. [(18)F]fluorodeoxyglucose PET/CT predicts response to steroid therapy in constrictive pericarditis. Journal of the American College of Cardiology. 2017;**69**:750-752

[42] Hoit BD, Shaw D. The paradoxical pulse in tamponade: Mechanisms and echocardiographic correlates. Echocardiography. 1994;**11**:477-487

[43] Imazio M, Bobbio M, Cecchi E, et al. Colchicine as first-choice therapy for recurrent pericarditis: Results of the CORE (COlchicine for REcurrent pericarditis) trial. Archives of Internal Medicine. 2005;**165**:1987-1991

[44] Cooper Jr. L.T. Treatment and Prognosis of Myocarditis in Adults. In: UpToDate. Mckenna WJ, editor. Wolter Kluwer. Waltham, USA; 2022

[45] Imazio M, Brucato A, Spodick DH, Adler Y. Prognosis of myopericarditis as determined from previously published reports. Journal of Cardiovascular Medicine (Hagerstown Md). 2014;**15**(12):835-839

[46] Manda YR, Baradhi KM. Myopericarditis. In: StatPearls [Internet]. Treasure Island (FL): StatPearls Publishing; 2024. Available from: http://www.ncbi.nlm.nih.gov/books/NBK534776/ [Accessed: May 27, 2024]

Chapter 6

Advanced Imaging in Myocarditis and Pericarditis

Sarah Keller, Jan Herzberg, Ernest Tsiaze, Gerrit Hellige and Nisha Arenja

Abstract

The aim of this review is to provide an overview of multimodality imaging in myocarditis (MC) and pericarditis (PC), which refer to the clinical and histological manifestation of a broad spectrum of pathological immune processes in the cardiomyocytes and pericardium. This review highlights and summarizes the diagnostic tools and their prognostic value. In general, the clinical presentation and the echocardiography are the first diagnostic steps in patients with suspected PC and MC. In cases of equivocal myocardial disease, various imaging modalities are available. Cardiac magnetic resonance imaging (CMR) is critical in the diagnosis of myocarditis, whereas cardiac computed tomography (cCT) is of secondary importance. Positron emission tomography (PET) and PET/CT are useful to detect underlying myocardial inflammatory activity. The data suggest that simultaneous cardiac PET/MR may have complementary and incremental value in the assessment of MC compared to PET/CT or CMR alone. Established guidelines and innovative recent publications are reviewed to further improve the diagnosis of PC and MC in the light of current treatment options.

Keywords: myocarditis, pericarditis, advanced imaging, echocardiography, cardiac magnetic resonance imaging, computed tomography, positron emission tomography

1. Introduction

Pericarditis (PC) is the most common pericardial syndrome, accounting for approximately 0.2% of all hospital admissions for cardiovascular causes and 5% of emergency department visits for chest pain [1–6]. Myocarditis (MC) has an overall incidence of 4–14 people per 100,000 each year and is associated with a mortality rate of approximately 1–7% [7, 8].

MC and PC are based on the clinical manifestation of a wide spectrum of pathological immune processes in the myocytes and the pericardium. The molecular and cellular pathophysiology may differ between the different aetiologies, but the consecutive cellular infiltration and necrosis results in structural and functional abnormalities such as oedema, fibrotic scarring leading to regional contractile impairment, ventricular stiffening, or conduction system disease [9, 10].

Both entities can be classified according to their cause, histology, clinicopathological (acute, subacute, chronic, recurrent) and clinical criteria [9]. The etiology of either MC or PC is multifactorial, depending on the epidemiological background, patient population and clinical setting [3, 11]. The causes can be broadly categorized as idiopathic, infectious (viral, bacterial, e.g. *Mycobacterium tuberculosis* is the most common cause in developing countries and often coexisting with HIV infection, fungal, parasitic) and non-infectious (autoimmune, neoplastic, which is often secondary due to leukemia, breast cancer, lung cancer, lymphoma and melanoma), metabolic, cardiovascular (e.g. Dressler's syndrome) and drug-related (e.g. isoniazid, doxorubicin, clozapine, ICI (immune checkpoints inhibitors)) [5, 7, 9, 10, 12–16].

Acute forms of MC and PC often present with non-specific symptoms of chest pain, dyspnoea, palpitations, presyncope or syncope, new-onset heart failure due to systolic or diastolic dysfunction, atrial or ventricular arrhythmias. However, in some cases acute viral MC causes cardiac damage without symptoms, thereby increases the risk of chronic inflammatory dilated cardiomyopathy (DCM) [7, 9].

In patients with clinical suspicion of MC or PC, the diagnosis should start with the analysis of serum biomarkers (cardiac troponin T (cTnT) or I (cTnI) and creatine kinase (CK)-MB). Non-specific serum markers of inflammation such as C-reactive protein (CRP) and white blood cell count (WBC) are often elevated in patients with MC or PC, but low specificity limits their diagnostic value [5, 9]. Most patients with MC have non-specific ECG findings, such as sinus tachycardia, ST- and T-wave abnormalities, atrioventricular or bundle branch block [9, 17, 18].

For the definitive diagnosis of MC and PC different imaging techniques are used. The aim of this review is to summarize recent developments in the available imaging modalities, highlight their advantages and drawbacks, make a statement about their diagnostic and prognostic value of MC and PC, and provide an insight into the recent work of various investigators.

2. Echocardiography

Transthoracic echocardiography (TTE) remains an indispensable and predominantly utilized initial diagnostic modality in patients with suspected PC and MC [9, 16, 19, 20]. Moreover, TTE is particularly efficacious in excluding differential diagnoses such as myocardial infarction, aortic dissection, and valvular heart disease [8, 9, 20]. The morphological and functional abnormalities observable in patients with PC and/or MC, along with advances in imaging techniques, are described here [8, 9, 20].

Regarding the diagnosis of PC, TTE offers critical insights into the presence and extent of pericardial effusion, including its volume and potential hemodynamic impacts such as cardiac tamponade and constrictive physiology. Additionally, TTE can detect pericardial thickening and increased echogenicity of the pericardial layers. Pericardial effusion is quantitatively classified as mild (<10 mm), moderate (10–20 mm), or large (>20 mm) based on its diastolic measurement [5, 21]. **Figure 1** illustrates a septated and partially fibrinous pericardial effusion in a patient suffering from constrictive pericarditis.

The echocardiographic characteristics of acute MC are generally non-specific and primarily involve left ventricular (LV) dysfunction attributable to focal or global inflammation with cellular necrosis and tissue oedema. This can result in a reduced LV ejection fraction (LVEF), LV wall thickness and/or regional dysfunction

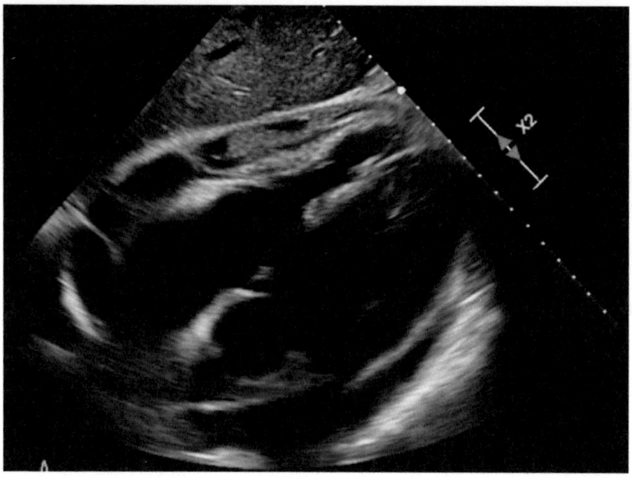

Figure 1.
A septated and partially fibrinous pericardial effusion in a patient suffering from constrictive pericarditis.

characterized by LV wall motion abnormalities. These abnormalities, which are not confined to a coronary artery distribution, serve as useful confirmatory and prognostic indicators. The regional wall motion abnormalities typically present as mild segmental hypokinesia, particularly affecting the inferior or inferolateral walls, though severe cases may exhibit extensive diffuse hypokinesia [7, 8, 20, 22–27].

LVEF remains preserved in approximately 75% of patients with MC; however, comprehensive assessment of both LV and right ventricular (RV) function is critical, as more severe ventricular dysfunction correlates with an increased risk of mortality or the need for heart transplantation [1, 7, 9, 11, 16, 19, 26, 28]. The LV typically appears normal or only mildly dilated in patients experiencing acute heart failure (AHF). Myocardial oedema may lead to increased ventricular wall thickness and abnormal (often granular) echogenicity, a phenomenon particularly common in fulminant MC [7, 27]. Furthermore, significant acute active MC may present with increased ventricular sphericity due to oedema [7, 9, 28]. It is important to note that a normal echocardiogram does not rule out the diagnosis of PC or MC [26].

Advanced imaging modalities such as strain and strain rate imaging via speckle tracking have emerged as valuable adjunctive echocardiographic parameters for assessing myocardial dysfunction. Research has demonstrated that reductions in LV fractional shortening, longitudinal strain, and strain rate are correlated with the histological degree of lymphocytic infiltration. Longitudinal and circumferential strain exhibit specificities for inflammation of 93 and 94%, respectively. LV global longitudinal strain (LV-GLS) has been shown to be the most effective measure for differentiating patients with MC from healthy controls, followed by LVEF and LV end-diastolic dimension (LVEDD). Numerous studies have indicated that impairment of LV-GLS is associated with adverse cardiovascular outcomes [7, 8, 20, 22–27]. Furthermore, TTE is a pivotal imaging modality for the precise identification of complications such as LV thrombus, and transient LV aneurysm [7, 22]. Tissue Doppler and colour M-mode echocardiography are valuable tools for distinguishing constrictive PC from restrictive cardiomyopathy [22].

The advantages of TTE include its widespread accessibility, affordability, and capability for urgent assessment. However, the limitations, as well as the inter- and intraobserver variability of TTE encompass its reliance on operator expertise and the quality of ultrasound equipment, occasional challenges associated with poor acoustic windows due to factors like obesity or pulmonary diseases (e.g., COPD), and limited tissue characterization [5, 29–31]. Recognizing these drawbacks, several alternative imaging modalities are used to aid in the diagnostic evaluation of patients with PC and MC.

Transesophageal echocardiography (TEE) is not routinely employed as a diagnostic tool for MC and PC.

3. Cardiovascular magnetic resonance

Cardiovascular magnetic resonance imaging (CMR) has emerged as the foremost modality for non-invasive imaging of MC due to its independence from acoustic window limitations with high reproducibility as well as its facilitation of optimal plane acquisitions, while also obviating radiation exposure [26, 32–34]. Nonetheless, the timing of CMR scans is critical; they should neither be too early (within 48 hours) nor too late after symptom onset to preserve sensitivity. Ideally, CMR should be conducted within 2–4 weeks of symptom onset and can serve as a valuable tool for monitoring disease progression and activity [8, 26, 27].

CMR not only aids in diagnosing myocarditis but also provides important prognostic information, helping to predict patient outcomes based on the extent of tissue damage [35].

Recent advancements in CMR hardware, software, and protocols have significantly improved the accurate visualization of tissue changes in patients with acute myocardial diseases. Consequently, CMR possesses unique features that make it the preferred imaging modality for in vivo tissue characterization in conditions such as myocarditis. The pathological cascade of MC, irrespective of its aetiology, entails the infiltration of immune cells into the myocardium, precipitating myocardial oedema, hyperaemia, necrosis, and eventual scar formation. All of these processes can be visualized by CMR [20, 32], which employs a protocol designed to evaluate both global and regional cardiac function and to identify primary imaging markers of inflammation, including oedema, hyperaemia, and necrosis. Additional indicators such as pericardial effusion, LV systolic function, or transient increase in wall thickness can further booster the diagnosis of active MC; as a result, CMR provides a comprehensive “all-in-one” imaging examination [5, 8, 23, 32, 36].

Cine short-axis images utilizing steady-state free precession (SSFP) have evolved into the reference standard for evaluating and quantifying cardiac volumes, myocardial mass, and ventricular function [8, 32, 37]. **Figure 2** illustrates cine-segmented short and long axis image in a patient with a constrictive pericarditis. T2-weighted sequences exhibit high sensitivity to oedema, stemming from inflammatory cell injury and the consequent augmented permeability of cellular membranes. The T2-weighted short tau triple inversion recovery (STIR) sequences have been validated for identifying epicardial, transmural, and global myocardial oedema, demonstrating a sensitivity of 84% and specificity of 74% [20, 32, 37]. The onset of myocardial inflammation prompts the release of inflammatory mediators, inducing regional dilation of the coronary microvasculature. This heightened blood flow to the affected segments results in augmented regional uptake of gadolinium contrast. Hyperaemia and the ensuing global relative enhancement of the myocardium are quantified by putting the myocardial signal into relation to that of skeletal muscle in both pre-contrast and post-contrast T1-weighted images [32].

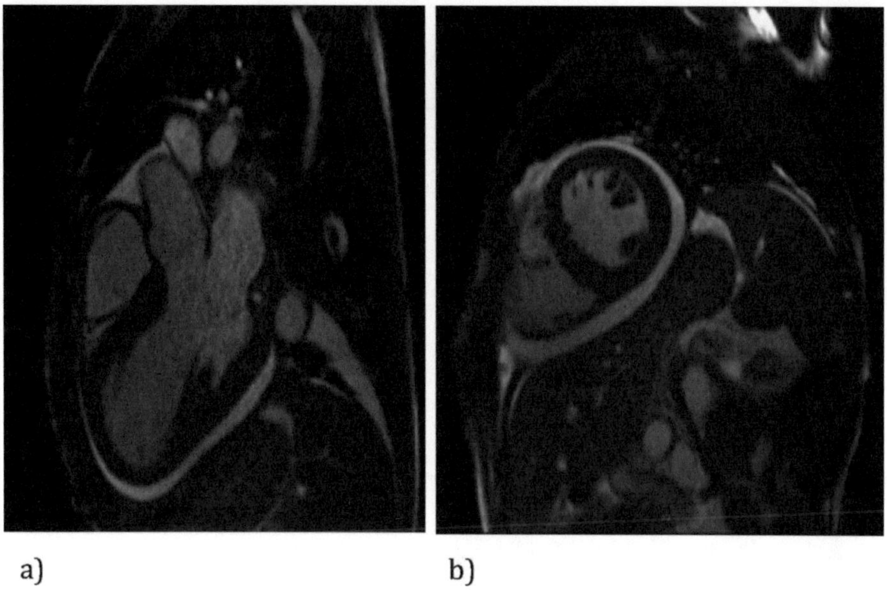

Figure 2.
Cine-segmented long (a) and short (b) axis image in a patient with constrictive pericarditis.

The Lake Louise Criteria (LLC) for CMR in diagnosing MC includes the presence of increased regional or global myocardial signal intensity on T2-weighted images, increased global myocardial early gadolinium enhancement (EGE) and at least one focal lesion with nonischaemic distribution in late gadolinium enhanced (LGE) T1 weighted images [3]. The LLC demonstrates an overall diagnostic accuracy of 78%, with a sensitivity ranging from 67–81% and a specificity ranging from 71–91% for acute MC. However, its diagnostic accuracy is not as reliable for chronic MC [10, 20, 26, 32, 33, 35]. A diagnosis of MC can be established when two out of the three primary inflammatory markers (see above) are present [20, 26, 32, 33] Bami et al. indicated that the inclusion of pericardial effusion in the diagnostic criteria did not significantly enhance diagnostic accuracy [20]. **Figure 3** illustrates CMR images showing typical inferolateral late gadolinium enhancement distribution in a patient with myocarditis.

A newer technique is the T1 and T2 mapping, which are parametric imaging tools that quantify tissue-specific magnetization characteristics for robust tissue characterization. Multiple images at fixed points in the cardiac cycle generate a relaxation curve for T1 or T2 [20, 26, 32]. T1 mapping provides information about longitudinal relaxation, for example, using a modified Look-Locker inversion recovery (MOLLI) sequence. Post-contrast T1 maps after gadolinium application can provide extracellular volume fraction maps [26, 32]. T1 mapping effectively assesses myocardial oedema and hyperaemia based on the hypothesis that T1 prolongation occurs due to increased water content. T1 values >990 ms indicate myocardial injury. As a result, T1 mapping is subsequently used to create a topographic map that allows visualization of the extent of myocardial involvement [20]. T2 mapping quantifies myocardial oedema and inflammation by providing information on transverse relaxation. T2 maps are generated using different echo times [26, 32]. In MC, T2 mapping identifies more extensive involvement than LGE, cine imaging, and T2-weighted short tau inversion recovery (STIR). Native T2 mapping has a higher diagnostic accuracy than

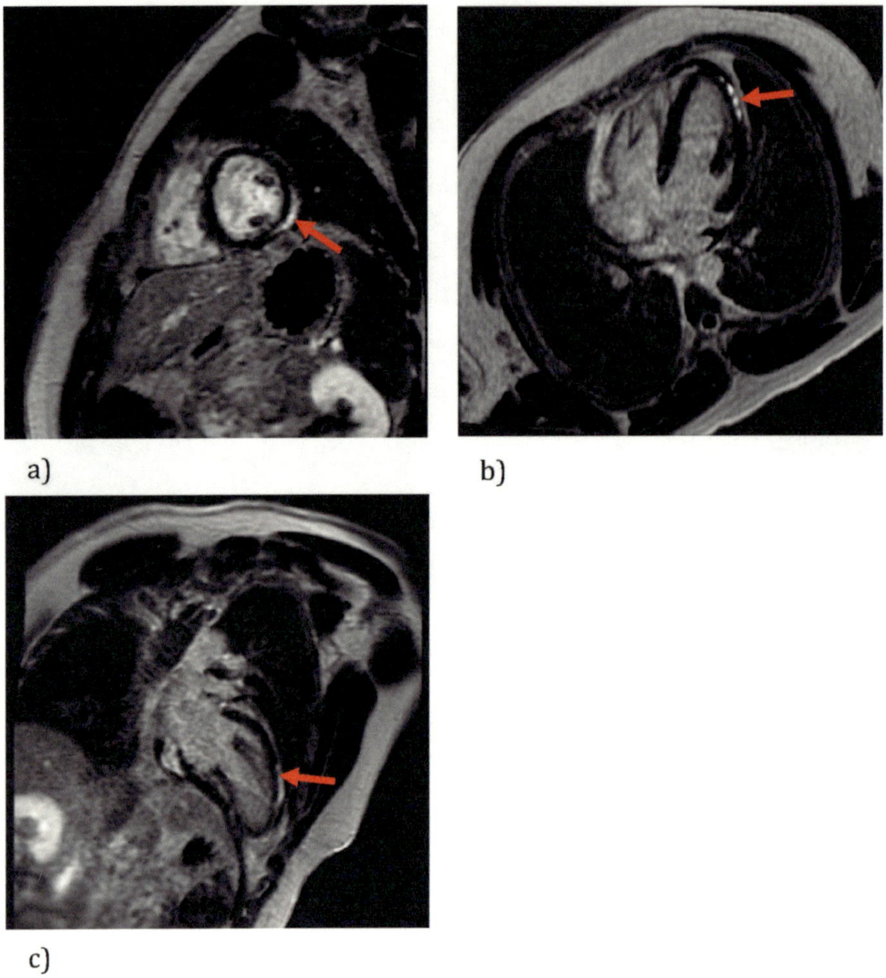

Figure 3.
CMR images showing typical inferolateral late gadolinium enhancement distribution (arrow) in a patient with myocarditis. (a) A short-axis view, (b) a four-chamber view, and (c) a two-chamber view.

the LLC for chronic myocarditis [32]. T1 and T2 mapping outperform the LLC in diagnosing myocardial inflammation, enhancing MRI's capability. T1 mapping alone has a diagnostic accuracy of 91%, which improves to 95% with T2-weighted imaging or LGE, achieving 92% sensitivity and 97% specificity [20, 32]. **Figure 4** illustrates CMR images in T1 mapping pre- (a) and post (b)-contrast agents administration in a patient with myocarditis.

The sensitivity and specificity of CMR for diagnosing acute MC vary depending on the sequences utilized. A combination of T2-weighted CMR and post-gadolinium early and late T1-weighted CMR yields the highest sensitivity (67%) and specificity (91%) for diagnosis. However, T1-weighted imaging after gadolinium contrast administration may not effectively differentiate acute MC from chronic scarring [8, 9, 38]. **Table 1** illustrates the sensitivity, specificity, and diagnostic accuracy of various combinations of CMR tissue criteria for MC diagnosis (T2-weighted imaging, EGE and LGE). This data is extracted from the Lancet Journal 2012 article "Myocarditis" authored by Sandeep et al. [8, 9].

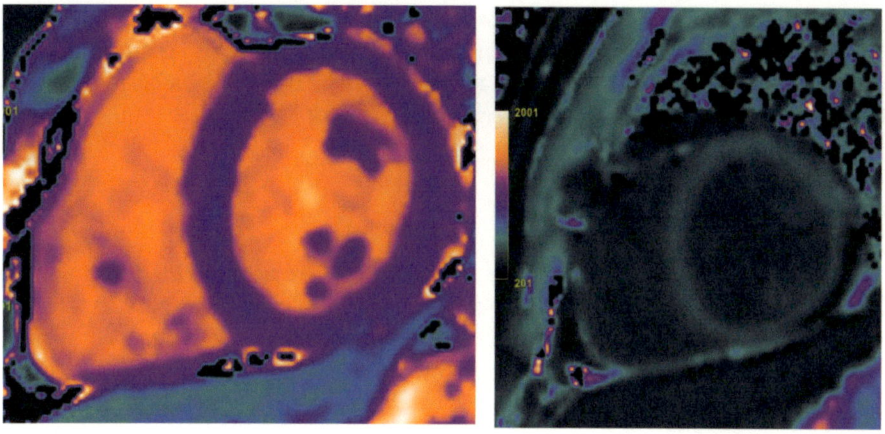

a) b)

Figure 4.
CMR images in T1 mapping pre- (a) and post (b)-contrast agents administration in a patient with myocarditis.

	Sensitivity (%)	Specificity (%)	Accuracy (%)	Positive predictive value (%)
T2-weighted MRI (T2) and LGE	25	95	56	86
T2, LGE or both	60	66	62	79
Any 1 of 3	88	48	70	68
Any 2 of 3	67	91	78	91
LGE = Late Gadolinium Enhancement.				

Table 1.
Diagnostic performance of various combinations of CMR tissue criteria (T2-weighted imaging, T1-weighted imaging, LGE) for the diagnosis of myocarditis.

A comprehensive CMR protocol for pericardial disease typically includes cine imaging, black-blood T1-weighted imaging of the heart and pericardium, myocardial tagging, phase-contrast sequences, and delayed enhancement imaging to assess late gadolinium enhancement (LGE) [5, 23]. Similar to CT imaging, in CMR, the pericardium appears on T1-weighted images as a thin hypodense (dark) curvilinear structure, surrounded by hyperintense (bright) mediastinal and epicardial fat. Normal pericardial thickness typically ranges from 0.7 to 2 mm [37]. CMR can accurately differentiate between mixed myopericardial diseases, such as mixed inflammatory forms (e.g. myopericarditis or perimyocarditis), and pericardial injury following myocardial infarction. Compared with CT, CMR offers the advantage of providing information regarding the hemodynamic consequences of a non-compliant pericardium on cardiac filling and the potential to visualize fibrotic fusion of pericardial layers [37].

The limitations of CMR include its restricted sensitivity, especially in instances of equivocal or borderline MC. Additionally, CMR struggles to ascertain the underlying cause and composition of MC accurately, the lack of widely used standardized scanner protocols, limited availability of CMR-capable MRI systems and shortage of experienced CMR imagers [20, 36]. While advancements in T1 and T2 mapping have aimed to mitigate some of these challenges, they have not entirely surmounted the limitations inherent to CMR [20]. Limiting patient characteristics related to the performance of CMR include implanted pacemakers [5, 29], claustrophobia or severe renal failure, which makes contrast administration difficult. It also requires good cooperation from the patient, as they have to hold their breath, which can be difficult if they are in pain or have a relevant pericardial effusion.

4. Computer tomography

Well-founded studies regarding the utilization of cardiac computed tomography (cCT) in the context of MC and PC are scarce. However, cCT holds potential for detecting pericardial calcifications and thickening, alongside evaluating comorbidities [5, 37]. In particular, acute coronary syndrome (ACS) stands as a primary differential diagnosis requiring exclusion, especially in patients presenting with chest pain and ST changes or segmental wall motion abnormalities, particularly those with increased cardiovascular risk factors [24].

The healthy pericardium typically acts as a barrier to inflammation and infection from adjacent mediatinal structures and limits the friction from cardiac motion within the mediastinum. On CT, it appears as a thin, dense line of > or = 2 mm thickness and is best visualized in the systole over the right ventricle. Intravenous administration of iodinated contrast is recommended to enhance blood density and visualize pericardial inflammation [37]. **Figure 5** illustrates a cCT image showing the compression of the left ventricle in a patient with constrictive pericarditis. **Figure 6** shows a cCT image illustrating the calcification of the pericardium in a patient with constrictive pericarditis.

Regarding MC, limited studies have indicated delayed myocardial enhancement (DME) with iodinated contrast or regions of low attenuation on cCT correlating with late gadolinium enhancement (LGE) areas observed on CMR imaging. Hence, non-localized delayed enhancement affecting the epicardial layer of the LV wall could serve as a cCT criterion for diagnosing MC [20, 39, 40]. Moreover, spectral/dual-energy CT – which utilizes different X-ray energy levels to acquire data, allowing differentiation of materials based on their energy-dependent attenuation characteristics – has demonstrated promising accuracy in evaluating inflamed myocardium in acute MC patients exhibiting typical subepicardial DME [26, 41].

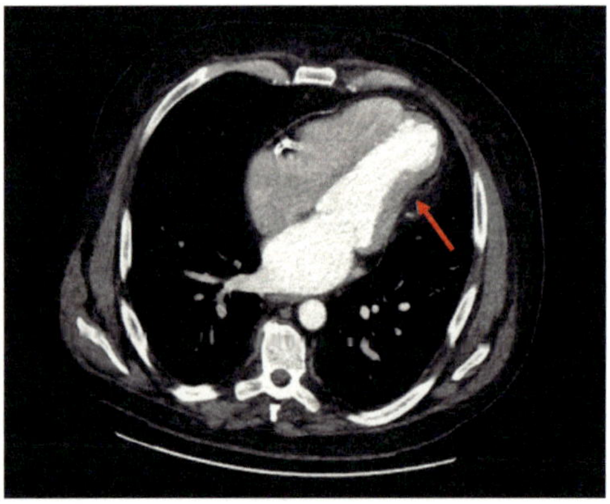

Figure 5.
A cCT image showing the compression of the left ventricle in a patient with constrictive pericarditis.

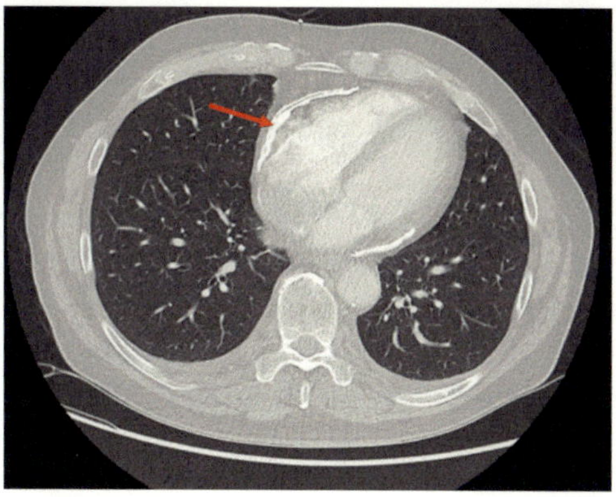

Figure 6.
A cCT image illustrating the calcification of the pericardium in a patient with constrictive pericarditis.

However, owing to inherent limitations of cCT, such as ionizing radiation exposure and the inability to assess unstable patients or those with arrhythmias, echocardiography and CMR are preferred modalities for evaluating pericardial and myocardial diseases in clinical practice [24, 29, 37].

5. Nuclear imaging

5.1 Positron emission tomography

Positron Emission Tomography (PET) employs 18F-fluorodeoxyglucose (18F-FDG), a fluorine-18-labelled glucose analogue, which accumulates in cells in proportion to their metabolic activity. Consequently, 18F-FDG PET serves as a reflection of metabolically active processes, including myocardial inflammation [20, 26]. A crucial prerequisite for optimal PET interpretation is meticulous patient preparation. Prior to 18F-FDG PET, patients are advised to adhere to a high-fat, low-carbohydrate diet followed by an extended fasting period (at least >12 hours) to suppress physiological myocardial glucose uptake. Under normal conditions, myocytes predominantly utilize fatty acids as their energy source; however, they can also metabolize glucose, leading to FDG uptake on PET, PET-CT, or PET-MR. The prescribed diet effectively mitigates physiological myocardial FDG uptake [24, 26, 32].

18F-FDG PET plays a pivotal role in detecting MC, particularly in the context of systemic autoimmune diseases such as cardiac sarcoidosis [26]. In cardiac sarcoidosis, focal or multifocal 18F-FDG uptake, distinct from normal myocardial uptake, is typically observed, often in conjunction with involvement of other affected organs such as the lungs and lymph nodes [24, 26]. Another field of application is for example pericardial 18F-FDG tracer uptake in patients with solid cancers and lymphoma, implying malignant pericardial involvement [37].

The integration of 18F-FDG PET with computed tomography (PET/CT) or magnetic resonance tomography (PET/MR) confers additional advantages. PET/CT or PET/MR amalgamates metabolic and functional information from PET with CT or the high soft tissue contrast and multi-parametric capabilities of MR imaging, facilitating a comprehensive evaluation of myocardial and pericardial inflammation. This synergistic combination enables simultaneous assessment of myocardial metabolism, perfusion, and tissue characterization, thereby augmenting diagnostic precision and therapeutic monitoring [32, 42–46].

5.2 PET/CT

In the realm of MC diagnosis, the utility of 18F-FDG PET/CT remains largely reliant on case-based observations due to the absence of prospective randomized trials or meticulously designed retrospective studies. Despite this limitation, available evidence suggests that 18F-FDG PET/CT exhibits promising capabilities in detecting and localizing active inflammation indicative of MC. The regional distribution of 18F-FDG uptake, characterized by patterns such as focal, diffuse, or focal-on-diffuse, along with the intensity of tracer uptake, can furnish valuable insights into the underlying pathophysiology of the disease. Notably, certain aetiologies, such as tuberculous pericarditis, may manifest with heightened FDG uptake compared to idiopathic forms, thereby aiding in differential diagnosis [32, 37]. Moreover, PET-CT holds potential as a tool for monitoring treatment response in MC cases [32].

5.3 PET/MR

18F-FDG PET/MR has emerged as a promising imaging modality for assessing MC and PC, offering distinct advantages over conventional techniques. Recent evidence suggests that simultaneous cardiac PET/MR provides complementary and incremental benefits compared to PET/CT or CMR alone. This integrated approach enhances the detection and characterization of myocardial inflammation and pericardial involvement [32].

18F-FDG PET performed on a hybrid 18F-FDG PET/MR platform holds promise for more effectively detecting MC (oedema, fibrosis, regional wall motion abnormalities) than 18F-FDG PET/CT. Clinical studies have shown that increased myocardial FDG uptake correlates well with CMR findings, enhancing sensitivity for mild or borderline myocarditis and enhancing specificity for chronic cases. Moreover, 18F-FDG PET complements CMR by providing metabolic information, which is particularly valuable in cases of diffuse myocardial damage undetectable by late gadolinium enhancement (LGE) in CMR [32].

For pericarditis assessment, 18F-FDG PET/MR offers superior soft tissue contrast, accurately evaluating disease extent and complications like constrictive PC [42–46].

Another advantage of PET/MR is its potential for reducing radiation exposure compared to PET/CT, making it particularly beneficial for radiation-sensitive populations like paediatric, pregnant patients and young patients with a higher incidence of myocarditis. However, PET/MR has a smaller inner bore, and limitations in patients with metal implants should be considered [32].

6. Coronary angiography and endomyocardial biopsy

Coronary angiography is not routinely used. Depending on the clinical context, coronary angiography may be used to exclude differential diagnoses, such as in patients with a high cardiovascular risk profile and ischaemic ECG changes, similar to CT. In addition, differentiation between constrictive pericarditis and restrictive cardiomyopathy is sometimes difficult and may require invasive testing [37].

DOI: http://dx.doi.org/10.5772/intechopen.1007301

Typical findings	Pericarditis	Myocarditis
Echocardiography	• Pericardial effusion (+/− pleural fluid, ascites) • Thickened and hyperreflective pericardial layers • +/− Intrapericardial fibrinous strands • Diastolic collapse of right atrium and right ventricle (in tamponade) • Respiratory variation in transvalvular flow velocities (in constrictive pericarditis; >25% fall in mitral inflow velocity, >40% increase in tricuspid velocity in the first beat after inspiration; opposite changes during expiration; normal or increased propagation velocity of early diastolic transmitral flow at color M-mode; decreased expiratory diastolic hepatic vein velocities with large reversals; normal or increased mitral annular velocity (>7 cm/sec) at tissue Doppler; annulus reversus (e' septal > e'lateral) • Inspiratory ventricular septal motion toward left ventricle (septal bounce; in constrictive pericarditis) • Marked dilation and absent or diminished collapse of the V. cava inferior and hepatic veins (in constrictive pericarditis) • Premature opening of the pulmonary valve (in constrictive pericarditis)	• Normal-sized or mildly dilated left ventricle • Systolic and diastolic dysfunction • Increased cardiac wall thickness • Increased echogenicity of the myocardium (mostly granular) • Wall motion abnormalities (generally mild segmental hypokinesia; especially in the inferior/inferolateral walls; in severe forms diffuse hypokinesia) • Impaired global longitudinal strain (LV-GLS)
Cardiac magnetic resonance	• Thickened pericardial layers • Strong pericardial LGE following contrast administration • Pericardial effusion • Signs of constriction such as septal bounce and exaggerated interventricular dependence • Combination of sequences with different weighting yield information with regard to the nature of the effusion	• Enhancement of Late gadolinium enhancement (LGE) in a non-ischaemic pattern • Myocardial oedema (T2 weighted imaging; hyperintensity) • T1 and T2 mapping abnormalities • Left ventricular wall thickening • Pericardial effusion • Increased extracellular volume (ECV)

Typical findings	Pericarditis	Myocarditis
Computed tomography	• Thickened pericardial layers enhancing after contrast administration (constrictive pericarditis: abnormalities usually most pronounced at the base of the ventricles (RV > LV), atrioventricular grooves and atria) • Calcifications in chronic cases • Pericardial effusion and effusion characterization (attenuation values of pericardial fluid (HU); simple effusion: 0–20 HU; proteinaceous/haemorrhagic: > 20 HU; chylopericardium: negative HU values; pneumopericardium: air) • Pericardial masses • Contrast enhancement of the pericardium (inflammation)	• Coronary artery disease (Calcification) • Pericardial effusion • LV and RV dysfunction
Positron emission tomography	• Increased FDG uptake in the pericardium	• Increased FDG uptake in myocardium • Heterogeneous distribution of FDG uptake • Assessment of LV function • Detection of extracardiac inflammation
Positron emission tomography/computed tomography	• Combined findings of CT and PET: Pericardial thickening, effusion, and increased FDG uptake indicating active inflammation	• Increased myocardial FDG uptake • Detection of coronary artery disease and evaluation of its burden • Evaluation of extracardiac pathology
Positron emission tomography/magnetic resonance	• Combined findings of MRI and PET: Detailed pericardial anatomy with thickening, effusion, LGE, and increased FDG uptake indicating active inflammation	• Increased myocardial FDG uptake • Assessment of coronary artery disease • Evaluation of extracardiac pathology

Table 2.
Typical findings of pericarditis and myocarditis in different imaging modalities.

Endomyocardial biopsy (EMB) is a widely accepted method for diagnosing MC based on the 1987 Dallas criteria. It is employed to obtain histological or immunohistological evidence of inflammatory cell infiltration, with or without myocyte damage, and to use molecular techniques for identifying viral genomes [7, 9]. However, the risks and low sensitivity associated with EMB limit its current diagnostic utility in acute DCM, confining its use primarily to research purposes or to exclude giant cell myocarditis. In chronic DCM, EMB remains crucial for confirming the presence of viral genomes and guiding treatment for persistent viral infections [7–10]. Additionally, EMB is important in patients with immune checkpoint inhibitor-associated MC [8, 10].

7. Conclusion

In the diagnostic landscape of MC and PC, a multimodal imaging approach is essential for accurate diagnosis and effective patient management. TTE remains the primary imaging modality due to its accessibility and utility in initial assessment and exclusion of differential diagnoses despite its limited specificity. Complementary imaging modalities, including CMR, PET, PET/CT, PET/MR, and cCT, are frequently employed to enhance diagnostic accuracy [26, 37]. Coronary angiography and endomyocardial biopsy are rarely used. The selection of imaging modalities is contingent upon the clinical context and the patient's condition [37]. CMR has emerged as a crucial secondary imaging tool, providing high sensitivity and specificity, especially with advancements in mapping techniques and the adoption of the Lake Louise Criteria [20, 26]. Nuclear Imaging, including PET, PET/CT, and PET/MR, offers significant benefits in detecting inflammatory processes with enhanced diagnostic accuracy when used in conjunction with CMR or CT [26]. cCT, while secondary in the diagnostic hierarchy, is particularly valuable for identifying calcifications associated with PC [37]. **Table 2** summarizes the typical imaging findings in PC and MC.

These complementary imaging modalities collectively enhance diagnostic accuracy, guiding appropriate therapeutic strategies and follow-up for patients with MC and PC. The integration of these advanced imaging techniques into clinical practice is supported by robust guidelines and evidence, underscoring their pivotal role in the comprehensive evaluation of these conditions.

Author details

Sarah Keller[1], Jan Herzberg[1], Ernest Tsiaze[1], Gerrit Hellige[1] and Nisha Arenja[1,2]*

1 Kardiologie Solothurner Spitäler AG, Solothurn, Switzerland

2 Faculty of Medicine, University of Basel, Basel, Switzerland

*Address all correspondence to: nisha.arenja@spital.so.ch

References

[1] Heidecker B, Kittleson MM, Kasper EK, Wittstein IS, Champion HC, Russell SD, et al. Transcriptomic biomarkers for the accurate diagnosis of myocarditis. Circulation. 2011;**123**(11):1174-1184

[2] Imazio M. Contemporary management of pericardial diseases. Current Opinion in Cardiology. 2012;**27**(3):308-317

[3] LeWinter MM. Clinical practice. Acute pericarditis. New England Journal of Medicine. 2014;**371**(25):2410-2416

[4] Imazio M, Gaita F. Diagnosis and treatment of pericarditis. Heart. 2015;**101**(14):1159-1168

[5] Xanthopoulos A, Skoularigis J. Diagnosis of acute pericarditis. ESC Guidelines. 6 Sep 2017;**15**(15-16)

[6] Klein AL, Abbara S, Agler DA, Appleton CP, Asher CR, Hoit B, et al. American Society of Echocardiography clinical recommendations for multimodality cardiovascular imaging of patients with pericardial disease: Endorsed by the Society for Cardiovascular Magnetic Resonance and Society of Cardiovascular Computed Tomography. Journal of the American Society of Echocardiography. 2013;**26**(9):965-1012.e15

[7] Skouri HN, Dec GW, Friedrich MG, Cooper LT. Noninvasive imaging in myocarditis. Journal of the American College of Cardiology. 2006;**48**(10):2085-2093

[8] Ammirati E, Moslehi JJ. Diagnosis and treatment of acute myocarditis: A review. Journal of the American Medical Association. 2023;**329**(13):1098-1113

[9] Sagar S, Liu PP, Cooper LT. Myocarditis. The Lancet. 25-February-2 March 2012;**379**(9817):738-747

[10] Lombardi M. Cardiovascular MR to diagnose myocarditis. ESC Council for Cardiology Practice. 2009;**8**

[11] Kühl U, Pauschinger M, Seeberg B, Lassner D, Noutsias M, Poller W, et al. Viral persistence in the myocardium is associated with progressive cardiac dysfunction. Circulation. 2005;**112**(13):1965-1970

[12] Mavrouli MD, Spanakis N, Levidiotou S, Politi C, Alexiou S, Tseliou P, et al. Serologic prevalence of coxsackievirus group B in Greece. Viral Immunology. 2007;**20**(1):11-18

[13] Kühl U, Lassner D, Pauschinger M, Gross UM, Seeberg B, Noutsias M, et al. Prevalence of erythrovirus genotypes in the myocardium of patients with dilated cardiomyopathy. Journal of Medical Virology. 2008;**80**(7):1243-1251

[14] Markel G, Imazio M, Koren-Morag N, Galore-Haskel G, Schachter J, Besser M, et al. CEACAM1 and MICA as novel serum biomarkers in patients with acute and recurrent pericarditis. Oncotarget. 2016;**7**(14):17885-17895

[15] Imazio M, Brucato A, Maestroni S, Cumetti D, Dominelli A, Natale G, et al. Prevalence of C-reactive protein elevation and time course of normalization in acute pericarditis: Implications for the diagnosis, therapy, and prognosis of pericarditis. Circulation. 2011;**123**(10):1092-1097

[16] Pinamonti B, Alberti E, Cigalotto A, Dreas L, Salvi A, Silvestri F, et al. Echocardiographic findings in

myocarditis. The American Journal of Cardiology. 1988;**62**(4):285-291

[17] Nakashima H, Katayama T, Ishizaki M, Takeno M, Honda Y, Yano K. Q wave and non-Q wave myocarditis with special reference to clinical significance. Japanese Heart Journal. 1998;**39**(6):763-774

[18] Ukena C, Mahfoud F, Kindermann I, Kandolf R, Kindermann M, Böhm M. Prognostic electrocardiographic parameters in patients with suspected myocarditis. European Journal of Heart Failure. 2011;**13**(4):398-405

[19] Imazio M, Spodick DH, Brucato A, Trinchero R, Markel G, Adler Y. Diagnostic issues in the clinical management of pericarditis. International Journal of Clinical Practice. 2010;**64**(10):1384-1392

[20] Bami K, Haddad T, Dick A, Dennie C, Dwivedi G. Noninvasive imaging in acute myocarditis. Current Opinion in Cardiology. 2016;**31**(2):217-223

[21] Snyder MJ, Bepko J, White M. Acute pericarditis: diagnosis and management. American Family Physician. 2014;**89**(7):553-560

[22] Troughton RW, Asher CR, Klein AL. Pericarditis. Lancet. 2004;**363**(9410):717-727

[23] Khanna S, Li C, Amarasekera AT, Bhat A, Chen HHL, Gan GCH, et al. Echocardiographic parameters of cardiac structure and function in the diagnosis of acute myocarditis in adult patients: A systematic review and meta-analysis. Echocardiography. 2024;**41**(2):e15760

[24] Ammirati E, Frigerio M, Adler ED, Basso C, Birnie DH, Brambatti M, et al. Management of acute myocarditis and chronic inflammatory cardiomyopathy: An expert consensus document. Circulation. Heart Failure. 2020;**13**(11):e007405

[25] Ammirati E, Cipriani M, Moro C, Raineri C, Pini D, Sormani P, et al. Clinical presentation and outcome in a contemporary cohort of patients with acute myocarditis: Multicenter lombardy registry. Circulation. 2018;**138**(11):1088-1099

[26] Bière L, Piriou N, Ernande L, Rouzet F, Lairez O. Imaging of myocarditis and inflammatory cardiomyopathies. Archives of Cardiovascular Diseases. 2019;**112**(10):630-641

[27] Lampejo T, Durkin SM, Bhatt N, Guttmann O. Acute myocarditis: Aetiology, diagnosis and management. Clinical Medicine (London, England). 2021;**21**(5):e505-e510

[28] Mendes LA, Dec GW, Picard MH, Palacios IF, Newell J, Davidoff R. Right ventricular dysfunction: An independent predictor of adverse outcome in patients with myocarditis. American Heart Journal. 1994;**128**(2):301-307

[29] Imazio M, Brucato A, Barbieri A, Ferroni F, Maestroni S, Ligabue G, et al. Good prognosis for pericarditis with and without myocardial involvement: Results from a multicenter, prospective cohort study. Circulation. 2013;**128**(1):42-49

[30] Bhardwaj R, Berzingi C, Miller C, Hobbs G, Gharib W, Beto RJ, et al. Differential diagnosis of acute pericarditis from normal variant early repolarization and left ventricular hypertrophy with early repolarization: An electrocardiographic study. The American Journal of the Medical Sciences. 2013;**345**(1):28-32

[31] Imazio M, Spodick DH, Brucato A, Trinchero R, Adler Y. Controversial issues in the management of pericardial diseases. Circulation. 2010;**121**(7):916-928

[32] Chen W, Jeudy J. Assessment of myocarditis: Cardiac MR, PET/CT, or PET/MR? Current Cardiology Reports. 2019;**21**(8):76

[33] Childs H, Friedrich MG. Cardiovascular magnetic resonance imaging in myocarditis. Progress in Cardiovascular Diseases. 2011;**54**(3):266-275

[34] American College of Cardiology Foundation Task Force on Expert Consensus Documents, Hundley WG, Bluemke DA, Finn JP, Flamm SD, Fogel MA, et al. ACCF/ACR/AHA/NASCI/SCMR 2010 expert consensus document on cardiovascular magnetic resonance: A report of the American College of Cardiology Foundation Task Force on Expert Consensus Documents. Circulation. 2010;**121**(22):2462-2508

[35] Friedrich MG, Sechtem U, Schulz-Menger J, Holmvang G, Alakija P, Cooper LT, et al. Cardiovascular magnetic resonance in myocarditis: A JACC white paper. Journal of the American College of Cardiology. 2009;**53**(17):1475-1487

[36] Friedrich MG, Calgary F. Tissue Characterization of Acute Myocardial Infarction and Myocarditis by Cardiac Magnetic Resonance. JACC Cardiovasc Imaging; Sep 2008;**1**(5):652-662

[37] Adler Y, Charron P, Imazio M, Badano L, Barón-Esquivias G, Bogaert J, et al. 2015 ESC guidelines for the diagnosis and management of pericardial disease. European Heart Journal. 2015;**36**:2940. DOI: 10.1093/euheartj/ehv318

[38] Mahrholdt H, Wagner A, Deluigi CC, Kispert E, Hager S, Meinhardt G, et al. Presentation, patterns of myocardial damage, and clinical course of viral myocarditis. Circulation. 2006;**114**(15):1581-1590

[39] Brett NJ, Strugnell WE, Slaughter RE. Acute myocarditis demonstrated on CT coronary angiography with MRI correlation. Circulation. Cardiovascular Imaging. 2011;**4**(3):e5-e6

[40] Brooks MA, Sane DC. CT findings in acute myocarditis: 2 cases. Journal of Thoracic Imaging. 2007;**22**(3):277-279

[41] Bouleti C, Baudry G, Iung B, Arangalage D, Abtan J, Ducrocq G, et al. Usefulness of late iodine enhancement on spectral CT in acute myocarditis. JACC: Cardiovascular Imaging. 2017;**10**(7):826-827

[42] Aquaro GD, Ghebru Habtemicael Y, Camastra G, Monti L, Dellegrottaglie S, Moro C, et al. Prognostic value of repeating cardiac magnetic resonance in patients with acute myocarditis. Journal of the American College of Cardiology. 2019;**74**(20):2439-2448

[43] Lurz P, Luecke C, Eitel I, Föhrenbach F, Frank C, Grothoff M, et al. Comprehensive cardiac magnetic resonance imaging in patients with suspected myocarditis: The MyoRacer-trial. Journal of the American College of Cardiology. 2016;**67**(15):1800-1811

[44] Ferreira VM, Schulz-Menger J, Holmvang G, Kramer CM, Carbone I, Sechtem U, et al. Cardiovascular magnetic resonance in nonischemic myocardial inflammation: Expert recommendations. Journal of the American College of Cardiology. 2018;**72**(24):3158-3176

[45] Francone M, Chimenti C, Galea N, Scopelliti F, Verardo R, Galea R, et al.

CMR sensitivity varies with clinical presentation and extent of cell necrosis in biopsy-proven acute myocarditis. JACC: Cardiovascular Imaging. 2014;7(3):254-263

[46] Lagan J, Schmitt M. The role of cardiac magnetic resonance in pericardial disease. Cardiology Clinics. Jul 2012;**9**:559-572. Article 877364

Chapter 7

The Role of Imaging Modalities in the Evaluation of Myocarditis

Marquis Griffin, Gift Echefu, Derek Geeslin and Adedayo Adeboye

Abstract

Myocarditis is a clinical condition characterized by inflammation of cardiac myocytes caused by various factors, which can potentially result in cardiomyopathy, morbidity, and mortality. The clinical presentations vary from asymptomatic to fulminant disease and cardiogenic shock. Therefore, it is prudent for physicians to identify this disease process early, and accurately. Unfortunately, diagnosis and treatment is often challenging. Currently, biopsy is the gold standard for the diagnosis of myocarditis with direct visualization of inflamed myocardial tissues being necessary. Endomyocardial biopsy is invasive; therefore, it is imperative to obtain additional information prior to pursuing this approach. There have been considerable breakthroughs in cardiovascular imaging that can provide valuable insights and improve diagnostic accuracy.

Keywords: myocarditis, fulminant myocarditis, dilated cardiomyopathy, imaging modalities in myocarditis, cardiac magnetic resonance imaging, transthoracic echocardiography, cardiac computed tomography angiography, nuclear scintigraphic imaging

1. Introduction

Myocarditis is an inflammatory condition of cardiac myocytes caused by a wide range of infectious agents, systemic disorders, medications, and toxins (**Table 1**) [1]. The immunohistochemical characterization of infiltrates in relation to LV dysfunction has resulted in the World Health Organization (WHO) recognizing inflammatory cardiomyopathies (DCMi) as a distinct category of secondary cardiomyopathies. Genetic susceptibility is thought to play a significant role in the development of viral and/or autoimmune myocarditis and its progression to dilated cardiomyopathy (DCM) in humans [2–5]. Patients with histologically verified chronic inflammation who are unable to eradicate culprit infectious organisms or those who acquire injurious cardiac autoantibodies against myocardial structural, sarcoplasmic, or sarcolemmal proteins appear to be at the greatest risk of progression to DCM [6, 7]. Persistent viral infection and intramyocardial inflammation confirmed with endomyocardial biopsy (EMB) have been linked to an unfavorable prognosis in DCM, with a higher risk of cardiac mortality or the requirement for cardiac transplantation [8].

	Etiology of myocarditis	Comments
1.	*Infectious myocarditis*: Viral, bacterial, spirochetal, fungal, protozoal, rickettsia	Histological evidence for myocarditis associated with appropriate positive serology/antigen testing
2.	*Immune mediated*: Allergens (tetanus toxoid, serum sickness), alloantigens (heart transplant rejection), autoantigens (infective negative lymphocytic, infection-negative giant cell) autoimmune disorders (systemic lupus erythematosus, rheumatoid arthritis, inflammatory bowel disease)	Histological evidence of myocarditis with negative viral PCR, with or without serum cardiac autoantibodies
3.	*Toxic Myocarditis*: Drugs (monoclonal antibodies; trastuzumab, interleukin-2), drugs of abuse (amphetamines, cocaine), heavy metals (copper and iron), scorpion sting, snake and spider venoms	Histological myocarditis with negative viral PCR, with history and laboratory evidence of specific culprit drugs and toxin

Table 1.
Etiologies of myocarditis.

The clinical presentations vary widely, presenting as subclinical illness in its mildest form and in severe cases, acute heart failure, arrhythmias, cardiogenic shock, and sudden cardiac death [1]. Diagnostic testing for clinically suspected myocarditis includes history of symptoms, cardiac biomarkers, electrocardiograms (ECGs) and advanced imaging. Nevertheless, none of these modalities are specific, relative to endomyocardial biopsy. Endomyocardial biopsy, which combines the application of the Dallas criteria with the inclusion of histochemical evidence of viral infection, is the gold-standard approach for diagnosing suspected myocarditis [9]. However, EMB is invasive and less frequently used especially in patients with highly unstable hemodynamic conditions because of the significant procedural risks. Further, sampling error is a limitation in cases of focal myocarditis and involvement of areas that are inaccessible to the bioptome, contributing to false-negative results [10]. It then becomes appealing that diagnosis of myocarditis, even by biopsy be supplemented and guided by multimodal and advanced imaging. In this chapter, we will review the various imaging modalities in the diagnosis of myocarditis, including the indications, specific findings, prognostic value, and limitations of each modality.

2. Imaging modalities in the assessment of myocarditis

2.1 Echocardiography

All patients with clinically suspected myocarditis should be evaluated with transthoracic echocardiography (TTE) as a safe and readily available test. Guideline statements by several societies including the American College of Cardiology, American Heart Association, and the European Society of Cardiology provide recommend performing transthoracic echocardiography for all patients presenting with suspected myocarditis for early characterization of cardiac structures and function [11–13]. They offer crucial diagnostic and prognostic insights and can help exclude other conditions, including primary valvular or pericardial diseases. TTE is highly sensitive for detecting pathologic changes to the cardiac structure associated with myocarditis; however, the echocardiographic features can often be subtle and occur in a variety of cardiac pathologies which limits the specificity of echocardiographic findings [11–13].

Myocarditis can lead to clinically and echocardiographically evident cardiomyopathy with varying and non-specific features such as diastolic or systolic dysfunction of either or both ventricles, myocardial thickening, global or regional wall motion abnormalities, pericardial effusion, and focal interstitial edematous changes to the myocardium [2, 12, 13]. Myocarditis can mimic ischemic heart disease and appear as dilated, hypertrophic, and restricted cardiomyopathies on echocardiogram [14].

The role of enhanced echocardiographic technologies including 3D imaging, speckle tracking, contrast echocardiography, and tissue Doppler imaging remains investigative and can detect modest ventricular function abnormalities that may aid in diagnosing myocarditis.

2.2 Two-dimensional transthoracic echocardiography

2-D TTE has been applied in distinguishing myocarditis sub-types, specifically fulminant and acute myocarditis [15, 16]. In this instance, patients with acute myocarditis demonstrate significant left ventricular dilatation, normal LV thickness, and diminished LV function, while those with fulminant myocarditis present with non-dilated, thickened, and hypocontractile left ventricles. Fulminant phenotype is associated with considerable improvement in left ventricular percentage fractional shortening at 6-month follow-up, while acute myocarditis portends poor prognosis. To distinguish between fulminant myocarditis from other forms of acute myocarditis, it is crucial to conduct a prompt assessment using echocardiography, followed by EMB. Viral myocarditis can be marked by echocardiographic evidence of elevated left ventricular (LV) wall thickness,

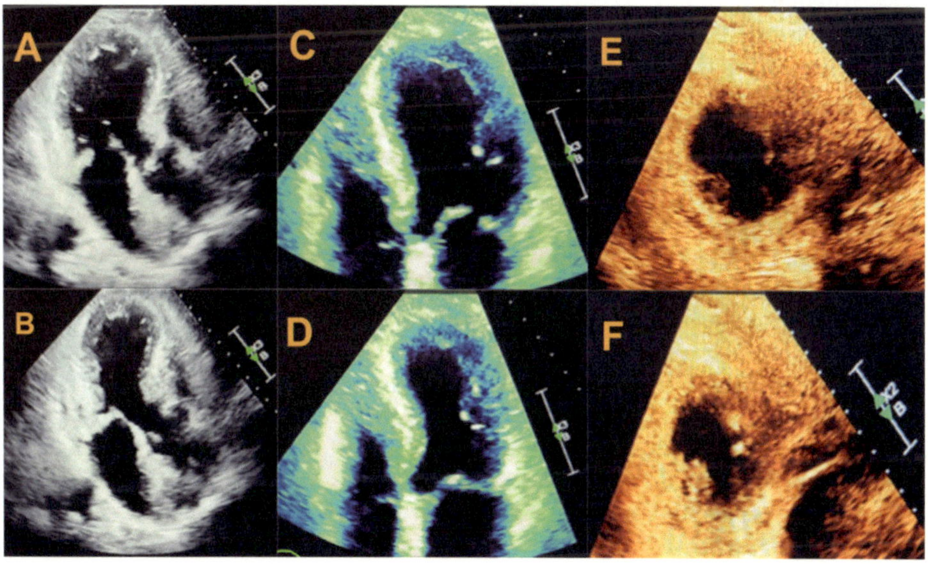

Figure 1.
These are images taken from an echocardiogram of a 62 year old patient presenting with fever and chest pain, found to have elevated troponin on work-up. Due to concerns for acute coronary syndrome, he underwent. Cardiac catheterization which showed no obstructive coronary artery disease. He was subsequently diagnosed with myocarditis. The top row Labeled A, C, and E show diastolic still images. The bottom row labeled B, D, F shows systolic still images. A and B depict the apical 3 chamber view showing diffuse apical hypokinesis which is also appreciated in images E and F which is the short axis view at the apex. Images C and D are the apical 4 chamber views showing apical hypokinesis.

LV mass index, and reduced contractility [8, 15, 16]. These changes are triggered by interstitial edema stemming from the infiltration of acute inflammatory cells (**Figure 1**).

2.3 Contrast echocardiography

In acute myocarditis, contrast echocardiography can enable the precise evaluation of regional wall motion abnormalities and left ventricular function [17]. Intravenous administration of echocardiographic contrast agents results in a significant increase in opacification of the left cardiac chambers. They are composed of microspheres containing a perfluorocarbon gas and have a size comparable to that of red blood cells. The quantities of contrast required for achieving left ventricle opacification are modest (0.1–0.3 ml) in comparison to other imaging techniques, such as X-ray [17, 18]. Myocardial contrast has been applied to conventional 2-D echocardiography in a multimodal approach to diagnose acute viral myocarditis. In this case, real-time low-mechanical-index myocardial contrast echocardiography (RTMCE) was conducted using harmonic imaging and commercially available lipid-encapsulated microbubble Definity (perflutren lipid microspheres). Time intensity curves were sampled offline using the EchoPAC workstation, with regions of interest measuring 6.0 × 3.0 mm. Affected regions had reduced perfusion and delayed contrast replenishment on real-time myocardial contrast echocardiography [19]. This was indicative of a reduction in the area of the myocardial capillary bed and compromised microvascular integrity in the affected segments. The abnormalities identified on echocardiography were subsequently verified by gadolinium-enhanced CMR. However, the perfusion use of contrast echocardiography remains experimental.

2.4 Strain/speckle tracking echocardiography

Speckle tracking imaging shows great potential as a noninvasive technique for detecting intramyocardial inflammation, even in the absence of wall motion abnormalities. Research has demonstrated that speckle tracking echocardiography (STE) can effectively diagnose early, subclinical ventricular dysfunction and provide valuable prognostic information. It is capable of identifying subtle LV dysfunction in patients with acute or subacute viral myocarditis, even when conventional TTE demonstrated preserved LV function. Combined with precise evaluations of regional contractility, STE may be extremely valuable in the diagnosis of myocarditis. Speckle tracking imaging can correlate with EMB-proven inflammation in patients with acute myocarditis and inflammatory cardiomyopathies, and is a supplemental tool for a comprehensive investigation of structural and functional alterations in the left ventricular myocardium [8]. Strain analysis has shown superiority in identifying subtle myocardial changes associated with myocarditis, specifically interstitial edema in the acute phase not detectable by conventional echocardiography [20, 21].

Among the parameters derived from myocardial deformation analyses, systolic strain rate is commonly considered the most significant indicator of left ventricular contractility [8]. Novel quantitative indicators of intrinsic cardiac deformation in real time, strain and strain rate measurements, are considered to be uninfluenced by translational motion and other through-plane motion and provide accurate assessment of regional contractility. The specific methodology for application of speckle tracking imaging has been suggested [8]. The apical four-chamber and the two-chamber views are used to record three cardiac cycles as three-beat cine-loop segments. The conventional ECHOPAC application for two-dimensional strain analysis can be used to generate a global longitudinal strain (GLS) and strain rate curve in each view, which encompasses all LV myocardial segments [8].

2.5 Tissue doppler imaging

Tissue doppler imaging (TDI) measures the velocity of myocardial tissue motion rather than blood flow. Tissue Doppler echocardiographic imaging is highly sensitive to myocardial contractility and appears to be beneficial in the identification of changes associated with myocardial inflammation and edema [22]. Tissue velocity (doppler) imaging has been applied in the diagnosis of myocarditis [23]. In this instance, TDI alone was diagnostic of myocarditis relative to normal findings on 2D, doppler echocardiogram and CMR in diagnosing myocarditis. TDI revealed a net decrease in systolic regional wall motion velocity which was later confirmed by EMB [23]. TDI exhibits potential; however, additional investigation is necessary to ascertain its role in acute myocarditis. Adsett et al. documented a case of eosinophilic myocarditis confirmed by biopsy [24]. The TD parameters in this study were evaluated and indicated anomalies in both systolic and diastolic functions. Color M-mode TD of the LV posterior wall demonstrated a decrease in both average myocardial velocities and myocardial velocity gradient during systole and diastole TD. The full dimensions and application of TDI in multimodal echocardiographic imaging remains investigational.

2.6 Three-dimensional transthoracic echocardiography

The application of 3-D transthoracic echocardiography in myocarditis remains unclear. The existing knowledge on the accuracy of these advanced echocardiographic techniques in detecting viral myocarditis is limited, therefore additional research is needed to compare them to cardiac magnetic resonance imaging (CMR) and endo myocardial biopsy [25]. Real-time two- and three-dimensional echocardiography were applied to myocarditis evaluation in a 13-year-old man with a dilated and hypokinetic left ventricle and bi-ventricular thrombosis which was reportedly better assessed by real-time, three-dimensional transthoracic echocardiogram [26].

3. Cardiac computed tomography angiography

Coronary computed tomographic angiography (CCTA) has been an emerging field in the detection of various cardiovascular diseases. Advancements in software and the introduction of newer multi-detector computed tomography (MDCT) have allowed for increased diagnostic performance, decreased time, and lower contrast volume [27]. The clinical manifestation of acute viral myocarditis varies widely, and MDCT has been shown to aid in differentiating it from imitating conditions like aortic dissection, acute coronary syndrome (ACS), acute pulmonary embolism (PE), congestive heart failure, and pneumonia [28, 29]. Increased permeability and myocyte rupture during myocardial inflammation in acute myocarditis lead to increased accumulation of radiographic contrast agents [30]. The Iodine and Gadolinium based contrast agents used with MDCT and CMR respectively, share similar pharmacokinetics. These similarities play a role in delayed contrast imaging techniques that both modalities use in the evaluation of acute myocarditis. Evaluating myocarditis using MDCT provides two phases of results each potentially showing alterations in the myocardium. During immediate contrast delivery, first pass features of acute myocarditis on MDCT include diffuse hyperenhancement of the myocardium. The first pass phase of MDCT evaluates blood flow and perfusion to the myocardium, which explains why hypo-enhancements are seen in the setting of myocardial infarction. The delayed contrast phase of MDCT as in CMR, is performed a designated amount of time after contrast has been delivered, and evaluates more for myocyte cell damage. During this second phase of MDCT, acute myocarditis is associated with late hyperenhancement of the myocardial wall. This finding can vary from subepicardial to transmural involvement, with a band like or nodular appearance of contrast material [30, 31]. While evaluating acute myocarditis, MDCT is able to simultaneously collect additional information of ventricular wall motion abnormalities, coronary artery disease/stenosis, pulmonary arteries, and lung tissue [28, 31].

In the evaluation of acute myocarditis and myocardial inflammation, CMR has been considered the primary imaging modality [32]. MDCT provides several advantages compared to CMR, which include not only accessibility and availability to patients, but the time needed for the examination itself. MDCT can also be a consideration in scenarios such as claustrophobic patients, non-MRI compatible devices, or any fixed indwelling metal. During MDCT evaluation of acute myocarditis, coronary vessels are also examined which can aid in ruling out ACS [27, 32, 33]. There also remains some downsides to MDCT evaluation of acute myocarditis, despite advances in software development, multi detectors, wide detectors, and increased slice count. Dependent on which generation of MDCT is available, these include variations in acquisition time, imaging artifacts, heart rate variability, and contrast dose [27].

There have been small studies comparing CMR to CT. One study examined 20 patients who were diagnosed with acute myocarditis using standard CMR protocols, and when compared, CT reported 95% accuracy [34]. Another small study showed correlation between the abnormalities detected using each modality [30]. There remains a paucity of data evaluating the efficacy and utility of CT in the diagnosis of acute myocarditis. However, the limited studies have shown promising results for its useful application.

4. Cardiac magnetic resonance imaging

Cardiac magnetic resonance (CMR) imaging has the greatest ability to characterize the myocardial tissues, and in the setting of myocarditis, observers are capable of identifying myocardial edema, hyperemia, necrosis, and fibrosis associated with inflammatory processes with acceptable interobserver variability and quantitative accuracy [35–38]. As such criteria has been developed to define acute myocarditis on MRI. The Lake Louise Criteria (LLC), revised in 2018 (**Table 1**), combines multiple criteria, and some supportive signs to diagnose myocarditis [32, 39]. Inherent to this criteria is a combination of T2 based, T1 based, and gadolinium contrast enhanced imaging each with ability to detect different tissue abnormalities that serve as signs of edema, hyperemia, necrosis, and fibrosis **Figure 2**. Depicts the findings of late gadolinium enhancement, T1 enhancement suggestive of edema, and an example of mapping performed to identify abnormal myocardial tissue relaxation.

In comparison to the 2009 criteria, the 2018 criteria now requires 2 out of 2 main criteria to be satisfied; however, changes to the main criteria are intended to improve the sensitivity of detection of acute myocardial inflammation without compromising specificity [39]. A validation study was published since these updates occurred which

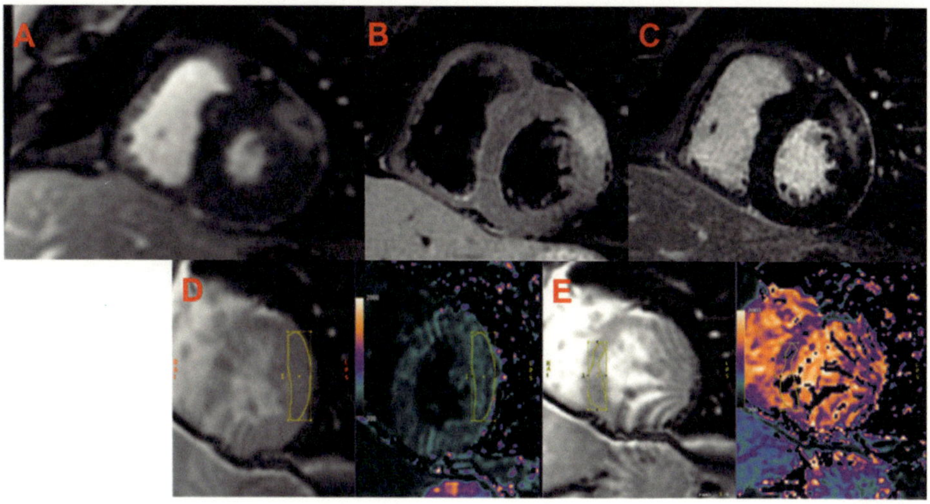

Figure 2.
These are MRI images of a patient who met the 2018 Lake Louise Diagnostic criteria for Myocarditis. A. During early gadolinium infusion, T1 images are showing enhancement of the anterolateral wall and the adjacent pericardium which is suggestive of hyperemia, edema, and inflammation. B. T2 double inversion recovery sequences demonstrate focal edema in the anterolateral wall of the mid left ventricle. Edema is also demonstrated in the adjacent pericardium. C. Delayed gadolinium-enhanced imaging demonstrates corresponding patchy subepicardial and mid myocardial enhancement, as well as abnormal enhancement of the pericardium along the anterior and lateral left ventricular wall. D and E T1 mapping has accurately identified the region of interest, and additionally, there is an infero-septal region of interest which was not well seen on the initial T1 and T2 sequences. Images courtesy of Neeraja Yedlapati, MD, FACC, FASE, FSCCT.

included 40 patients with clinical myocarditis, and 26 healthy patients as a control group, testing each criteria to determine sensitivity and specificity [40]. They found that the 2018 criteria accomplished its goal with an increased sensitivity in direct comparison to the 2009 criteria with equivalent specificity. Of the 40 patients with myocarditis the 2009 criteria identified 29 out of 40 cases (72.5%) with 1 false positive, and the 2018 criteria identified 35 out of 40 patients (87.5%) with 1 false positive. Further studies and meta analysis of large pools of data will likely be necessary to determine the true sensitivity and specificity with more accuracy (**Table 2**).

4.1 T2 based imaging

T2 based imaging, typically relying on black-blood spin-echo techniques, provides the ability to identify myocardial edema. The details and physics are beyond the scope of this book chapter; however, the goal is to make blood appear black such that more static tissues adjacent to blood flow, in this case the heart, are more easily visualized [41]. Edematous myocardium causes prolonged T2 decay times which appears as hyperintense signals on T2-weighted images [39, 42, 43]. The 2018 LLC criteria for myocarditis notes one semi-quantitative method to determine the signal intensity T2 enhancement in comparison to skeletal muscle with a Ratio of ≥ 2.0 being a significant finding of edematous changes. No imaging technique is without limitations, and notably the reference region of interest, skeletal muscle, could also be inflamed in the setting of systemic inflammatory conditions leading to false negative results [43–45]. Nonetheless, T2 weighted imaging has a sensitivity of 84%, and specificity of 74%, with an overall accuracy of 79% for the detection of myocarditis as seen in multiple studies [43, 46].

Main criteria		
T2 Based Imaging	Regional* high T2 signal intensity (SI) Or Global T2 SI ratio ≥ 2.0 in T2-weighted CMR images Or Regional or global increase of myocardial T2 relaxation time	Target: Myocardial edema
T1 based imaging	Regional or global increase of native myocardial T1 relaxation time or extracellular volume Or Areas with high SI in a nonischemic distribution pattern in Late Gadolinium Enhancement (LGE) images.	Targets: 1. Increase T1: edema(intra or extracellular), hyperemia/capillary leak, necrosis, fibrosis 2. Early Gadolinium enhancement: hyperemia, capillary leak 3. Late Gadolinium Enhancement: necrosis, fibrosis (extracellular acute edema) 4. Increased Extracellular volume: edema (extracellular, hyperemia/capillary leak, necrosis, fibrosis).
Supportive criteria		
Pericardial abnormalities	Pericardial effusion in cine CMR images Or High Signal Intensity of the pericardium in LGE images, T1-mapping or T2-mapping Or T1-mapping or T2- mapping	Target: Pericardial inflammation
LV dysfunction	Systolic LV wall motion abnormality in cine CMR images	Target: LV dysfunction

**Regional is defined as an area of at least 10 continuous pixels. SI Ratio: Signal intensity ratio is defined as the signal intensity of the myocardium compared to the signal intensity of skeletal muscle.*

Table 2.
2018 Lake Louise criteria for identification of myocardial inflammation.

4.2 T1 based imaging

T1 based imaging, using spin-echo techniques, is also capable of detecting myocardial edema and in addition, combination with gadolinium based contrast allows the detection of hyperemia, necrosis, and tissue fibrosis. T1 weighted images similarly show hyperintense signals in the setting of tissue edema. Semi-quantitative methods also exist for the determination of myocardial to skeletal muscle signal intensity before and after administering gadolinium contrast.

There are a variety of gadolinium based contrast agents which have different tissue affinity and pharmacokinetics. The role of gadolinium lies in its paramagnetic properties. It is susceptible to magnetic fields and this property can be exploited during magnetic resonance imaging. Like many metals, Atomic gadolinium is toxic to humans. Fortunately, gadolinium is a chelating metal with several unpaired electrons available to form covalent bonds with organic compounds. The combination of gadolinium and a variety of chelating ligands form soluble contrast agents for use in combination with magnetic resonance. In the case of myocarditis, contrast agents that have affinity for extracellular spaces will predominate as they will be tailored towards identifying inflammation, and hyperemia [47].

4.3 Early gadolinium enhancement

Inflamed tissues experience many changes including hyperemia, expansion of the extracellular space, increased free water content, and increased vascular permeability [39]. When gadolinium enhancement in tissue is seen within 1 minute during T1 weighted imaging, hyperemia and leaky capillaries are suspected to be present within the tissues due to its rapid uptake of gadolinium contrast [39, 42]. Early gadolinium enhancement is no longer included in the Lake louise criteria for myocarditis, and data have shown that this does not affect the diagnostic accuracy of the Lake Louise Criteria in identifying myocarditis [39, 42, 48].

4.4 Late gadolinium enhancement

T1 weighted images, taken 10 minutes after gadolinium based contrast is administered, is used to evaluate for late gadolinium enhancement. Over time, gadolinium finds its way into extracellular spaces, and when in the presence of myocardium that has been extensively damaged, gadolinium based contrast is able to enter the intercellular spaces of myocytes that are injured or necrotic. If fibrosis or scarring is present, there is an increased amount of extracellular space available for the diffusion and accumulation of contrast. Under these circumstances, gadolinium contrast enhances the signal within these tissues [39, 42, 43].

The patterns of late gadolinium enhancement (LGE) seen during CMR are heterogenous. The most common distribution of LGE is seen in the mid and subepicardial regions. The most common myocardial distribution is in the septal, and basal to mid inferolateral walls [39, 42, 43, 49]. These patterns occur in a non coronary distribution, and in addition inflammation related to ischemia tends to have a subendocardial distribution owing to the endocardial to epicardial progression of myocardial ischemia [39]. While the distribution of LGE differs from ischemia, there are some exceptions: Severe inflammation may cause subendocardial extension of LGE, and hypereosinophilic syndromes may cause circumferential LGE [39]. Another limitation is the inability for LGE images alone to distinguish active myocarditis from chronic changes due to necrosis and fibrosis. T2 weighted images can be compared to LGE as T2 weighted images which has a tendency to show early signs of inflammation such as edema as opposed to fibrosis and scarring [42, 50, 51].

4.5 T1 and T2 mapping and extracellular volume quantification

T1, and T2 mapping as well as extracellular volume quantification are novel techniques used to characterize tissue changes seen in myocarditis. As seen in the 2018 Lake Louise criteria for myocarditis, T1 and T2 mapping can be used in addition to LGE to characterize both myocardial tissues and pericardial disease as a supportive feature [39, 52]. Intrinsically T1, and T2 weighted images look for relaxation of tissues exposed to a strong magnetic field along the transverse (T2), and longitudinal (T1) planes. Each tissue within the body is thought to have a "normal" T1 and T2 relaxation time. Mapping is the process of calculating these relaxation times for each pixel and displaying the values as a map which circumvents the limitations of visual assessment, signal intensity ratios, and early gadolinium enhancement. Thereafter, global or regional relaxation times can be established and allows the ability to discern more subtle tissue edema even without the use of contrast agents. Extracellular volume quantification utilizes T1 mapping techniques applied pre and post administration of gadolinium based contrast to estimate the extracellular volume [39, 52]. ECV mapping is also useful for detecting diffuse more mild and myocardial fibrosis, and complements LGE in this regard which is good at identifying focal fibrosis. Overall, multiple studies have shown good sensitivity, specificity, and accuracy of mapping techniques for the identification of myocarditis [39].

5. Nuclear scintigraphic imaging

Myocardial scintigraphy relies on using radioactive isotopes that target the myocardium to gain information regarding the perfusion or state of the myocardial tissues. Inflammation-sensitive radioisotopes were developed and used to diagnose myocarditis including: gallium-67 (Ga-67), indium-111 (In-111) monoclonal antimyosin antibody, and technetium-99 m (Tc-99 m)-labeled methoxy-isobutyl isonitrile (MIBI) single-photon emission computed tomography (SPECT), and technetium-99 m depreotide [53]. In the era of CMR the use of nuclear scintigraphy has declined as CMR provides much better spatial resolution, no radiation exposure, and better correlation with histopathology [22, 54–58].

5.1 Gallium-67

Lymphocyte labeling techniques using gallium-67 scintigraphy allows for the detection and localization of inflammation in myocarditis. Some studies have also shown that gallium-67 scintigraphy is capable of differentiating myocarditis from acute myocardial infarctions as well [59–61]. There has been a study comparing Gallium-67 scintigraphic imaging against endomyocardial biopsy in a case sarees for the diagnosis of myocarditis in patients with dilated cardiomyopathy, and determined that five out of six cases of biopsy proven myocarditis showed a dense uptake of gallium-67. This suggested that screening patients with Gallium-67 scintigraphy could increase the yield of biopsy by showing the areas of inflamed myocardium [60].

5.2 Antimyosin

Antimyosin is a monoclonal antibody that targets cardiac myosin proteins. Once radiolabeled with Indium-111, it can be used in nuclear scintigraphy [62–65]. Antimyosin scintigraphy has been studied in pediatric patients with clinical myocarditis. Antimyosin uptake in the myocardium correlated well with biopsy and histological diagnosis of myocarditis. Furthermore, persistence of antimyosin uptake was associated with increased morbidity which added some prognostic value to this technique [66]. Another study was performed in 65 patients with clinical myocarditis using antimyosin labeled with indium-111, and showed that uptake correlated well with biopsy findings. While uptake of indium-11 was highly specific, this study reported poor sensitivity for the detection of myocarditis compared to biopsy [67].

5.3 Technetium-99 m-labeled methoxy-isobutyl isonitrile

Technetium-99 m labeled Methoxy-isobutyl Isonitrile is a widely used radiotracer in nuclear stress testing to determine myocardial perfusion. Tc-99 m is taken up and cleared by myocardium at varying rates depending on the viability and integrity of the tissues. In the setting of myocardial inflammation and necrosis, there will be reduce uptake of Tc-99 m [68]. Tc-99 m scintigraphy was used to investigate 46 children with coxsackie viral myocarditis, and found that areas of "hypoperfusion" were present [69].

5.4 Combined positron emission tomography and computed tomography (PET-CT)

18F-fluorodeoxyglucose (18F-FDG) positron emission tomography (PET) with computed tomography (CT) is another tool which can be used for cardiac imaging. In comparison to CMR, PET-CT has the potential to quantify the degree of myocardial inflammation which could be useful for disease monitoring. PET-CT can be considered as an alternative to CMR when there are contraindications to MRI [70].

Some investigators have studied simultaneous PET-CT and CMR imaging and found complementary benefits in the evaluation for myocarditis that could not be achieved by either alone [71]. There have been several case reports demonstrating the use of PTE-CT to diagnose cardiac sarcoidosis, viral myocarditis, giant cell myocarditis, and post-infarction myocarditis [72–78].

There has been a prospective feasibility study comparing CMR and PET/CT as well as investigating feasibility of integrated PET/MRI. 65 patients were included in the study and they found that the sensitivity and specificity of PET-CT was 74 and 97%, respectively. Pet findings were in overall agreement with CMR findings [79]. The ongoing STREAM trial aims to assess patients with clinically suspected myocarditis using TTE, nuclear SPECT imaging, and 18F-FDG PET-CT. Endomyocardial biopsies will be performed as the gold standard for diagnosis, and the trial is designed to determine the sensitivity and specificity of 18F-FDG PET-CT imaging in diagnosing acute myocarditis [80].

6. The role of imaging in determining prognosis in acute myocarditis

The majority of patients with myocarditis recover, and their disease regresses with minor damage to the myocardium. The exception being patients with fulminant myocarditis who have a worse prognosis overall [15, 81]. Rates of major cardiac adverse events (MACE) have been studied in patients with myocarditis. MACE, all cause mortality, recurrence of myocarditis, heart failure, and sustained ventricular tachycardia was examined in a retrospective, single-center, observational study including 112 patients with myocarditis diagnosed by CMR. MACE was significantly higher in patients with extensive LGE as defined by LGE more than 17 g (71 vs. 4%, p-value = 0.005). Additionally, symptoms of chest pain, ST elevation on ECG, and elevated cardiac troponin were also associated with MACE, recurrence of myocarditis, and sustained ventricular tachycardia. During the subsequent 16 months of follow up, LGE more than 17 g and New York Heart Association functional classification III or IV were independent predictors of MACE in this population [82]. However, using cut-off values of LGE (17 g or 13% of myocardial mass) is not currently a validated approach to be used in clinical practice routinely [82, 83]. Additionally, another study showed that different patterns of LGE may have prognostic significance. In 374 patients with myocarditis, patients with LGE in the mid anteroseptum had a worse prognosis than LGE seen in other locations [84].

7. Advances in artificial intelligence and multimodality imaging

The use of artificial intelligence and machine learning has rapidly expanded, including the realm of imaging modalities, and their use for cardiovascular disease could have significant implications. This technology is being studied and applied to multiple imaging modalities including cardiac magnetic resonance, cardiac computed tomography, echocardiography, and nuclear imaging. The use of Artificial Intelligence enhanced imaging has shown promise in terms of accuracy compared to traditional methods in all modalities. Most of these technologies and their applications in the clinical setting remain experimental, and there is need for further refinement and clinical trials for validation. Additionally, positive clinical outcomes would be necessary, analysis of cost effectiveness, and security of data are all barriers that will need to be overcome for practical use [85].

8. Conclusion

Numerous technologies and diagnostic tools exist that can provide direction for the accurate identification of myocarditis in both acute and chronic phases. The optimized acquisition protocol, enhanced by contemporary mapping techniques, facilitates noninvasive diagnosis with high diagnostic accuracy. Clinical features and initial investigations may indicate myocarditis; however, many presenting characteristics overlap with other cardiac conditions. Endomyocardial biopsy has historically served as the reference standard for diagnosis, while cardiac magnetic resonance imaging (CMR) continues to be an essential non-invasive diagnostic technique. Therefore, clinical guidelines and expert consensus statements can be excellent resources to leverage for information to direct appropriate testing and management.

Author details

Marquis Griffin[1,2,3], Gift Echefu[1,2,3], Derek Geeslin[1,2] and Adedayo Adeboye[1,2]*

1 University of Tennessee Health Sciences Center, Memphis, Tennessee, USA

2 Lt. Col. Luke Weathers, Jr. VA Medical Center, Memphis, Tennessee, USA

3 Methodist University Hospital, Memphis, Tennessee, USA

*Address all correspondence to: aadeboye@uthsc.edu

References

[1] Blauwet LA, Cooper LT. Myocarditis. Progress in Cardiovascular Diseases. 2010;**52**(4):274-288. DOI: 10.1016/j.pcad.2009.11.006

[2] Caforio ALP et al. Current state of knowledge on aetiology, diagnosis, management, and therapy of myocarditis: A position statement of the European Society of Cardiology Working Group on myocardial and pericardial diseases. European Heart Journal. 2013;**34**(33). pp. 2636-2648, 2648a–2648d. DOI: 10.1093/eurheartj/eht210

[3] Lim JK, Murphy PM. Chemokine control of West Nile virus infection. Experimental Cell Research. 2011;**317**(5):569-574. DOI: 10.1016/j.yexcr.2011.01.009

[4] Caforio ALP et al. Evidence from family studies for autoimmunity in dilated cardiomyopathy. The Lancet. 1994;**344**(8925):773-777. DOI: 10.1016/S0140-6736(94)92339-6

[5] Caforio ALP et al. Prospective familial assessment in dilated cardiomyopathy: Cardiac autoantibodies predict disease development in asymptomatic relatives. Circulation. 2007;**115**(1):76-83. DOI: 10.1161/CIRCULATIONAHA.106.641472

[6] Kühl U et al. Viral persistence in the myocardium is associated with progressive cardiac dysfunction. Circulation. 2005;**112**(13):1965-1970. DOI: 10.1161/CIRCULATIONAHA.105.548156

[7] Kindermann I et al. Predictors of outcome in patients with suspected myocarditis. Circulation. 2008;**118**(6):639-648. DOI: 10.1161/CIRCULATIONAHA.108.769489

[8] Escher F et al. New echocardiographic findings correlate with intramyocardial inflammation in endomyocardial biopsies of patients with acute myocarditis and inflammatory cardiomyopathy. Mediators of Inflammation. 2013;**2013**:1-9. DOI: 10.1155/2013/875420

[9] Aretz HT et al. Myocarditis. A histopathologic definition and classification. The American Journal of Cardiovascular Pathology. 1987;**1**(1):3-14

[10] Hauck AJ, Kearney DL, Edwards WD. Evaluation of postmortem endomyocardial biopsy specimens from 38 patients with lymphocytic myocarditis: Implications for role of sampling error. Mayo Clinic Proceedings. 1989;**64**(10):1235-1245. DOI: 10.1016/s0025-6196(12)61286-5

[11] McDonagh TA et al. 2021 ESC guidelines for the diagnosis and treatment of acute and chronic heart failure. European Heart Journal. 2021;**42**(36):3599-3726. DOI: 10.1093/eurheartj/ehab368

[12] Heidenreich PA et al. 2022 AHA/ACC/HFSA guideline for the Management of Heart Failure: A report of the American College of Cardiology/American Heart Association joint committee on clinical practice guidelines. Circulation. 2022;**145**(18):e913-e915. DOI: 10.1161/CIR.0000000000001063

[13] Douglas PS et al. ACCF/ASE/ACEP/ASNC/SCAI/SCCT/SCMR 2007 appropriateness criteria for transthoracic and transesophageal echocardiography developed in accordance with the principles and methodology outlined by ACCF: Patel MR, Spertus JA, Brindis RG, Hendel RC, Douglas PS, Peterson E, Wolk MJ, Allen JM, Raskin IE. ACCF

proposed method for evaluating the appropriateness of cardiovascular imaging. J Am Coll Cardiol 2005;46:1606-13 (1). Journal of the American College of Cardiology. 2007;**50**(2):187-204. DOI: 10.1016/j.jacc.2007.05.003

[14] Angelini A. Myocarditis mimicking acute myocardial infarction: Role of endomyocardial biopsy in the differential diagnosis. Heart. 2000;**84**(3):245-250. DOI: 10.1136/heart.84.3.245

[15] Felker GM et al. Echocardiographic findings in fulminant and acute myocarditis. Journal of the American College of Cardiology. 2000;**36**(1):227-232. DOI: 10.1016/S0735-1097(00)00690-2

[16] Pinamonti B et al. Echocardiographic findings in myocarditis. The American Journal of Cardiology. 1988;**62**(4):285-291. DOI: 10.1016/0002-9149(88)90226-3

[17] Olszewski R et al. The clinical applications of contrast echocardiography. European Journal of Echocardiography. 2007;**8**(3):S13-S23. DOI: 10.1016/j.euje.2007.03.021

[18] Becher BH. Contrast agents for echocardiography: Principles and instrumentation. In: Handbook of Contrast Echocardiography. LV Function and Myocardial Perfusion. Berlin: Springer-Verlag; 2000. Available from: www.sunnybrook.utoronto.ca/EchoHandbook/

[19] Afonso L, Hari P, Pidlaoan V, Kondur A, Jacob S, Khetarpal V. Acute myocarditis: Can novel echocardiographic techniques assist with diagnosis? European Heart Journal - Cardiovascular Imaging. 2010;**11**(3):E5-E5. DOI: 10.1093/ejechocard/jep183

[20] Di Bella G et al. Strain Doppler echocardiography can identify longitudinal myocardial dysfunction derived from edema in acute myocarditis. International Journal of Cardiology. 2008;**126**(2):279-280. DOI: 10.1016/j.ijcard.2007.01.110

[21] Di Bella G et al. Myocardial deformation in acute myocarditis with normal left ventricular wall motion--a cardiac magnetic resonance and 2-dimensional strain echocardiographic study. Official Journal of the Japanese Circulation Society. 2010;**74**(6):1205-1213. DOI: 10.1253/circj.cj-10-0017

[22] Skouri HN, Dec GW, Friedrich MG, Cooper LT. Noninvasive imaging in myocarditis. Journal of the American College of Cardiology. 2006;**48**(10):2085-2093. DOI: 10.1016/j.jacc.2006.08.017

[23] Urhausen A, Kindermann M, Böhm M, Kindermann W. Diagnosis of myocarditis by cardiac tissue velocity imaging in an olympic athlete. Circulation. 2003;**108**(4):e21-e22. DOI: 10.1161/01.CIR.0000075302.23631.D1

[24] Adsett M, West MJ, Galbraith A, Duhig E, Lange A, Palka P. Eosinophilic heart: Marked left ventricular wall thickening and myocardial dysfunction improving with corticosteroid therapy. Echocardiography (Mount Kisco, N.Y.). 2003;**20**(4):369-374. DOI: 10.1046/j.1540-8175.2003.03043.x

[25] Jeserich M, Konstantinides S, Pavlik G, Bode C, Geibel A. Non-invasive imaging in the diagnosis of acute viral myocarditis. Clinical Research in Cardiology. 2009;**98**(12):753-763. DOI: 10.1007/s00392-009-0069-2

[26] Thuny F et al. Images in cardiovascular medicine. Massive biventricular thrombosis as a consequence of myocarditis: Findings from 2-dimensional

and real-time 3-dimensional echocardiography. Circulation. 2006;**113**(25):e932-e933. DOI: 10.1161/CIRCULATIONAHA.105.599167

[27] Choi SI, George RT, Schuleri KH, Chun EJ, Lima JAC, Lardo AC. Recent developments in wide-detector cardiac computed tomography. The International Journal of Cardiovascular Imaging. 2009;**25**(1):23-29. DOI: 10.1007/s10554-009-9443-4

[28] Budoff MJ et al. Diagnostic performance of 64-multidetector row coronary computed tomographic angiography for evaluation of coronary artery stenosis in individuals without known coronary artery disease: Results from the prospective multicenter ACCURACY (assessment by coronary computed tomographic angiography of individuals undergoing invasive coronary angiography) trial. Journal of the American College of Cardiology. 2008;**52**(21):1724-1732. DOI: 10.1016/j.jacc.2008.07.031

[29] Burrill J, Dabbagh Z, Gollub F, Hamady M. Multidetector computed tomographic angiography of the cardiovascular system. Postgraduate Medical Journal. 2007;**83**(985):698-704. DOI: 10.1136/pgmj.2007.061804

[30] Dambrin G, Laissy JP, Serfaty JM, Caussin C, Lancelin B, Paul JF. Diagnostic value of ECG-gated multidetector computed tomography in the early phase of suspected acute myocarditis. A preliminary comparative study with cardiac MRI. European Radiology. 2007;**17**(2):331-338. DOI: 10.1007/s00330-006-0391-2

[31] Schuleri KH, George RT, Lardo AC. Applications of cardiac multidetector CT beyond coronary angiography. Nature Reviews. Cardiology. 2009;**6**(11):699-710. DOI: 10.1038/nrcardio.2009.172

[32] Friedrich MG et al. Cardiovascular magnetic resonance in myocarditis: A JACC white paper. Journal of the American College of Cardiology. 2009;**53**(17):1475-1487. DOI: 10.1016/j.jacc.2009.02.007

[33] le Polain J-B, de Waroux A-C, Pouleur C, Goffinet A, Pasquet J-LV, Gerber BL. Combined coronary and late-enhanced multidetector-computed tomography for delineation of the etiology of left ventricular dysfunction: Comparison with coronary angiography and contrast-enhanced cardiac magnetic resonance imaging. European Heart Journal. 2008;**29**(20):2544-2551. DOI: 10.1093/eurheartj/ehn381

[34] Bouleti C et al. Usefulness of late iodine enhancement on spectral CT in acute myocarditis. JACC: Cardiovascular Imaging. 2017;**10**(7):826-827. DOI: 10.1016/j.jcmg.2016.09.013

[35] Chetrit M, Friedrich MG. The unique role of cardiovascular magnetic resonance imaging in acute myocarditis. F1000Research. 2018;**7**:1153. DOI: 10.12688/f1000research.14857.1

[36] Karamitsos TD, Francis JM, Neubauer S. The current and emerging role of cardiovascular magnetic resonance in the diagnosis of nonischemic cardiomyopathies. Progress in Cardiovascular Diseases. 2011;**54**(3):253-265. DOI: 10.1016/j.pcad.2011.08.007

[37] Huttin O et al. Acute myocarditis presenting with ventricular arrhythmias: The role of CMR in the differential diagnosis of ARVD. Internal Medicine. 2013;**52**(17):1915-1918. DOI: 10.2169/internalmedicine.52.0462

[38] Liu PP, Mason JW. Advances in the understanding of myocarditis.

Circulation. 2001;**104**(9):1076-1082. DOI: 10.1161/hc3401.095198

[39] Ferreira VM et al. Cardiovascular magnetic resonance in nonischemic myocardial inflammation. Journal of the American College of Cardiology. 2018;**72**(24):3158-3176. DOI: 10.1016/j.jacc.2018.09.072

[40] Luetkens JA et al. Comparison of original and 2018 Lake Louise criteria for diagnosis of acute myocarditis: Results of a validation cohort. Radiology: Cardiothoracic Imaging. 2019;**1**(3):e190010. DOI: 10.1148/ryct.2019190010

[41] Henningsson M, Malik S, Botnar R, Castellanos D, Hussain T, Leiner T. Black blood contrast in cardiovascular MRI. Journal of Magnetic Resonance Imaging. 2022;**55**(1):61-80. DOI: 10.1002/jmri.27399

[42] Mirakhur A, Anca N, Mikami Y, Merchant N. T2-weighted imaging of the heart—A pictorial review. European Journal of Radiology. 2013;**82**(10):1755-1762. DOI: 10.1016/j.ejrad.2013.06.005

[43] Lurz P et al. Diagnostic performance of CMR imaging compared with EMB in patients with suspected myocarditis. JACC: Cardiovascular Imaging. 2012;**5**(5):513-524. DOI: 10.1016/j.jcmg.2011.11.022

[44] Abdel-Aty H et al. Diagnostic performance of cardiovascular magnetic resonance in patients with suspected acute myocarditis. Journal of the American College of Cardiology. 2005;**45**(11):1815-1822. DOI: 10.1016/j.jacc.2004.11.069

[45] Lewis AJM, Burrage MK, Ferreira VM. Cardiovascular magnetic resonance imaging for inflammatory heart diseases. Cardiovascular Diagnosis and Therapy. 2020;**10**(3):598-609. DOI: 10.21037/cdt.2019.12.09

[46] Guglin M, Nallamshetty L. Myocarditis: Diagnosis and treatment. Current Treatment Options in Cardiovascular Medicine. 2012;**14**(6):637-651. DOI: 10.1007/s11936-012-0204-7

[47] Ibrahim MA, Hazhirkarzar B, Dublin AB. Gadolinium magnetic resonance imaging. In: StatPearls. Treasure Island (FL): StatPearls Publishing; 2004. Available from: https://www.ncbi.nlm.nih.gov/books/NBK482487/

[48] Ferreira VM et al. T1 mapping for the diagnosis of acute myocarditis using CMR. JACC: Cardiovascular Imaging. 2013;**6**(10):1048-1058. DOI: 10.1016/j.jcmg.2013.03.008

[49] Abdel-Aty H, Cocker M, Strohm O, Filipchuk N, Friedrich MG. Abnormalities in T2-weighted cardiovascular magnetic resonance images of hypertrophic cardiomyopathy: Regional distribution and relation to late gadolinium enhancement and severity of hypertrophy. Journal of Magnetic Resonance Imaging. 2008;**28**(1):242-245. DOI: 10.1002/jmri.21381

[50] Verhaert D et al. Direct T2 quantification of myocardial edema in acute ischemic injury. JACC: Cardiovascular Imaging. 2011;**4**(3):269-278. DOI: 10.1016/j.jcmg.2010.09.023

[51] Wagner A et al. Contrast-enhanced MRI and routine single photon emission computed tomography (SPECT) perfusion imaging for detection of subendocardial myocardial infarcts: An imaging study. The Lancet. 2003;**361**(9355):374-379. DOI: 10.1016/S0140-6736(03)12389-6

[52] Liguori C, Farina D, Vaccher F, Ferrandino G, Bellini D,

Carbone I. Myocarditis: Imaging up to date. La Radiologia Medica (Torino). 2020;**125**(11):1124-1134. DOI: 10.1007/s11547-020-01279-8

[53] Alexander C, Oberhausen E. Myocardial scintigraphy. Seminars in Nuclear Medicine. 1995;**25**(2):195-201. DOI: 10.1016/S0001-2998(95)80026-3

[54] Javadi H et al. The role of gated myocardial perfusion scintigraphy (GMPS) in myocarditis: A case report and review of the literature. 2012;**14**(2):112-115

[55] Kiratli PO, Tuncel M, Ozkutlu S, Caglar M. Gated myocardial perfusion scintigraphy in children with myocarditis: Can it be considered as an indicator of clinical outcome? Nuclear Medicine Communications. 2008;**29**(10):907-914. DOI: 10.1097/MNM.0b013e328303359f

[56] Boccara F, Blanchard-Lemoine B, Sarda L, Bardet J, Le Guludec D, Cohen A. Diagnostic strategy in acute myocarditis. Archives des Maladies du Coeur et des Vaisseaux. 1998;**91**(9):1151-1158

[57] Hoey ETD, Gulati GS, Ganeshan A, Watkin RW, Simpson H, Sharma S. Cardiovascular MRI for assessment of infectious and inflammatory conditions of the heart. American Journal of Roentgenology. 2011;**197**(1):103-112. DOI: 10.2214/AJR.10.5666

[58] Dec GW et al. Antimyosin antibody cardiac imaging: Its role in the diagnois of myocarditis. Journal of the American College of Cardiology. 1990;**16**(1):97-104. DOI: 10.1016/0735-1097(90)90463-Y

[59] Moralidis E, Mantziari L, Gerasimou G, Styliadis IH, Gotzamani-Psarrakou A. Somatostatin analogue scintigraphy in a patient with viral myocarditis. Hellenic Journal of Nuclear Medicine. 2012;**15**(2):144-146. DOI: 10.1967/s002449910031

[60] O'Connell JB, Henkin RE, Robinson JA, Subramanian R, Scanlon PJ, Gunnar RM. Gallium-67 imaging in patients with dilated cardiomyopathy and biopsy-proven myocarditis. Circulation. 1984;**70**(1):58-62. DOI: 10.1161/01.CIR.70.1.58

[61] Strain JE, Fine E, Grose RM, Kramer DC, Cho S, Factor SM. Comparison of myocardial biopsy and gallium-67 imaging for diagnosing myocarditis. Circulation. 1983;**68**(Suppl.111):208

[62] Hung M-Y, Hung M-J, Cheng C-W. Use of gallium 67 scintigraphy to differentiate acute myocarditis from acute myocardial infarction. Texas Heart Institute Journal. 2007;**34**(3):305-309

[63] Narula J et al. Diagnostic accuracy of antimyosin scintigraphy in suspected myocarditis. Journal of Nuclear Cardiology. 1996;**3**(5):371-381. DOI: 10.1016/S1071-3581(96)90070-7

[64] Yasuda T et al. Indium 111-monoclonal antimyosin antibody imaging in the diagnosis of acute myocarditis. Circulation. 1987;**76**(2):306-311. DOI: 10.1161/01.CIR.76.2.306

[65] Le Guludec D, Sarda L, Rouzet F, Merlet P, Slama MS, Lebtahi R. Imaging inflammatory cardiomyopathies. Journal of Nuclear Cardiology. 2005;**12**(6):731-739. DOI: 10.1016/j.nuclcard.2005.09.005

[66] Martin MER et al. Role of noninvasive antimyosin imaging in infants and children with clinically suspected myocarditis. The Journal of Nuclear Medicine. 2004;**45**(3):429-437

[67] Kühl U, Lauer B, Souvatzoglu M, Vosberg H, Schultheiss H-P. Antimyosin

scintigraphy and immunohistologic analysis of endomyocardial biopsy in patients with clinically suspected myocarditis—Evidence of myocardial cell damage and inflammation in the absence of histologic signs of myocarditis. Journal of the American College of Cardiology. 1998;**32**(5):1371-1376. DOI: 10.1016/S0735-1097(98)00397-0

[68] Bière L, Piriou N, Ernande L, Rouzet F, Lairez O. Imaging of myocarditis and inflammatory cardiomyopathies. Archives of Cardiovascular Diseases. 2019;**112**(10):630-641. DOI: 10.1016/j.acvd.2019.05.007

[69] Sun Y et al. 99mTc-MIBI myocardial perfusion imaging in myocarditis. Nuclear Medicine Communications. 2003;**24**(7):779-783. DOI: 10.1097/01.mnm.0000080254.50447.5a

[70] Yilmaz A, Klingel K, Kandolf R, Sechtem U. Imaging in inflammatory heart disease: From the past to current clinical practice. Hellenic Journal of Cardiology. 2009;**50**(6):449-460

[71] Lawal I, Sathekge M. F-18 FDG PET/CT imaging of cardiac and vascular inflammation and infection. British Medical Bulletin. 2016;**120**(1):55-74. DOI: 10.1093/bmb/ldw035

[72] Chen W, Jeudy J. Assessment of myocarditis: Cardiac MR, PET/CT, or PET/MR? Current Cardiology Reports. 2019;**21**(8):76. DOI: 10.1007/s11886-019-1158-0

[73] Schneider S, Batrice A, Rischpler C, Eiber M, Ibrahim T, Nekolla SG. Utility of multimodal cardiac imaging with PET/MRI in cardiac sarcoidosis: Implications for diagnosis, monitoring and treatment. European Heart Journal. 2014;**35**(5):312. DOI: 10.1093/eurheartj/eht335

[74] Genovesi D et al. The role of positron emission tomography in the assessment of cardiac sarcoidosis. The British Journal of Radiology. 2019;**92**(1100):20190247. DOI: 10.1259/bjr.20190247

[75] von Olshausen G, Hyafil F, Langwieser N, Laugwitz K-L, Schwaiger M, Ibrahim T. Detection of acute inflammatory myocarditis in Epstein Barr virus infection using hybrid 18F-fluoro-deoxyglucose-positron emission tomography/magnetic resonance imaging. Circulation. 2014;**130**(11):925-926. DOI: 10.1161/CIRCULATIONAHA.114.011000

[76] Nensa F, Poeppel TD, Krings P, Schlosser T. Multiparametric assessment of myocarditis using simultaneous positron emission tomography/magnetic resonance imaging. European Heart Journal. 2014;**35**(32):2173-2173. DOI: 10.1093/eurheartj/ehu086

[77] Lamacie MM et al. Serial ^{18}F-fluorodeoxyglucose positron emission tomography imaging in a patient with giant cell myocarditis. Circulation. Cardiovascular Imaging. 2020;**13**(2):e009940. DOI: 10.1161/CIRCIMAGING.119.009940

[78] Prato FS et al. Can the inflammatory response be evaluated using ^{18}F-FDG within zones of microvascular obstruction after myocardial infarction? Journal of Nuclear Medicine. 2015;**56**(2):299-304. DOI: 10.2967/jnumed.114.147835

[79] Nensa F et al. Feasibility of FDG-PET in myocarditis: Comparison to CMR using integrated PET/MRI. Journal of Nuclear Cardiology. 2018;**25**(3):785-794. DOI: 10.1007/s12350-016-0616-y

[80] Evaluation of the feaSibility of FDG-PET/CT Images Comparing to MRI and Endomyocardial Biopsy Findings in clinicAlly Suspected Myocarditis. 2019.

Available from: https://clinicaltrials.gov/study/NCT04085718 [Accessed: September 01, 2019]

[81] Ammirati E et al. Acute and fulminant myocarditis: A pragmatic clinical approach to diagnosis and treatment. Current Cardiology Reports. 2018;**20**(11):114. DOI: 10.1007/s11886-018-1054-z

[82] Chopra H et al. Prognostic value of the infarct- and non-infarct like patterns and cardiovascular magnetic resonance parameters on long-term outcome of patients after acute myocarditis. International Journal of Cardiology. 2016;**212**:63-69. DOI: 10.1016/j.ijcard.2016.03.004

[83] Mewton N et al. Myocardial biomarkers and delayed enhanced cardiac magnetic resonance relationship in clinically suspected myocarditis and insight on clinical outcome. Journal of Cardiovascular Medicine. 2015;**16**(10):696. DOI: 10.2459/JCM.0000000000000024

[84] Aquaro GD et al. Cardiac MR with late gadolinium enhancement in acute myocarditis with preserved systolic function. Journal of the American College of Cardiology. 2017;**70**(16):1977-1987. DOI: 10.1016/j.jacc.2017.08.044

[85] Lim LJ, Tison GH, Delling FN. Artificial intelligence in cardiovascular imaging. Methodist DeBakey Cardiovascular Journal. 2020;**16**(2):138. DOI: 10.14797/mdcj-16-2-138

Chapter 8

Cardiac Magnetic Resonance in Progressive Systemic Sclerosis (Scleroderma)

Gonzalo J. Prado Bustamante and Alicia M. Maceira

Abstract

Progressive systemic sclerosis, or scleroderma, is a complex autoimmune disorder that frequently affects the cardiovascular system, which increases morbidity and mortality. Cardiovascular magnetic resonance (CMR) has emerged as a crucial diagnostic tool for detecting myocardial involvement in patients with scleroderma, even in the initial stages, offering advantages such as superior tissue characterization and functional evaluation for both diagnosis and prognostic assessment. In this chapter, a pathophysiologic description of the disease from a CMR perspective, along with a description of characteristic CMR findings, is presented. Finally, indications for CMR in scleroderma, CMR protocols and acquisition techniques, as well as the role of artificial intelligence in improving diagnostic accuracy, are summarized.

Keywords: scleroderma, progressive systemic sclerosis, CMR, late gadolinium enhancement, autoimmune disease, artificial intelligence

1. Introduction

Progressive systemic sclerosis (PSS), also known as scleroderma, is a chronic autoimmune disease characterized by progressive fibrosis of the skin and various organs, along with vascular abnormalities and an altered immune response. This process begins with the abnormal activation of T lymphocytes and the release of pro-inflammatory cytokines, such as tumor necrosis factor-alpha (TNF-α), interleukin 6 (IL-6), and interleukin 1 (IL-1). These cytokines activate fibroblasts, key cells in the production of collagen and other extracellular matrix components. In PSS, fibroblasts become hyperactive, leading to excessive accumulation of collagen in tissues, including the cardiac muscle [1].

This chronic inflammatory process also affects small blood vessels, causing severe endothelial dysfunction. The endothelium, responsible for regulating vascular tone and preventing clot formation, among other functions, becomes dysfunctional, favoring a pro-inflammatory and pro-fibrotic state. The release of molecules such as transforming growth factor-beta (TGF-β) plays a crucial role in this process, stimulating collagen production and the activation of myofibroblasts, the cells that generate fibrosis [2].

Over time, the chronic damage resulting from inflammation and endothelial dysfunction leads to myocardial fibrosis, in which normal cardiac tissue is replaced by collagen and extracellular matrix proteins. This decreases the heart's elasticity, compromising its ability to contract and eventually leading to cardiac dysfunction. This process can progress silently, without evident clinical symptoms, until fibrosis reaches a level that significantly impairs cardiac function.

In addition, the microvascular dysfunction that accompanies systemic sclerosis contributes to subclinical myocardial ischemia. This means that the small vessels in the heart cannot supply enough oxygen to the myocardial tissue, exacerbating cardiac damage. Although ischemia may not manifest with typical symptoms such as chest pain, its contribution to fibrosis development increases the risk of arrhythmias and severe events, such as sudden death [1, 2]. Although the skin is the most visibly affected organ, systemic sclerosis also frequently affects internal organs, which significantly contributes to its morbidity and mortality.

Systemic sclerosis presents in two main forms: diffuse and limited. The former is characterized by rapid progression and more extensive involvement of the skin and internal organs, affecting key organs, such as the lungs, heart, and kidneys. In contrast, the limited form has a slower progression and is associated with CREST syndrome, which includes calcinosis, Raynaud's phenomenon, esophageal dysmotility, sclerodactyly, and telangiectasias [2]. This classification is essential for prognosis and disease management, as the diffuse form tends to have worse clinical outcomes due to more extensive visceral involvement [2, 3].

The prevalence of systemic sclerosis varies geographically, with estimates ranging between 50 and 300 cases per million inhabitants, being significantly more common in women, with an approximate ratio of 4:1 compared to men [1]. Although it is a rare disease, its impact on patients' quality of life is significant due to multisystemic complications. The most frequently affected organs are the lungs, kidneys, heart, and gastrointestinal system, contributing to the morbidity and mortality of the disease. In particular, lung involvement occurs in about 70% of patients and is the main cause of scleroderma-related death [3]. Pulmonary fibrosis is the most common manifestation and significantly contributes to the high mortality rate [4].

Although renal involvement is less common, it can present as the renal crisis in systemic sclerosis, a severe complication occurring in 5–10% of patients that requires immediate medical attention to prevent fatal outcomes. Scleroderma renal crisis (SRC) is characterized by a rapid decline in renal function, typically due to a vasculopathy affecting the small renal vessels. This condition can lead to malignant hypertension and acute renal failure, which, if not treated promptly, can result in irreversible renal insufficiency. Approximately 25% of patients with SRC are diagnosed with systemic sclerosis at the time of renal presentation. Despite its severity, early detection of renal crisis can significantly improve prognosis, as appropriate intervention can partially reverse renal damage and prevent fatal consequences. About two-thirds of SRC cases require renal replacement therapy, such as dialysis, and of these, half may recover enough renal function to discontinue dialysis after 24 months. This potential for delayed renal recovery distinguishes SRC from other causes of end-stage renal failure. Historically, SRC was the most common cause of death associated with scleroderma, although advances in treatment, such as the use of angiotensin-converting enzyme (ACE) inhibitors, have dramatically improved short-term outcomes [5–7].

Cardiac involvement is another critical aspect of systemic sclerosis, as it represents a key risk factor for adverse outcomes. Cardiac manifestations include cardiomyopathy, arrhythmias, heart failure, and pulmonary hypertension (**Figure 1**). In severe cases,

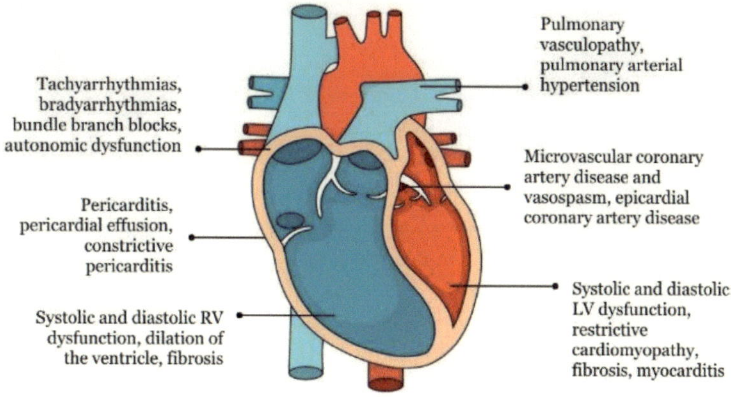

Figure 1.
Cardiovascular disease in systemic sclerosis.

myocardial fibrosis and microvascular dysfunction can lead to serious events, such as sudden death [8, 9]. Myocardial fibrosis, a common feature of cardiac involvement in scleroderma, results from a chronic inflammatory process and associated vasculopathy that compromises cardiac function. Myocardial fibrosis is detected in 15–50% of patients, depending on the diagnostic methods used [8]. Moreover, microvascular dysfunction and subclinical myocardial ischemia exacerbate cardiac damage and further promote myocardial fibrosis, complicating disease management [10].

As many of these cardiac manifestations are subclinical in the early stages, early detection is crucial to improve long-term outcomes. Cardiac Magnetic Resonance Imaging (CMR) has emerged as an invaluable diagnostic tool for the detailed characterization of the myocardium. CMR is the gold standard method for quantification of ventricular volumes, mass, and ejection fraction, particularly for the right ventricle, given its high accuracy and reproducibility. Also, CMR provides a unique capability of tissue characterization, allowing the detection of focal fibrosis through late gadolinium enhancement (LGE) [11]. This is crucial for a comprehensive view of the cardiac status in patients with systemic sclerosis, facilitating not only diagnosis but also monitoring and risk stratification (**Figure 2**) [12].

Recent studies have shown that myocardial fibrosis detected by CMR is associated with a higher risk of adverse cardiac events, including heart failure and arrhythmias in a wide range of cardiac conditions [11, 12]. This underlines the relevance of CMR not only in diagnosis but also its potential utility in risk stratification and long-term monitoring of disease progression, enabling a more personalized and targeted approach to their care [9, 13]. Despite its utility, the implementation of CMR in clinical guidelines is still limited, but its role is likely to expand with the use of advanced imaging techniques and artificial intelligence in the near future [11–13].

In addition to CMR, advanced imaging techniques such as T1 and T2 mapping allow for the detection of myocardial edema, interstitial fibrosis, and infiltration with substances such as amyloid. T1 mapping is particularly useful in cases of diffuse fibrosis that may not be detected by conventional late gadolinium enhancement techniques [14]. In addition, CMR allows the assessment of valvular function, noninvasive estimation of ventricular pressures and pulmonary vascular resistance, along with accurate depiction of aortic and pulmonary artery dimensions. Finally, stress CMR provides an accurate, noninvasive assessment of myocardial perfusion and the function of the microcirculation. Thus, CMR offers a comprehensive assessment of

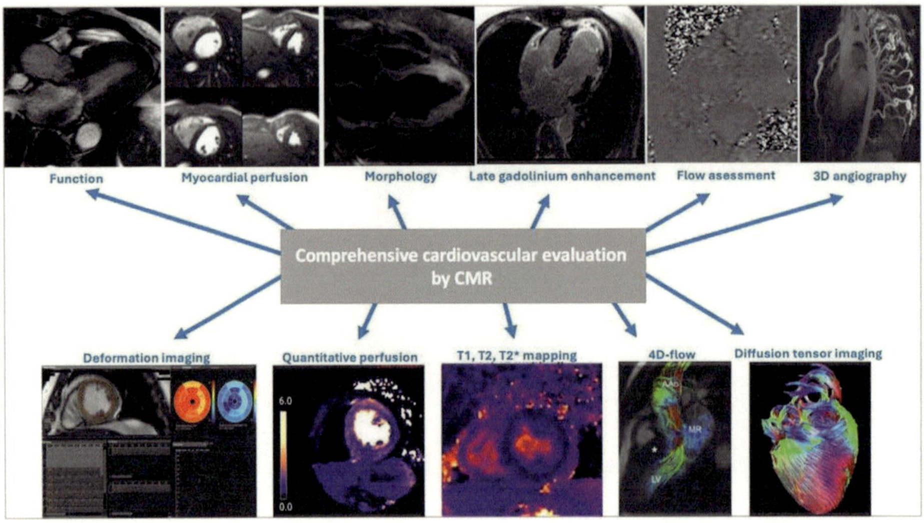

Figure 2.
Comprehensive evaluation of the cardiovascular system by cardiovascular magnetic resonance. The availability of several sequences (top) allows for a comprehensive evaluation of the cardiovascular system, including assessment of morphology, function, valve function, stress and rest myocardial perfusion, myocardial tissue characterization, and angiography. In recent years new sequences (bottom) have been implemented for further cardiovascular quantification, including deformation imaging, quantitative perfusion, parametric imaging, 4D Flow assessment, and diffusion tensor imaging.

the heart and great vessels in PSS for more precise diagnosis and effective monitoring of disease progression.

In summary, the growing evidence supports the use of CMR as an essential tool not only for the early diagnosis of cardiac involvement in PSS but also as a guide to treatment and long-term monitoring. By detecting myocardial fibrosis early, more effective and personalized interventions can be made, potentially improving clinical outcomes and reducing mortality [15].

2. Typical findings in cardiac magnetic resonance imaging (CMR) in scleroderma

Scleroderma is a multisystemic disease that affects numerous organs, including the heart, which significantly contributes to the morbidity and mortality of patients. Since cardiac involvement can be subclinical in the early stages, Cardiac Magnetic Resonance (CMR) has emerged as a cutting-edge tool for the comprehensive assessment of myocardial involvement. CMR provides a detailed, multimodal view of the myocardium, offering essential information on structure, ventricular function, fibrosis, edema, and myocardial perfusion, allowing for a noninvasive and precise evaluation [13]. In particular, CMR is a unique technique for myocardial tissue characterization (**Figures 3** and **4**).

2.1 Myocardial fibrosis

The most characteristic and clinically relevant finding on CMR in patients with scleroderma is myocardial fibrosis, detected through late gadolinium

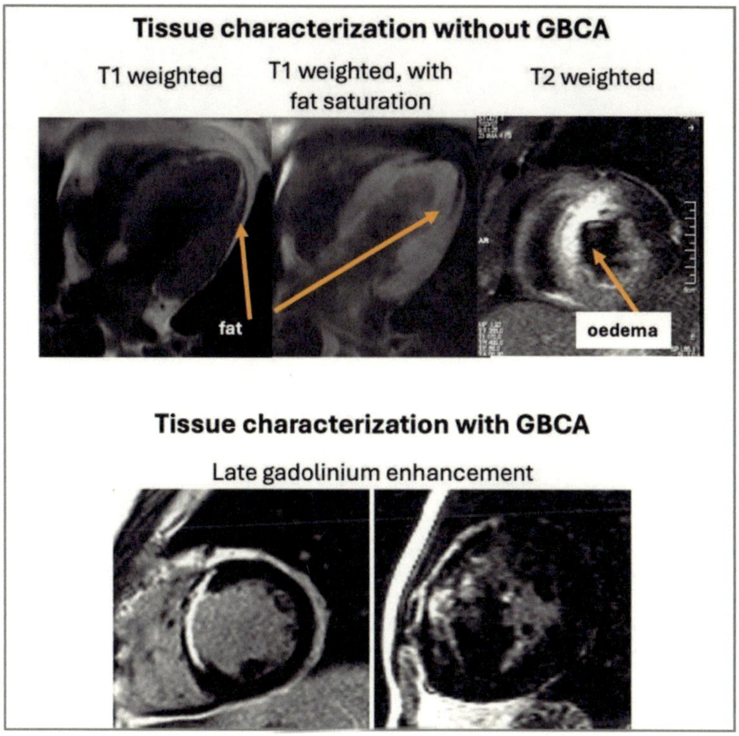

Figure 3.
CMR for myocardial tissue characterization. T1 and T2-weighted spin-echo sequences provide tissue characterization without the administration of gadolinium-based contrast agent (GBCA), mainly the detection of fat and water within the myocardium. Late gadolinium enhancement sequences allow for the detection of myocardial focal fibrosis as a white region inside the healthy myocardium, which in turn appears black.

enhancement (LGE). This myocardial fibrosis is one of the main contributors to cardiac dysfunction in scleroderma. Unlike fibrosis observed in ischemic heart disease, where LGE distribution follows vascular territories, in scleroderma, fibrosis tends to be patchy, subendocardial, or even diffuse, without following a clear ischemic pattern (**Figures 2** and 5) [16, 17].

Recent studies have shown that the presence of LGE in scleroderma patients is associated with a worse prognosis, as it reflects irreversible myocardial damage. Fibrosis detected by LGE increases the risk of developing ventricular arrhythmias and sudden death, highlighting the importance of CMR for risk stratification in these patients [18]. Additionally, the extent and pattern of fibrosis observed on LGE provide valuable information for predicting long-term outcomes and guiding therapeutic decisions [17]. Along with the progression of myocardial fibrosis ventricular function becomes compromised, emphasizing the importance of early detection through CMR.

2.2 Myocardial edema

In addition to fibrosis, identifying myocardial edema through CMR is crucial for detecting active myocardial inflammation. Myocardial edema is a marker of acute inflammation and can be visualized on CMR using T2-weighted sequences, which are sensitive to water content in tissues. Detecting areas of active inflammation is essential, since myocardial edema may precede the development of irreversible fibrosis,

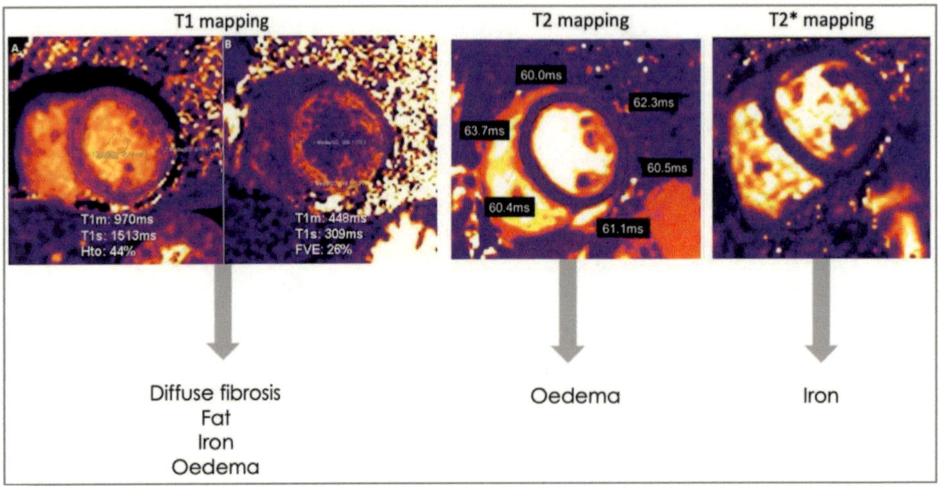

Figure 4.
CMR parametric techniques for further tissue characterization. Parametric techniques have been developed recently for tissue characterization beyond late gadolinium enhancement. T1 mapping allows for a direct measure of the longitudinal relaxation time, which increases in diffuse fibrosis and edema, and decreases when there is fat or iron infiltration in the myocardium. T2 mapping measures the transverse relaxation time and increases in the presence of myocardial edema. T2 mapping measures the inhomogeneity of the myocardium due to iron deposition.*

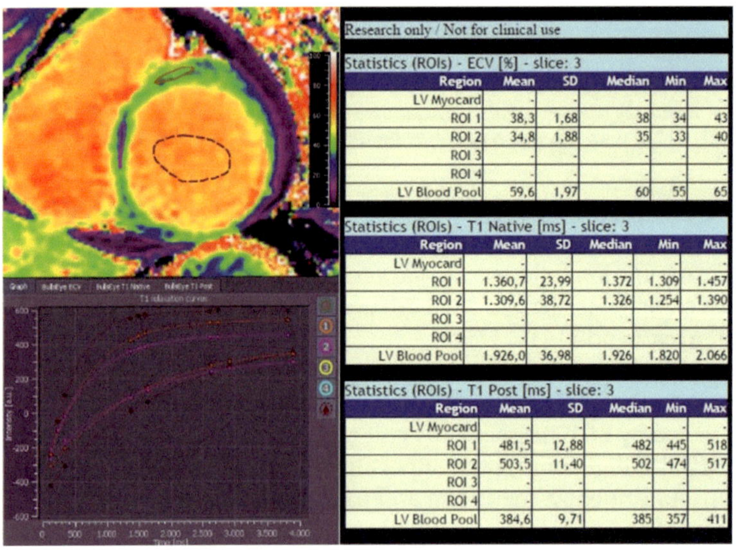

Figure 5.
Diffuse fibrosis in a patient with scleroderma.

representing a stage of the disease where damage could still be reversible with therapeutic intervention [16]. In scleroderma, myocardial edema can present.

subclinically, making CMR a crucial tool for early detection and preventing progression to permanent myocardial fibrosis.

It is important to note that the presence of myocardial edema without evidence of LGE suggests an early stage of cardiac involvement, offering a therapeutic window

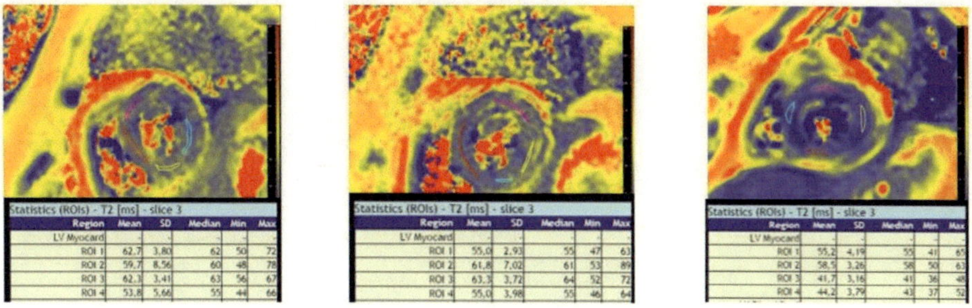

Figure 6.
Improvement of the T2 mapping parameter in a patient with subclinical disease. A patient whose treatment was intensified. The CRMs were carried out 6 months apart.

where intervention could prevent the progression to irreversible fibrosis (**Figure 2**). This information is essential for guiding clinical management, especially in asymptomatic patients or those with mild symptoms (**Figure 6**) [19, 20].

2.3 Microvascular dysfunction and myocardial perfusion

Another key aspect of cardiac involvement in scleroderma is microvascular dysfunction, which contributes to subclinical myocardial ischemia and fibrosis progression. CMR allows for the detailed evaluation of myocardial perfusion using perfusion sequences, essential for detecting microvascular alterations that may go unnoticed in other imaging modalities, such as echocardiography or computed tomography. These perfusion abnormalities often reflect extensive microvascular compromise, contributing not only to myocardial ischemia but also to the progression of myocardial fibrosis [21].

In scleroderma patients, microvascular dysfunction can be present even in the absence of overt cardiac symptoms, reinforcing the importance of CMR in comprehensive cardiovascular risk assessment. Detecting myocardial perfusion abnormalities through CMR allows for the identification of patients at risk of adverse cardiac events and could influence the decision to initiate preventive therapies [22, 23].

2.4 Assessment of ventricular function

CMR cine sequences are fundamental for the precise evaluation of ventricular function. These sequences allow for detailed measurement of ventricular volumes, ejection fraction, and abnormal ventricular wall motion patterns, all of which are crucial for assessing heart functionality. In scleroderma patients, ventricular dysfunction is common and often results from a combination of myocardial fibrosis, microvascular dysfunction, and even secondary pulmonary hypertension (**Figure 7**).

Early detection of ventricular dysfunction through CMR is paramount, as it can precede the onset of clinical symptoms. This allows for more timely therapeutic intervention, which could slow down or even prevent the progression of heart failure [24, 25].

2.5 Pericardial effusion and pericardial involvement

Pericardial effusion is another common finding on CMR in scleroderma patients. Although it is a less specific finding, its presence is often related to systemic inflammation and microvascular dysfunction. CMR not only allows for the precise

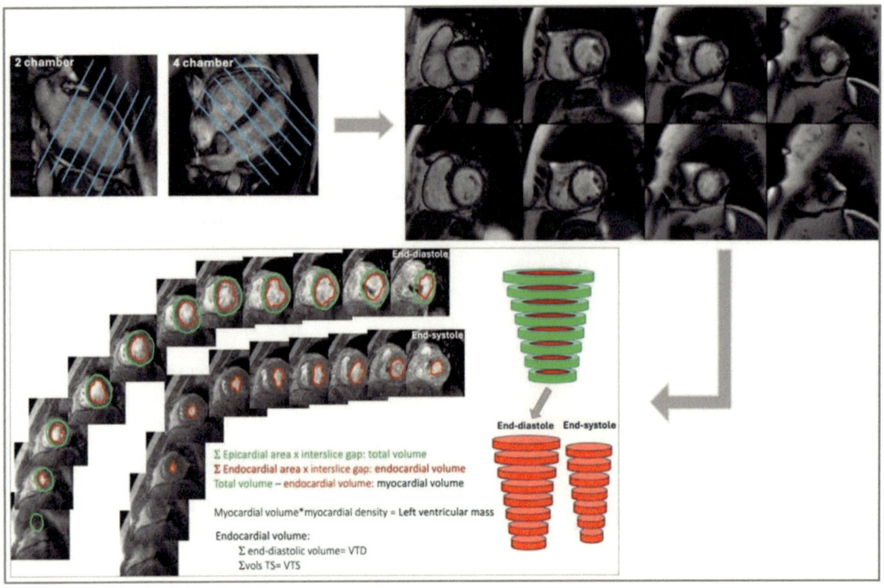

Figure 7.
CMR for quantification of ventricular dimensions and function. CMR is the most accurate and reproducible technique for the measurement of left and right ventricular dimensions and function. These parameters are obtained by Simpson's rule as depicted in the figure. A short axis stack of parallel cine sequences is obtained from the atrioventricular groove to the apex with a fixed interslice gap. Endocardial and epicardial boundaries are drawn to obtain the surface area of each slice from which volumes are obtained as shown.

evaluation of the amount of fluid in the pericardium but also the identification of pericardial thickening, which may indicate an underlying chronic inflammatory process.

Detailed pericardial assessment provided by CMR is crucial, as some patients may require additional interventions, such as fluid drainage or targeted anti-inflammatory therapy. The ability of CMR to detect these complications allows for appropriate monitoring and adjustment of therapies based on clinical evolution [26] (**Figures 3** and **8**).

2.6 Right ventricular dysfunction

Many patients with systemic sclerosis present with right ventricular dysfunction due to associated pulmonary arterial hypertension (PAH). It is crucial to detect dysfunction in this population, as it may be an even stronger predictor of mortality than pulmonary hypertension detected by cardiac catheterization [27].

In a multicenter study of 570 systemic sclerosis patients, only 1.4% had left ventricular systolic dysfunction on echocardiography, though 22.6% had left ventricular hypertrophy and 17.7% had left ventricular diastolic dysfunction. In the European League Against Rheumatism (EULAR) database, the prevalence of reduced left ventricular ejection fraction was 5.4% [28, 29].

Though traditional echocardiographic screening suggests the prevalence of right ventricular dysfunction in systemic sclerosis patients is low, CMR is the most accurate technique for the evaluation of the right ventricle and may be more sensitive than echocardiography for detecting subclinical myocardial involvement [30].

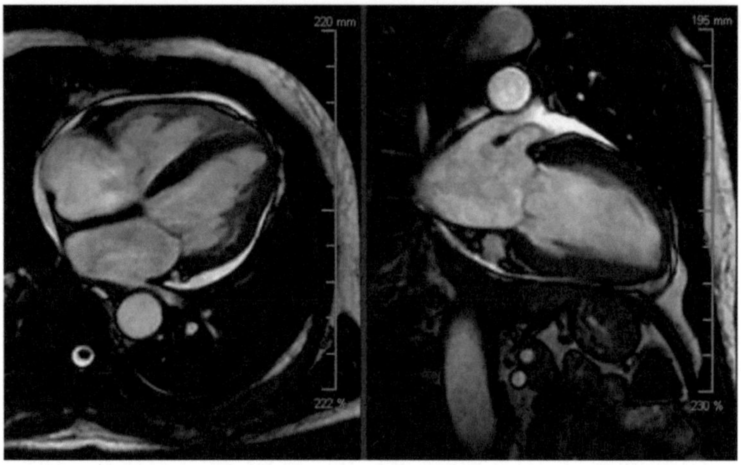

Figure 8.
Patient with light-moderate circumferential pericardial effusion. Recently diagnosed with systemic sclerosis with lung, kidney, and heart disease.

2.7 Other relevant findings

Another relevant finding is the detection of intracavitary thrombi, especially in patients with severe ventricular dysfunction. While these thrombi may go unnoticed in other imaging modalities, CMR has the ability to detect them with greater sensitivity, which is important for preventing embolic events [31, 32].

In summary, Cardiac Magnetic Resonance offers a comprehensive and detailed view of cardiac involvement in scleroderma. Its ability to assess fibrosis, edema, perfusion, and ventricular function makes it an essential tool for risk stratification and therapeutic planning. CMR not only enables the early detection of subclinical alterations but also facilitates continuous monitoring of disease progression, helping to optimize treatment and improve long-term outcomes in patients with scleroderma.

3. Indications for cardiac magnetic resonance imaging (CMR) in scleroderma

While echocardiography is the gold standard for monitoring patients with systemic sclerosis, cardiovascular Magnetic Resonance Imaging (CMR) can play a role in identifying those patients at higher cardiovascular risk. Currently, there is no consensus on how CMR should be used to guide treatment in systemic sclerosis. However, due to its ability to detect early changes such as myocardial fibrosis, inflammation, and ventricular dysfunction, CMR enables early intervention that may alter the course of the disease. Below, the main clinical indications for CMR in the context of scleroderma are outlined, addressing both subclinical involvement and more advanced manifestations [33].

3.1 Evaluation of subclinical cardiac involvement

One of the main challenges in managing scleroderma is the early detection of cardiac involvement, which may be subclinical in the early stages of the disease.

CMR could be indicated in patients with scleroderma even when they do not have obvious cardiac symptoms, as structural and functional changes may precede the appearance of clinical symptoms. This is particularly relevant in patients with long-standing scleroderma or extensive skin involvement, who are at an increased risk of developing cardiac complications. Early detection of myocardial fibrosis or edema by CMR allows timely intervention, which may delay disease progression and improve long-term prognosis [11, 13, 23].

3.2 Nonspecific cardiac symptoms

In patients with scleroderma presenting with nonspecific cardiac symptoms such as exertional dyspnea, fatigue, palpitations, or atypical chest pain, CMR may be indicated to rule out underlying myocardial involvement that cannot be detected with other diagnostic modalities [3]. These symptoms may be related to processes such as myocardial fibrosis, microvascular dysfunction, or pulmonary hypertension, all of which are accurately detectable by CMR [4]. CMR allows differentiation between cardiac and noncardiac causes of symptoms, which is crucial to guide appropriate therapeutic management and avoid unnecessary treatments (**Figure 9**) [23, 30].

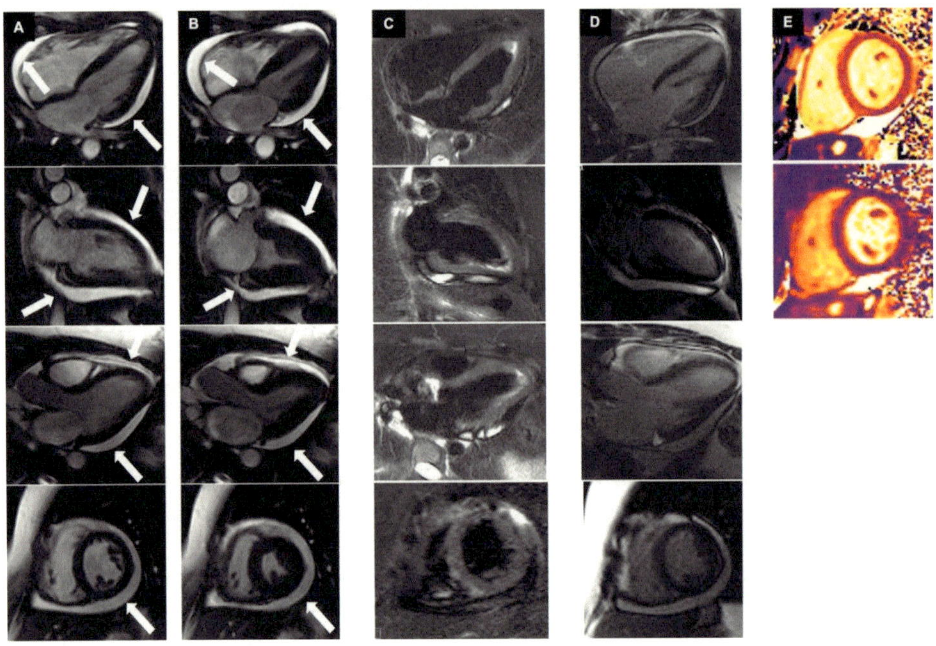

Figure 9.
CMR study at 3 T of a 41 y.o. woman with PSS and pericardial effusion saw in follow-up transthoracic echocardiography. CMR was requested to rule out acute myocardial inflammation. Cine images in (top to bottom) the 4-chamber, 2-chamber, 3-chamber, and mid-short axis views (A) and corresponding end-systolic cine (B), STIR (C) and late gadolinium (D) images. Native T1 (top) and T2 (bottom) maps are shown in (E). Left and right ventricular volumes were normal as well as left ventricular mass without any regional wall motion abnormalities. No myocardial edema was detected. No late gadolinium enhancement was seen. The pericardium of normal thickness and signal intensity but mild pericardial effusion was observed (arrows) with transudate characteristics (native T1 3565ms) and no signs of hemodynamic compromise.

3.3 Abnormalities in previous diagnostic studies

Another important indication for CMR in scleroderma is the presence of abnormal findings on previous diagnostic studies, such as echocardiography or electrocardiogram, that suggest cardiac involvement but do not provide sufficient information for a definitive diagnosis. For example, a new conduction disturbance on the electrocardiogram in a patient with scleroderma should be followed by CMR to assess for the presence of myocardial fibrosis or edema, which is a known risk factor for arrhythmias and sudden death (**Figure 2**). Similarly, in patients with scleroderma and preserved ejection fraction on echocardiography but with clinical signs of heart failure, CMR can detect subendocardial fibrosis or microvascular dysfunction that could be contributing to the symptoms (**Figure 10**) [33].

3.4 Risk stratification in asymptomatic patients

CMR plays an essential role in the risk stratification of asymptomatic patients with scleroderma, especially in those with additional risk factors such as pulmonary hypertension or renal involvement. CMR can identify patients who, despite

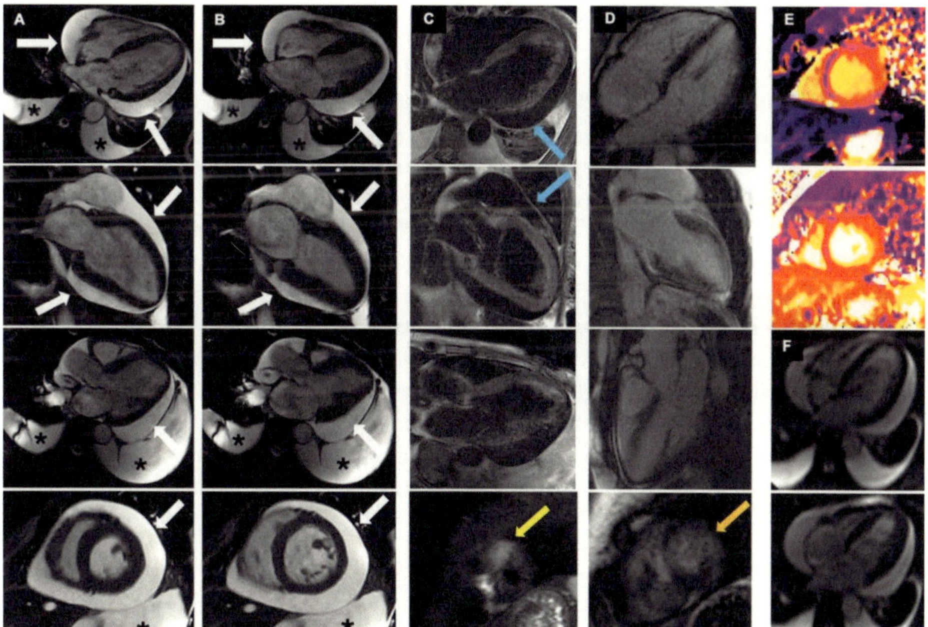

Figure 10.
CMR study at 3 T of a 47 y.o. woman with PSS of 13 yrs. admitted 15 days previous with acute renal failure and acute pulmonary edema. CMR was requested after discharge to rule out myocardial involvement. Cine images in (top to bottom) the 4-chamber, 2-chamber, 3-chamber, and mid-short axis views (A) and corresponding end-systolic cine (B), STIR (C), and late gadolinium (D) images. Native T1 (top) and T2 (bottom) maps are shown in (E). The left ventricle appears mildly dilated and with mild systolic dysfunction. The right ventricle is of normal size and function. Spin-echo sequences show myocardial edema in the anteroapical wall (yellow arrow) with corresponding late gadolinium enhancement (orange arrow) and T1 and T2maps. Overall high signal intensity was observed in the pericardium (blue arrow) with severe pericardial effusion (White arrows). The presence of diastolic right atrial collapse in real-time cine sequences (F) along with dilated inferior vena cava is indicative of hemodynamic compromise. Bilateral pleural effusion was also seen (stars).

not presenting symptoms, have significant myocardial involvement, which places them at an increased risk of developing serious cardiac complications such as heart failure, ventricular arrhythmias, or even sudden death. This proactive approach allows for early therapeutic interventions, including the use of immunosuppressants or treatments targeting fibrosis, aiming to prevent disease progression and improve survival [16, 19].

3.5 Pre-treatment evaluation and monitoring therapeutic response

Before initiating immunosuppressive therapy in patients with scleroderma, CMR is useful to establish a baseline on the extent of myocardial involvement. This is critical for selecting the most appropriate therapeutic regimen and for monitoring response to treatment. CMR allows for accurate assessment of changes in myocardial fibrosis and ventricular function over time, providing crucial information on the effectiveness of treatment and the need for treatment adjustments. Furthermore, in patients undergoing treatment, CMR is valuable for detecting disease progression or the emergence of new cardiac complications, which may indicate the need to intensify or change therapy [11].

3.6 Monitoring disease progression

In patients with scleroderma and known cardiac involvement, CMR is the tool of choice for long-term follow-up. This monitoring is crucial for assessing the progression of myocardial fibrosis, ventricular dysfunction, or cardiac disease [14].

3.7 Follow-up on pulmonary involvement

CMR monitoring is not only useful for assessing the progression of fibrosis but also for detecting the progression of pulmonary hypertension, which often affects the right ventricle. Detailed follow-up of right ventricular function *via* CMR is essential for predicting and preventing additional complications. With this technique, it is possible to measure not only right ventricular volume and systolic function but also parameters such as flow measurement, pulmonary artery velocities, and estimates of pulmonary vascular resistance, among other signs of pulmonary hypertension [34].

4. Conclusion

CMR is a fundamental tool in the evaluation and management of cardiac involvement in scleroderma, offering a detailed and accurate view that surpasses other imaging modalities. Its ability to detect myocardial fibrosis, assess ventricular function, and monitor disease progression makes it an indispensable technique in managing these patients. The implementation of CMR in clinical practice allows for better risk stratification, early intervention, and effective monitoring of therapeutic response, contributing to improved long-term outcomes in patients with scleroderma. With advances in technology, including developments in artificial intelligence and acquisition protocols, the diagnostic accuracy and clinical utility of CMR are expected to continue improving, offering an even more personalized and effective approach to managing cardiac disease in scleroderma [35].

Conflict of interest

The authors declare no conflict of interest. All figures included in the manuscript are edited and original by the authors, not previously published.

Author details

Gonzalo J. Prado Bustamante and Alicia M. Maceira*
Ascires, Valencia, España

*Address all correspondence to: amaceira@ascires.com

References

[1] Lee K-I, Manuntag LJ, Kifayat A, Manuntag SE, Sperber K, Ash JY, et al. Cardiovascular manifestations of systemic sclerosis: An overview of pathophysiology, screening modalities, and treatment options. Cardiology in Review. 2023;**31**(1):22-27

[2] Zanin-Silva DC, Santana-Gonçalves M, Kawashima-Vasconcelos MY, Oliveira MC. Management of Endothelial Dysfunction in systemic sclerosis: Current and developing strategies. Frontiers in Medicine. 2021;**8**:788250. DOI: 10.3389/fmed.2021.788250

[3] LeRoy EC, Black C, Fleischmajer R, Jablonska S, Krieg T, Medsger TA Jr, et al. Scleroderma (systemic sclerosis): Classification, subsets and pathogenesis. The Journal of Rheumatology. 1988;**15**(2):202-205

[4] McNearney TA et al. Pulmonary involvement in systemic sclerosis: Associations with genetic, serologic, sociodemographic, and behavioural factors. Arthritis and Rheumatism. 2007;**57**(2):318-326

[5] Denton CP. Renal manifestations of systemic sclerosis--clinical features and outcome assessment. Rheumatology (Oxford, England). 2008;**47**(Suppl. 5): v54-v56. DOI: 10.1093/rheumatology/ken307

[6] Penn H, Howie AJ, Kingdon EJ, et al. Scleroderma renal crisis: Patient characteristics and long-term outcomes. The Quarterly Journal of Medicine. 2007;**100**:485-494

[7] Steen VD, Medsger TA. Changes in causes of death in systemic sclerosis, 1972-2002. Annals of the Rheumatic Diseases. 2007;**66**:940-944

[8] Steen V. The heart in systemic sclerosis. Current Rheumatology Reports. 2004;**6**:137-140

[9] Nihtyanova SI, Schreiber BE, Ong VH, Rosenberg D, Moinzadeh P, Coghlan JG, et al. Prediction of pulmonary complications and long-term survival in systemic sclerosis. Arthritis & Rhematology. 2014;**66**:1625-1635. DOI: 10.1002/art.38390

[10] Ross L, Costello B, Brown Z, Hansen D, Lindqvist A, Stevens W, et al. Myocardial fibrosis and arrhythmic burden in systemic sclerosis. Rheumatology (Oxford, England). 2022;**61**(11):4497-4502. DOI: 10.1093/rheumatology/keac065

[11] Glynn P, Hale S, Hussain T, Freed BH. Cardiovascular imaging for systemic sclerosis monitoring and management. Frontiers in Cardiovascular Medicine. 2022;**9**:846213. DOI: 10.3389/fcvm.2022.846213

[12] Poindron V, Chatelus E, Canuet M, Gottenberg JE, Arnaud L, Gangi A, et al. T1 mapping cardiac magnetic resonance imaging frequently detects subclinical diffuse myocardial fibrosis in systemic sclerosis patients. Seminars in Arthritis and Rheumatism. 2020;**50**(1):128-134. DOI: 10.1016/j.semarthrit.2019.06.013. Epub 2019 Jun 19

[13] Fairley JL, O'Rourke R, Puranik R, Nikpour M. Cardiac magnetic resonance imaging in systemic sclerosis: Heart involvement in high-resolution. Rheumatology and Immunology Research. 2024;**5**(2):83-92. DOI: 10.1515/rir-2024-0011

[14] Haaf P, Garg P, Messroghli DR, Broadbent DA, Greenwood JP, Plein S.

Cardiac T1 mapping and extracellular volume (ECV) in clinical practice: A comprehensive review. Journal of Cardiovascular Magnetic Resonance. 2016;**18**(1):89. DOI: 10.1186/s12968-016- 0308-4

[15] Bing R. Dweck MR myocardial fibrosis: Why image, how to image and clinical implications. Heart. 2019;**105**:1832-1840

[16] Ambale-Venkatesh B, Lima JA. Cardiac MRI: a central prognostic tool in myocardial fibrosis. Nature Reviews. Cardiology. 2015;**12**:18-29

[17] Hundley WG, Bluemke D, Bogaert JG, et al. Society for cardiovascular magnetic resonance guidelines for reporting cardiovascular magnetic resonance examinations. Journal of Cardiovascular Magnetic Resonance. 2009;**11**:5.s

[18] De Luca G, Bombace S, Monti L. Heart involvement in systemic sclerosis: The role of magnetic resonance imaging. Clinical Reviews in Allergy and Immunology. 2023;**64**(3):343-357. DOI: 10.1007/s12016-022-08923-3. Epub 2022 Jan 24

[19] Mavrogeni SI, Bratis K, Karabela G, et al. Cardiovascular magnetic resonance imaging clarifies cardiac pathophysiology in early, asymptomatic diffuse systemic sclerosis. Inflammation and Allergy Drug Targets. 2015;**14**:29-36

[20] De Luca G, Palmisano A, Campochiaro C, et al. Cardiac magnetic resonance in systemic sclerosis myocarditis: The value of T2 mapping to detect myocardial inflammation. Rheumatology (Oxford, England). 2022;**61**:4409-4419

[21] Kellman P, Hansen MS, Nielles-Vallespin S, et al. Myocardial perfusion cardiovascular magnetic resonance: Optimized dual sequence and reconstruction for quantification. Journal of Cardiovascular Magnetic Resonance. 2017;**19**:43

[22] Follansbee WP, Curtiss EI, Medsger TA Jr, et al. Physiologic abnormalities of cardiac function in progressive systemic sclerosis with diffuse scleroderma. The New England Journal of Medicine. 1984;**310**:142-148

[23] Dumitru RB, Bissell LA, Erhayiem B, et al. Subclinical systemic sclerosis primary heart involvement by cardiovascular magnetic resonance shows No significant interval change. ACR Open Rheumatology. 2023;**5**:71-80

[24] Kramer CM, Barkhausen J, Bucciarelli-Ducci C, et al. Standardized cardiovascular magnetic resonance imaging (CMR) protocols: 2020 update. Journal of Cardiovascular Magnetic Resonance. 2020;**22**:17

[25] Captur G, Manisty C, Moon JC. Cardiac MRI evaluation of myocardial disease. Heart. 2016;**102**:1429-1435

[26] Antonopoulos AS, Vrettos A, Androulakis E, et al. Cardiac magnetic resonance imaging of pericardial diseases: A comprehensive guide. European Heart Journal Cardiovascular Imaging. 2023;**24**:983-998

[27] Tennøe AH, Murbræch K, Andreassen JC, et al. Left ventricular diastolic dysfunction predicts mortality in patients with systemic sclerosis. Journal of the American College of Cardiology. 2018;**72**(15):1804-1813. DOI: 10.1016/j.jacc.2018.07.068

[28] Groote P, Gressin V, Hachulla E, et al. Evaluation of cardiac abnormalities by Doppler echocardiography in a large nationwide multicentric cohort of patients with systemic sclerosis.

Annals of the Rheumatic Diseases. 2008;**67**(1):31-36. DOI: 10.1136/ard.2006.057760

[29] Allanore Y, Meune C, Vonk MC, et al. Prevalence and factors associated with left ventricular dysfunction in the EULAR scleroderma trial and research group (EUSTAR) database of patients with systemic sclerosis. Annals of the Rheumatic Diseases. 2010;**69**(1):218-221

[30] Hachulla AL, Launay D, Gaxotte V, et al. Cardiac magnetic resonance imaging in systemic sclerosis: A cross-sectional observational study of 52 patients. Annals of the Rheumatic Diseases. 2009;**68**(12):1878-1884

[31] Barkhausen J, Hunold P, Eggebrecht H, et al. Detection and characterization of intracardiac thrombi on MR imaging. AJR. American Journal of Roentgenology. 2002;**179**:1539-1544

[32] Weinsaft J, Kim H, Shah DJ, et al. Detection of left ventricular thrombus by delayed-enhancement CMR: Prevalence and markers in patients with systolic dysfunction. Journal of the American College of Cardiology. 2008;**52**:148-157

[33] Mavrogeni SI, Sfikakis PP, Dimitroulas T, et al. Prospects of using cardiovascular magnetic resonance in the identification of arrhythmogenic substrate in autoimmune rheumatic diseases. Rheumatology International. 2018;**38**(9):1615-1621. DOI: 10.1007/s00296-018-4110-5

[34] Laffon E, Vallet C, Bernard V, et al. A computed method for noninvasive MRI assessment of pulmonary hypertension. Journal of Applied Physiology. 2004;**96**:463-468

[35] Fotaki A, Puyol-Antón E, Chiribiri A, et al. Artificial intelligence in cardiac MRI: Is clinical adoption forthcoming? Frontiers in Cardiovascular Medicine. 2022;**8**:818765

Section 3

Interventions for Inflammatory Myocardial Diseases

Chapter 9

Emergency Veno-Arterial Extracorporeal Membrane Oxygenation for Fulminant Myocarditis Complicated with Cardiogenic Shock

Mohamed Laimoud, Mosleh Alanazi, Rehan Qureshi, Emad Hakami, Khalid Hussein, Rozana Sadraldin and Ismail Raslan

Abstract

Fulminant myocarditis is a life-threatening condition that can rapidly progress to cardiogenic shock or cardiac arrest. Because of its rarity and different etiologies, it can be challenging to diagnose. It should be kept in the differential diagnosis, especially in patients without known cardiomyopathy. We present two cases with Fulminant myocarditis (FM) that were challenging for the medical team to diagnose and achieve successful outcomes. The first patient had systemic lupus erythematosus and had presented with cardiogenic shock. The second patient had FM after COVID-19 vaccination and presented with out-of-hospital cardiac arrest and required extracorporeal cardiopulmonary resuscitation (ECPR). Veno-arterial extracorporeal membrane oxygenation (VA-ECMO) is a life-saving short-term circulatory and ventilatory support that gives the medical team sufficient time to reach an accurate diagnosis and deliver definite management. Moreover, VA-ECMO can be a bridge to a durable ventricular assist device or heart transplantation in case of failed cardiac recovery.

Keywords: fulminant myocarditis, cardiogenic shock, extracorporeal membrane oxygenation, VA-ECMO, systemic lupus erythematosus, COVID-19

1. Introduction

Myocarditis refers to myocardial inflammation that can be caused due to infections, drugs, and autoimmune diseases, and the presentations vary from mild discomfort to severe conditions including sudden cardiac death [1]. Fulminant myocarditis (FM) is a severe myocardial injury that can rapidly progress to cardiogenic shock and ventricular arrhythmias with a high mortality in the absence of timely management

[2]. The estimated rates of acute myocarditis have been reported as 4.4 cases per 100,000 women and 6.1 cases per 100,000 men, and FM represented 5–10% of them [3]. There is under-reporting of myocarditis due to difficulty in getting the diagnosis without cardiac magnetic resonance imaging (MRI) and myocardial biopsy. Fulminant myocarditis is a rare, highly challenging clinical condition with high mortality rates if emergency support and definite treatment are not timely delivered. The studies that reported the outcomes of patients with FM who received mechanical circulatory support (MCS), mainly veno-arterial extracorporeal membrane oxygenation (VA-ECMO), were summarized in **Table 1** [4–24]. The aim of this chapter is to review the importance of early diagnosis of FM and potential benefits of early implementation of MCS, mainly VA-ECMO. We will present two challenging cases of FM of different etiologies with different presentations that have been successfully managed and survived after VA-ECMO and intra-aortic balloon pump (IABP) support.

2. VA-ECMO supported patients with FM

2.1 Fulminant myocarditis due to SLE

A 17-year-old female patient with a body surface area (BSA) 1.35 m^2 and a body mass index (BMI) 16.4 kg/m^2, presented with shortness of breath, arthralgia, and seizures, and she was diagnosed with Systemic lupus erythematosus (SLE) according to the clinical criteria and laboratory evidence: positive antinuclear antibody (ANA) and anti-Smith antibodies, low levels of serum compliments (C3&C4), and hemolytic anemia. Transthoracic echocardiography (TTE) revealed normal-sized left ventricle (LV) with ejection fraction (EF) 45–50%, mild global hypokinesia, normal right ventricle (RV), normal valves, and pulmonary artery systolic pressure (PASP) 25 mmHg without pericardial effusion. She received high-dose corticosteroid therapy, intravenous immunoglobulins (IVIG), maintenance prednisolone, and hydroxychloroquine therapy. Brain MRI excluded vascular insult and brain space-occupying lesions.

Two weeks after hospital discharge, she presented to the emergency department with shortness of breath and palpitations. She was lethargic without focal neurological manifestations. The vital signs: blood pressure 88/45 mmHg, sinus tachycardia: 159 bpm, temperature 38.2°C, respiratory rate (RR) 39 bpm, pulse oximetry saturation (SPO2%) 82% on ambient air. Arterial blood gases (ABG) revealed lactic acidosis and hypoxemia. Chest X-ray (CXR) revealed bilateral pulmonary infiltrates, suggesting pulmonary edema and possibility of right-sided infection (**Figure 1**).

Hemodynamic and respiratory support was done using vasopressors and invasive mechanical ventilation. There was no alveolar hemorrhage. Laboratory work-up revealed: white blood cell count of 12.9 (10^9/L), platelet count of 29 (10^9/L), hemoglobin 87 (g/L), serum Na 137 mmol/L, pro-BNP 47,347 ng/L, procalcitonin 1.7 mcg/L, serum creatinine 57 umol/L, serum bilirubin 6 umol/L, albumin 29 (g/L), alanine transaminase 33 unit/L, INR 1,4, fibrinogen 2 (g/L), haptoglobin 0.25(g/L). Septic and virology screening was done, including influenza, corona, coxsackie, Epstein-Barr, respiratory syncytial and adenoviruses, and COVID-19 PCR. TTE revealed LV dilatation with EF 20%, global hypokinesia, and moderate-sized circumferential pericardial effusion. Left ventricular outflow tract (LVOT) velocity time interval (VTI) 5.4 cm/m^2, PASP 30 mmHg, tricuspid annular plane

Studies	Patients' characteristics	Number of patients (MCS)	Study period	Outcomes
Tonna et al. [4]	4792 patients with ECLS for COVID-19, 88 patients had myocarditis with a mean age 47.6 ± 13.7 yrs., 65% were males, 24% had diabetes mellitus, and a mean SAVE score − 5.2 ± 3.5	88 (ECMO)	2020–2021	49% survival to discharge
Ammirati et al. [5]	54 patients with COVID-19 myocarditis, a median age 39 yrs., 39% were females, and 39% had cardiogenic shock.	10 patients (6 ECMO, 5 IABP,2 Impella, 1 Centrimag LVAD)	2020–2021	78.5% survival after 120 days
Nunez et al. [6]	850 patients with a mean age 40.9 ± 14.6 years, 51.6% of them were males, 82% had idiopathic myocarditis, 18% had viral myocarditis.	850 (ECMO), 20 patients upgraded to durable LVAD,	2011–2020	65.1% survival to discharge. 16 patients had HTx.
Tadokoro et al. [7]	70 patients received VA-ECMO, 57% of them were males, 75.7% of them had lymphocytic myocarditis. 8.6% had eosinophilic myocarditis, and 7.1% had giant cell myocarditis.	70 (ECMO), 48 patients upgraded to durable LVAD.	2006–2020	76% 5-year survival. 2 patients had HTx.
Chou et al. [8]	273 patients with myocarditis, 88 patients required VA-ECMO, with a mean age 41.8 years, and 60% were females.	88 (ECMO), 14 patients shifted to Centrimag LVAD, 1 had durable LVAD	2006–2018	48.9% survival to discharge without durable MCS. 7 patients had HTx
Danial et al. [9]	1254 patients with VA-ECMO, of them 47 patients had FM with a mean age 45.8 ± 14.4 years, 45% of them were females, and a mean SOFA score 12.4 ± 5.3.	47 (ECMO)	2015–2018	37.9% survival to discharge and 32.9% 5-year survival
Annamalai et al. [10]	34 patients with FM, with a mean age 42 ± 17 years, and 34% of them were males.	34 (Impella), 11 patients received IABP before Impella.	2009–2016	61.8% survival to discharge, 1 patient had HTx.
Saito et al. [11]	30 patients with FM, 8 patients of them received immunosuppressive therapy.	25 (23 ECMO, 2 temporary LVAD)	2009–2015	83.3% survival to discharge. 6 patients had permanent LVAD
Mody et al. [12]	260 patients received MCS, 11 patients had FM required MCS.	11 (3 ECMO,8 Centrimag BiVAD)	2007–2013	73% survival to discharge, 2 patients had durable LVAD. 1 patient had HTx
Lorusso et al. [13]	57 patients with FM, with a mean age 37.6 ± 11.8 years, 65% of them were females.	57 (ECMO)	2008–2013	72% survival to discharge. 1 patient had HTx.
Ting et al. [14]	134 patients with FM (93 adults and 41 pediatrics) required VA-ECMO.	93 (ECMO)	1994–2014	50.1% survival without HTx. 5% successful HTx.
Matsumoto et al. [15]	37 patients with FM received ECMO, 21 of them were males.	37 (37 ECMO, 28 IABP)	1995–2014	59% successful weaning off ECMO 2 patients had durable LVAD. 2 patients had HTx.

Studies	Patients' characteristics	Number of patients (MCS)	Study period	Outcomes
Chang et al. [16]	1145 patients with myocarditis, with a mean age 40.2 ± 14.8 years, 59% of them were males.	294 (99 IABP,195 ECMO)	1997–2011	81% and 61% survival to discharge with IABP and ECMO, respectively.
Wu et al. [17]	60 patients received ECMO without cardiac surgery. 16 patients with FM mostly viral myocarditis.	16 (ECMO)	2003–2010	87.5% survival to discharge. 1 patient had HTx.
Mirabel et al. [18]	41 patients with a median age of 38 years, had FM and received MCS	41 (35 ECMO; 6 BiVAD)	2002–2009	68.6% survival to discharge. 4 patients had HTx.
Beurtheret et al. [19]	87 patients with a mean age 46 ± 15 years, received VA-ECMO. 14 patients had FM.	14 (ECMO)	2005–2009	65% survival to discharge
Diddle et al. [20]	147 patients with a median age of 31 years, had FM and received MCS	147 (ECMO)	1995–2011	61% survival to discharge. 9 patients had HTx.
Ishida et al. [21]	20 patients with a median age of 50 years, had FM and received MCS.	20 (ECMO)	1995–2010	65% survival to discharge
Hsu et al. [22]	75 patients with a mean age of 29.6 ± 18.6 years had FM and received MCS.	75 (ECMO) 5 patients switched to LVAD; 1 patient switched to BiVAD.	1994–2009	61% survival to discharge. 3 patients had HTx.
Asaumi et al. [23]	27 patients with myocarditis, 14 patients with a median age of 38 years received MCS	14 (ECMO)	1993–2001	71.4% survival to discharge
Aoyama et al. [24]	52 patients with a median age of 48 years.	52 (ECMO)	1989–2000	57.7% survival to discharge

ECMO, extracorporeal membrane oxygenation; ECLS. extracorporeal life support; FM, fulminant myocarditis; IABP, intra-aortic balloon pump; HTx, heart transplantation; LVAD, left ventricular assist device.

Table 1.
Studies of FM supported with MCS mainly VA-ECMO.

systolic excursion (TAPSE) 1.8 cm. Progressive deterioration of hemodynamics and increased lactic acidosis happened. Bifemoral VA-ECMO was initiated, and intra-aortic balloon pump (IABP) was inserted for indirect LV unloading. Multidisciplinary management was done involving critical care, heart failure, and rheumatology teams. The patient received five sessions of plasmapheresis and corticosteroid therapy. Anticoagulation with unfractionated heparin infusion was done after an increase of platelet count >50 (10^9/L). Gradual improvement of cardiac function and weaning of vasopressors were done. The ECMO duration was 7 days, the IABP was used for 8 days, the ICU stay was 18 days, and invasive ventilation was used for 11 days. Follow-up TTE revealed cardiac recovery that was evident by normal-sized LV with EF 50–55%, normal valves, and no pericardial effusion. The patient received SLE-directed immunosuppressive therapy, including cyclophosphamide, and was discharged with regular follow-up with the rheumatology department (**Figure 2**).

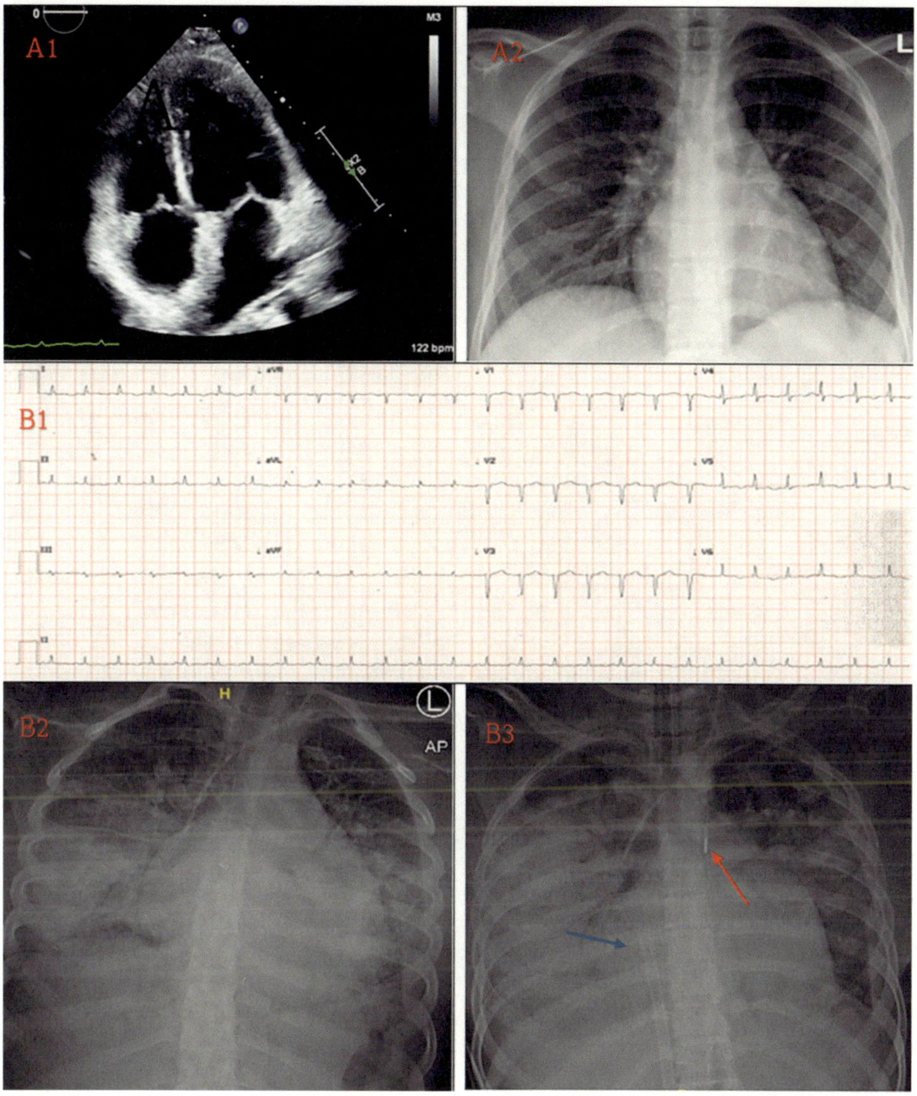

Figure 1.
Initial TTE showing normal-sized ventricles with LV EF 45–50% and no pericardial effusion (A1). A2 is the CXR during the initial diagnosis of SLE with a normal cardiothoracic ratio. The ECG during presentation with cardiogenic shock showed low voltage sinus tachycardia without ST segment deviation (B1). The CXR showed increased cardiac shadow with bilateral pulmonary congestion and right-sided consolidation (B2). B3 shows the CXR after invasive mechanical ventilation, IABP insertion (red arrow), and VA-ECMO insertion. The blue arrow points to the drainage venous cannula of ECMO.

2.2 Fulminant myocarditis after COVID-19 vaccination

A 45-year-old man without a medical history except for dyslipidemia for which he was receiving a small dose statin therapy. He fell down while attending an online business meeting, and his colleagues found him unresponsive without pulsations. They started cardiopulmonary resuscitation (CPR) for 10 minutes, and then the patient was transferred to the nearest hospital within 10 minutes. Initial pulse checking at the emergency department revealed ventricular fibrillation, CPR was continued according to the advanced cardiopulmonary life support (ACLS) protocol for 31 minutes,

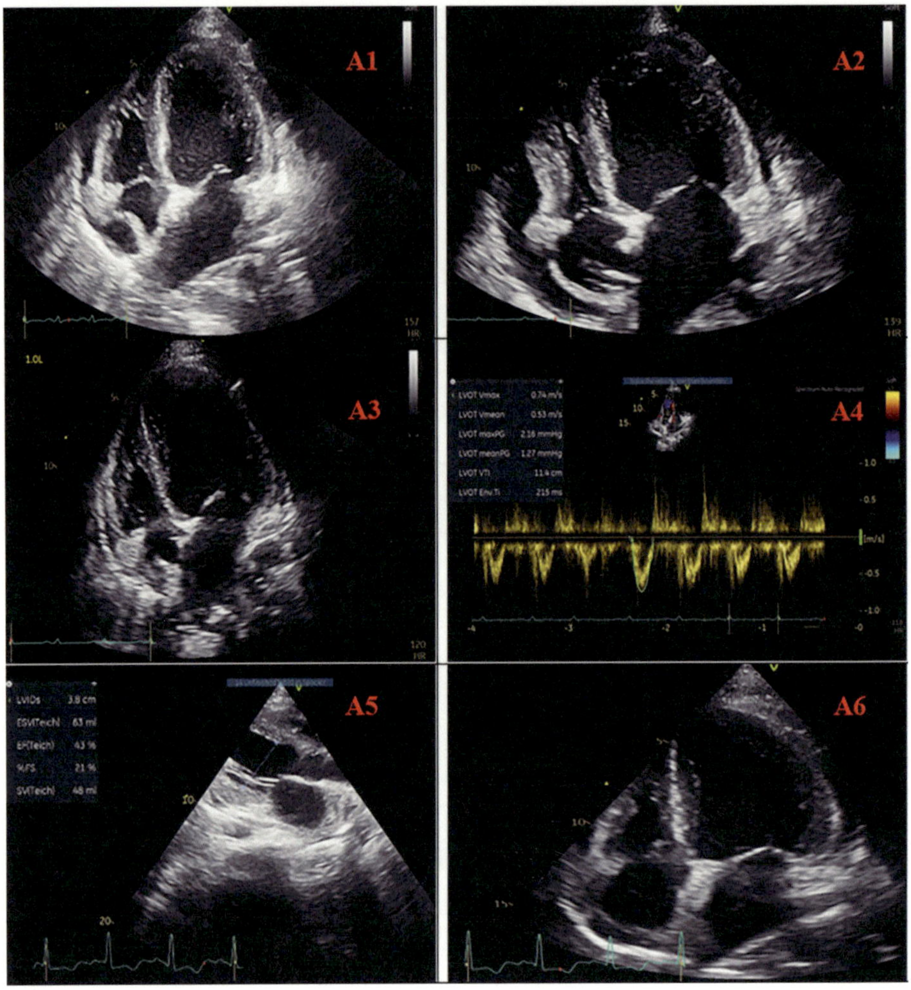

Figure 2.
Transthoracic echocardiography performed after admission with cardiogenic shock revealed left ventricle dilatation with LV EF 20%, LVOT VTI 5.4 cm/m², and circumferential pericardial effusion (A1,2). Echocardiography-guided ECMO weaning revealed LV EF 35%, LVOT VTI 11.4 cm/m², and minimal pericardial effusion (A3,4). One week later, TTE showed normal-sized LV with EDV 111 ml, ESV 63 ml, and LV EF 43% (A5). Pre-discharge TTE showed LV EF 50% (A6).

during which five defibrillation shocks were delivered. After achieving return of spontaneous circulation (ROSC) with a 60-minute CPR duration, ECG showed ST segment elevation in anterior chest leads. The patient was shifted to the catheterization laboratory, where coronary angiography was done and revealed normal coronary arteries with thrombolysis in myocardial infarction (TIMI) flow III. Toxicological screening was done and was negative for amphetamines, opiates, and cannabis. Emergency TTE revealed severely reduced ventricular function with LV EF 10%, global hypokinesia, and no pericardial effusion (**Figures 3** and **4**).

Progressive hemodynamic deterioration occurred and lactic acidosis increased; peripheral VA-ECMO was inserted via bifemoral approach. Therapeutic hypothermia was applied, and hemodynamic stabilization was gradually achieved. Brain computed tomography (CT) scan excluded acute cerebrovascular stroke. Multidisciplinary management was done involving cardiovascular critical care, heart failure, and neurology

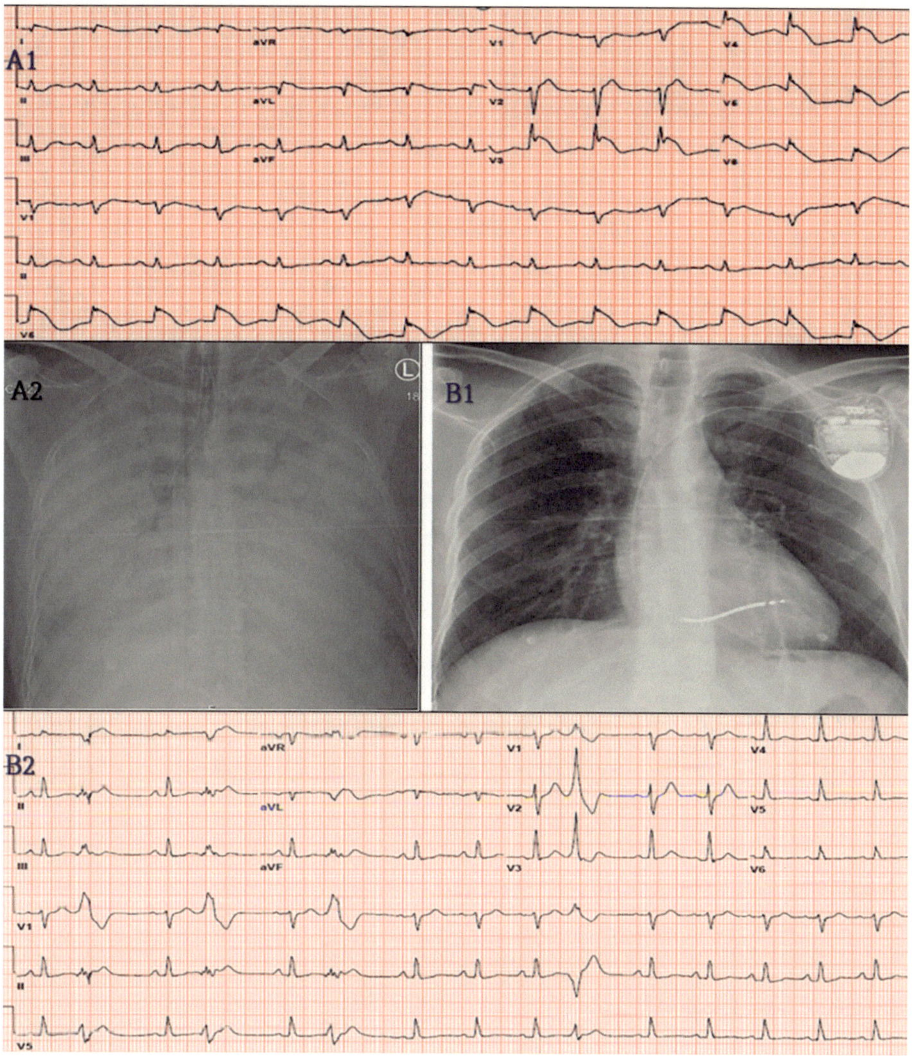

Figure 3.
Post-ROSC ECG (A1) showed ST segment elevation in anterior chest leads. Admission CXR (A2) showed bilateral white lungs with pulmonary edema. Pre-discharge CXR (B1) showed clear lung fields and a single lead ICD. ECG (B2) after cardiac recovery showed frequent PVCs despite optimal electrolytes and beta-blocker therapy.

teams. Autoimmune profile and virology screenings were done and were normal. Suspision of COVID-19-associated myocarditis was raised as the patient received the second dose of the messenger ribonucleic acid (mRNA) vaccine 3 weeks before the hospital admission. The patient received high-dose corticosteroid therapy. The patient developed acute kidney injury without the need for dialysis, acute ischemic hepatitis, and delayed neurological recovery. Electroencephalogram (EEG) excluded epileptic activity. Gradual improvement of hemodynamic profile and multi-organ function occurred, and the follow-up transesophageal echocardiography (TEE) revealed improved cardiac function with LVEF 40% and VTI 12.4 cm/m^2. Decannulation of the ECMO was done after 6 days of support. Brain MRI revealed scattered T2 hyperintense foci with mild diffusion restriction in the bilateral frontoparietal region and basal ganglia related to subacute ischemic changes and likely a sequela of prior hypoxic-ischemic

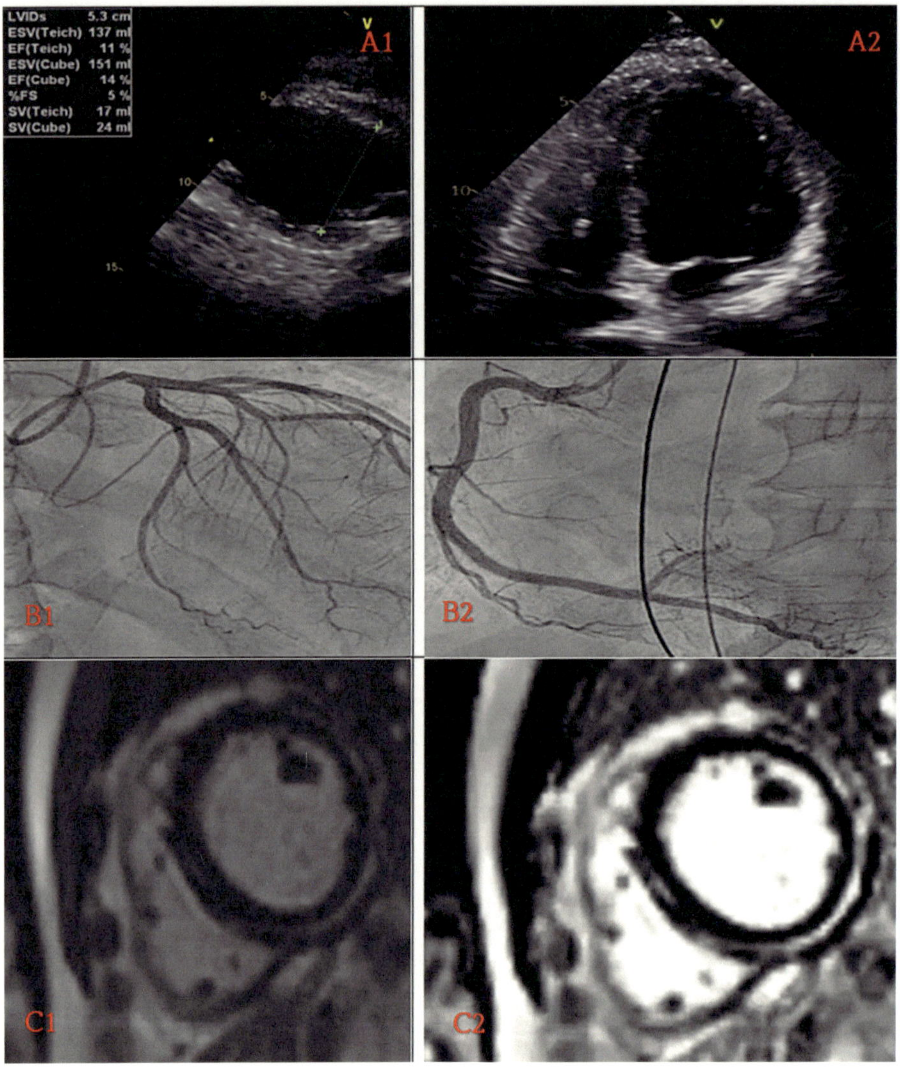

Figure 4.
Admission TTE (A1&2) showed severely reduced LV function with EF 11%, LV ESV 137 ml, global hypokinesia, and there was no pericardial effusion, pulmonary hypertension, or RV strain. Left coronary angiogram (B1) showed normal coronaries with TIMI III flow. Right coronary artery was normal with TIMI III flow (B2). Short-axis MRI images (C1 and 2) show myopericarditis changes with late epicardial gadolinium enhancement.

injury. After 11 days of admission, cardiac MRI was done, and it revealed normal size, shape, and function of the left and right ventricles with ejection fractions of 54% and 52%, respectively. The MRI showed late epicardial gadolinium enhancement involving the mid-anterolateral, inferolateral, and inferior walls, as well as apical lateral and inferior wall segments, and there was a subtle high T2 stair signal intensity involving the mid-lateral and inferior walls along with pericardial enhancement (**Figure 4**).

Gradual neurological recovery happened, and the removal of the invasive mechanical ventilation occurred after 16 days of support. Despite the cardiac recovery, there were frequent premature ventricular contractions (PVCs), so an internal cardioverter defibrillator (ICD) was implanted for secondary prevention of sudden cardiac death. The patient was discharged after 37 days of hospitalization.

3. Discussion

The presented two cases with cardiogenic shock and out-of-hospital cardiac arrest (OHCA) were challenging to reach the diagnosis. Emergency cardio-respiratory support with VA-ECMO was life-saving and gave the medical team vital time to reach the diagnosis and deliver the definite treatment waiting for cardiac recovery or assessment for durable mechanical support with ventricular assist devices (VADs) or heart transplantation.

The patient with SLE-associated myocarditis presented with hemodynamic instability, fever, and bilateral lung infiltrates with recent TTE showing good cardiac function. She might be easily misdiagnosed as a case of septic shock; however, the low voltage criteria of ECG and neck vein distension raised the suspicion of cardiac emergency. Repeating the TTE showed the severely reduced cardiac contractility. Getting a cardiac MRI was not possible in the life-threatening condition and during ECMO support. The heart failure team denied the benefit of getting an endomyocardial biopsy due to the possibility of false negative results, and the patient had already improved after the SLE-directed treatment. The cardiac involvement of SLE includes pericarditis, conduction disturbances, Liebman–Sacks endocarditis, vasculitis, and myocarditis [25]. While clinical myocarditis was reported in 5–10% of patients with SLE, subclinical myocarditis was reported in 57% of patients in postmortem studies [26]. The myocardial biopsy of patients with SLE usually reveals nonspecific inflammation and multifocal infiltration with lymphocytes and macrophages [27]. There is a lack of optimal therapy for patients with SLE-associated FM who received VA-ECMO support. High-dose corticosteroids and plasmapheresis sessions were effective in our case and were followed with cyclophosphamide therapy after ECMO decannulation. Raval et al. [28] reported a challenging case with SLE-associated FM that presented with heart failure and did not require MCS and achieved cardiac recovery with high-dose corticosteroid and immune-suppression therapy. Another patient was reported with SLE-associated FM, who presented with cardiogenic shock with ischemic hepatitis and acute kidney injury, for whom IABP was initially inserted but failed to achieve stable hemodynamics, then VA-ECMO was inserted [29]. The patient did not achieve cardiac recovery after steroids, rituximab, and intravenous immunoglobulins, and LVAD was inserted for 2 years, and then heart transplantation was done [29]. From the two reported cases, besides our case, we can propose that early diagnosis of myocarditis and delivering SLE-directed treatment can affect the outcome, and early initiation of VA-ECMO before the occurrence of multi-organ dysfunction can be associated with improved outcomes.

The patient with COVID-19 vaccine-associated myocarditis had another fatal presentation of FM that required extracorporeal cardiopulmonary resuscitation (ECPR). The diagnosis was made by the history of recent intake of the second dose of mRNA vaccine, severe LV dysfunction, and negative coronary angiography in a healthy young man without a significant medical history or drug abuse. While the COVID-19 infection was linked to the risk of myocarditis [30–32], a recent meta-analysis included seven studies reported that the people who received COVID-19 mRNA vaccines had a two-fold risk of developing myocarditis compared to the unvaccinated persons during the 30 days after second dose [33]. The molecular mimicry and immune-mediated process were hypothesized, and histopathological analysis revealed T lymphocytes infiltration [34]. There are no proven roles of corticosteroid and immunosuppressive therapies for vaccine-related myocarditis. Our patient received high-dose corticosteroid therapy and achieved full recovery, but we did not know what would happen without corticosteroid therapy.

The use of short-term MCS including VA-ECMO, Impella, and IABP has been reported in patients with FM but without clear recommendations. However, it was recommended that patients with life-threatening cardiac dysfunction should be transferred to specialized centers with facilities of MCS, advanced monitoring, and investigations, including cardiac MRI and myocardial biopsy [1, 35]. The guidelines recommended a team-based approach for managing patients with acute heart failure not specific to FM, including close hemodynamic monitoring, serial measurements of blood lactate with use of laboratory markers, and early use of MCS to achieve improved outcomes [36, 37]. Many studies revealed that early implementation of MCS before progressive hyperlactatemia in patients with cardiogenic shock, regardless of the etiology, was associated with better outcomes [38–43]. Considering the high recovery potential of myocarditis if the patient received cardiovascular support and specific therapy to the underlying etiology, temporary MCS should be considered. There are no randomized controlled trials comparing different MCS devices for managing patients with myocarditis. The choice of MCS is usually decided by many factors included need for uni-or-biventricular failure, need for ventilatory support, need for ventricular venting, the facilities and expertise of each center. VA-ECMO provided emergency cardio-ventilatory support, giving the medical team enough time to achieve multi-organ support get the diagnosis, and deliver the proper therapy to increase the chances of recovery.VA-ECMO allows biventricular and ventilatory support, while Impella allows univentricular support in patients without oxygenation problems. A combination of two Impella machines can be used in patients with biventricular failure without oxygenation issues and this was referred to as Bi-Pella [44]. The peripheral VA-ECMO increases the left ventricular afterload and wall stress, which could result in pulmonary edema and impaired myocardial recovery. The use of Impella helps in cardiovascular support and LV venting without ventilatory support [45]. The survival rates of FM were similar in patients supported with either VA-ECMO or Impella [10, 16].

A combination of VA-ECMO and Impella, known as ECPELLA, was reported to have reduced mortality and improved cardiac recovery in patients with cardiogenic shock, compared to VA-ECMO alone due to cardiopulmonary support and LV unloading allowing myocardial recovery [45–47]. The use of IABP in cardiogenic shock helps in ventricular unloading and improving coronary blood flow. There are no data about IABP in cardiogenic shock except in patients with cardiogenic shock due to acute coronary syndromes (IABP-SHOCK II trial) that revealed no mortality benefit compared to medical therapy alone [48].

In case of failed recovery of the cardiac function, the medical team should assess for eligibility to durable MCS with VADs or heart transplantation. There are no clear recommendations about the duration of short-term MCS,; however, most of the studies mentioned a median duration of 7 days was associated with good outcomes, while a duration of more than 14 days carried unfavorable outcomes [22, 49, 50].

4. Conclusions

Fulminant myocarditis is a serious life-threatening medical condition that requires timely management to reach the diagnosis and deliver disease-specific therapy. Early MCS, especially VA-ECMO is a salvage measure to stabilize the patient, preventing multi-organ failure and giving the medical team a crucial time to give the specific therapy enhancing the cardiac recovery.

Declarations

The authors declare no conflict of interest. The presented two cases gave informed consents to publish.

Additional information

The ORCIDs of authors:

Mohamed Laimoud:	0000-0002-5069-2813
Mosleh Alanazi:	0009-0006-9944-012X
Rehan Qureshi:	0009-0000-9238-052X
Emad Hakami:	0000-0002-8415-5901
Khalid Hussein:	0009-0002-4795-0321
Rozana Sadraldin:	0000-0002-2743-3047
Ismail Raslan:	0009-0001-8305-0817

Author details

Mohamed Laimoud[1,2*], Mosleh Alanazi[3], Rehan Qureshi[3], Emad Hakami[4], Khalid Hussein[5], Rozana Sadraldin[6] and Ismail Raslan[6,7]

1 Cardiovascular Critical Care department, Prince Sultan Cardiac Center, Riyadh, Saudi Arabia

2 Critical Care Medicine Department, Cairo University, Cairo, Egypt

3 Cardiovascular Critical Care Department, King Faisal Specialist Hospital and Research Center, Riyadh, Saudi Arabia

4 Cardiovascular Nursing Department, King Faisal Specialist Hospital and Research Center, Riyadh, Saudi Arabia

5 Nephrology Department, Dr. Sulaiman Al Habib hospital, Qassim, Saudi Arabia

6 Adult Cardiology Department, Prince Sultan Cardiac Center, Riyadh, Saudi Arabia

7 Department of Cardiac Sciences, King Fahad Cardiac Center, King Saud University, Riyadh, Saudi Arabia

*Address all correspondence to: m.laimoud@cu.edu.eg

References

[1] Caforio AL, Pankuweit S, Arbustini E, Basso C, Gimeno-Blanes J, Felix SB, et al. Current state of knowledge on aetiology, diagnosis, management, and therapy of myocarditis: A position statement of the European society of cardiology working group on myocardial and pericardial diseases. European Heart Journal. 2013;**34**(33):2636-2648

[2] Kociol RD, Cooper LT, Fang JC, Moslehi JJ, Pang PS, Sabe MA, et al. Recognition and initial management of fulminant myocarditis: A scientific statement from the American Heart Association. Circulation. 2020;**141**(6):e69-e92

[3] Mensah GA, Roth GA, Fuster V. The global burden of cardiovascular diseases and risk factors: 2020 and beyond. Journal of the American College of Cardiology. 2019;**74**(20):2529-2532

[4] Tonna JE, Tan CS, Hryniewicz K, Barbaro RP, Brodie D, MacLaren G. Outcomes after extracorporeal life support for COVID-19 myocarditis: An analysis of the extracorporeal life support organization registry. Critical Care. 2022;**26**(1):235

[5] Ammirati E, Lupi L, Palazzini M, Hendren NS, Grodin JL, Cannistraci CV, et al. Prevalence, characteristics, and outcomes of COVID-19–associated acute myocarditis. Circulation. 2022;**145**(15):1123-1139

[6] Nunez JI, Grandin EW, Reyes-Castro T, Sabe M, Quintero P, Motiwala S, et al. Outcomes with peripheral venoarterial extracorporeal membrane oxygenation for suspected acute myocarditis: 10-year experience from the extracorporeal life support organization registry. Circulation: Heart Failure. 2023;**16**(7):e010152

[7] Tadokoro N, Fukushima S, Minami K, Taguchi T, Saito T, Kawamoto N, et al. Efficacy of central extracorporeal life support for patients with fulminant myocarditis and cardiogenic shock. European Journal of Cardio-Thoracic Surgery. 2021;**60**(5):1184-1192

[8] Chou HW, Wang CH, Lin LY, Chi NH, Chou NK, Yu HY, et al. Prognostic factors for heart recovery in adult patients with acute fulminant myocarditis and cardiogenic shock supported with extracorporeal membrane oxygenation. Journal of Critical Care. 2020;**57**:214-219

[9] Danial P, Olivier ME, Bréchot N, Ponnaiah M, Schoell T, D'Alessandro C, et al. Association between shock etiology and 5-year outcomes after venoarterial extracorporeal membrane oxygenation. Journal of the American College of Cardiology. 2023;**81**(9):897-909

[10] Annamalai SK, Esposito ML, Jorde L, Schreiber T, Hall SA, O'Neill WW, et al. The impella microaxial flow catheter is safe and effective for treatment of myocarditis complicated by cardiogenic shock: An analysis from the global cVAD registry. Journal of Cardiac Failure. 2018;**24**(10):706-710

[11] Saito S, Toda K, Miyagawa S, Yoshikawa Y, Hata H, Yoshioka D, et al. Diagnosis, medical treatment, and stepwise mechanical circulatory support for fulminat myocarditis. Journal of Artificial Organs. 2018;**21**:172-179

[12] Mody KP, Takayama H, Landes E, Yuzefpolskaya M, Colombo PC, Naka Y, et al. Acute mechanical circulatory support for fulminant myocarditis complicated by cardiogenic shock. Journal of Cardiovascular Translational Research. 2014;7:156-164

[13] Lorusso R, Centofanti P, Gelsomino S, Barili F, Di Mauro M, Orlando P, et al. Venoarterial extracorporeal membrane oxygenation for acute fulminant myocarditis in adult patients: A 5-year multi-institutional experience. The Annals of Thoracic Surgery. 2016;**101**:919-926

[14] Ting M, Wang CH, Tsao CI, Huang SC, Chi NH, Chou NK, et al. Heart transplantation under mechanical circulatory support for acute fulminant myocarditis with cardiogenic shock: 10 years' experience of a single center. Transplantation Proceedings. Apr 2016;**48**(3):951-955. DOI: 10.1016/j.transproceed.2015.12.109. PMID: 27234777

[15] Matsumoto M, Asaumi Y, Nakamura Y, Nakatani T, Nagai T, Kanaya T, et al. Clinical determinants of successful weaning from extracorporeal membrane oxygenation in patients with fulminant myocarditis. ESC Heart Failure. 2018;**5**(4):675-684

[16] Chang JJ, Lin MS, Chen TH, Chen DY, Chen SW, Hsu JT, et al. Heart failure and mortality of adult survivors from acute myocarditis requiring intensive care treatment-a nationwide cohort study. International Journal of Medical Sciences. 2017;**14**(12):1241

[17] Wu MY, Lee MY, Lin CC, Chang YS, Tsai FC, Lin PJ. Resuscitation of non-postcardiotomy cardiogenic shock or cardiac arrest with extracorporeal life support: The role of bridging to intervention. Resuscitation. 2012;**83**(8):976-981

[18] Mirabel M, Luyt CE, Leprince P, Trouillet JL, Léger P, Pavie A, et al. Outcomes, long-term quality of life, and psychologic assessment of fulminant myocarditis patients rescued by mechanical circulatory support. Critical Care Medicine. 2011;**39**(5):1029-1035

[19] Beurtheret S, Mordant P, Paoletti X, Marijon E, Celermajer DS, Léger P, et al. Emergency circulatory support in refractory cardiogenic shock patients in remote institutions: A pilot study (the cardiac-RESCUE program). European Heart Journal. 2013;**34**(2):112-120

[20] Diddle JW, Almodovar MC, Rajagopal SK, Rycus PT, Thiagarajan RR. Extracorporeal membrane oxygenation for the support of adults with acute myocarditis. Critical Care Medicine. 2015;**43**(5):1016-1025

[21] Ishida K, Wada H, Sakakura K, Kubo N, Ikeda N, Sugawara Y, et al. Long-term follow-up on cardiac function following fulminant myocarditis requiring percutaneous extracorporeal cardiopulmonary support. Heart and Vessels. 2013;**28**:86-90

[22] Hsu KH, Chi NH, Yu HY, Wang CH, Huang SC, Wang SS, et al. Extracorporeal membranous oxygenation support for acute fulminant myocarditis: Analysis of a single center's experience. European Journal of Cardio-Thoracic Surgery. 2011;**40**(3):682-688

[23] Asaumi Y, Yasuda S, Morii I, Kakuchi H, Otsuka Y, Kawamura A, et al. Favourable clinical outcome in patients with cardiogenic shock due to fulminant myocarditis supported by percutaneous extracorporeal membrane oxygenation. European Heart Journal. 2005;**26**(20):2185-2192

[24] Aoyama N, Izumi T, Hiramori K, Isobe M, Kawana M, Hiroe M, et al. National survey of fulminant myocarditis in Japan therapeutic guidelines and long-term prognosis of using percutaneous cardiopulmonary support for fulminant myocarditis (special report from a

scientific committee). Circulation Journal. 2002;**66**(2):133-144

[25] Apte M, McGwin G Jr, Vilá LM, Kaslow RA, Alarcón GS, Reveille JD, et al. Associated factors and impact of myocarditis in patients with SLE from LUMINA, a multiethnic US cohort. Rheumatology. 2008;**47**(3):362-367

[26] Wijetunga M, Rockson S. Myocarditis in systemic lupus erythematosus. The American Journal of Medicine. 2002;**113**(5):419-423

[27] Gartshteyn Y, Tamargo M, Fleischer S, Kapoor T, Li J, Askanase A, et al. Endomyocardial biopsies in the diagnosis of myocardial involvement in systemic lupus erythematosus. Lupus. 2020;**29**(2):199-204

[28] Raval JJ, Ruiz CR, Heywood J, Weiner JJ. SLE strikes the heart! A rare presentation of SLE myocarditis presenting as cardiogenic shock. BMC Cardiovascular Disorders. 2021;**21**:1-2

[29] Tariq S, Garg A, Gass A, Aronow W. Myocarditis due to systemic lupus erythematosus associated with cardiogenic shock. Archives of Medical Science. 2018;**14**(2):460-462

[30] Patone M, Mei XW, Handunnetthi L, Dixon S, Zaccardi F, Shankar-Hari M, et al. Risks of myocarditis, pericarditis, and cardiac arrhythmias associated with COVID-19 vaccination or SARS-CoV-2 infection. Nature Medicine. 2022;**28**(2):410-422

[31] Seeherman S, Suzuki YJ. Viral infection and cardiovascular disease: Implications for the molecular basis of COVID-19 pathogenesis. International Journal of Molecular Sciences. 2021;**22**(4):1659

[32] Rathore SS, Rojas GA, Sondhi M, Pothuru S, Pydi R, Kancherla N, et al. Myocarditis associated with Covid-19 disease: A systematic review of published case reports and case series. International Journal of Clinical Practice. 2021;**75**(11):e14470

[33] Alami A, Krewski D, Farhat N, Mattison D, Wilson K, Gravel CA, et al. Risk of myocarditis and pericarditis in mRNA COVID-19-vaccinated and unvaccinated populations: A systematic review and meta-analysis. BMJ Open. 2023;**13**(6):e065687

[34] Lenz M, Krychtiuk KA, Zilberszac R, Heinz G, Riebandt J, Speidl WS. Mechanical circulatory support Systems in Fulminant Myocarditis: Recent advances and outlook. Journal of Clinical Medicine. 2024;**13**(5):1197

[35] Ammirati E, Frigerio M, Adler ED, Basso C, Birnie DH, Brambatti M, et al. Management of acute myocarditis and chronic inflammatory cardiomyopathy: An expert consensus document. Circulation: Heart Failure. 2020;**13**(11):e007405

[36] Basir MB, Kapur NK, Patel K, Salam MA, Schreiber T, Kaki A, et al. Improved outcomes associated with the use of shock protocols: Updates from the national cardiogenic shock initiative. Catheterization and Cardiovascular Interventions. 2019;**93**(7):1173-1183

[37] Tehrani BN, Truesdell AG, Sherwood MW, Desai S, Tran HA, Epps KC, et al. Standardized team-based care for cardiogenic shock. Journal of the American College of Cardiology. 2019;**73**(13):1659-1669

[38] Lee HH, Kim HC, Ahn CM, Lee SJ, Hong SJ, Yang JH, et al. Association between timing of extracorporeal membrane oxygenation and clinical outcomes in refractory cardiogenic

shock. Cardiovascular Interventions. 2021;**14**(10):1109-1119

[39] Laimoud M, Hakami E, Machado P, Lo MG, Maghirang MJ. Appropriate timing of veno-arterial extracorporeal membrane oxygenation initiation after cardiac surgery. The Cardiothoracic Surgeon. 2024;**32**(1):2

[40] Wang J, Han J, Jia Y, Zeng W, Shi J, Hou X, et al. Early and intermediate results of rescue extracorporeal membrane oxygenation in adult cardiogenic shock. The Annals of Thoracic Surgery. 2009;**88**(6):1897-1903

[41] Biancari F, Kaserer A, Perrotti A, Ruggieri VG, Cho SM, Kang JK, et al. Hyperlactatemia and poor outcome after postcardiotomy veno-arterial extracorporeal membrane oxygenation: An individual patient data meta-analysis. Perfusion. 2024;**39**(5):956-965

[42] Laimoud M, Machado P, Lo MG, Maghirang MJ, Hakami E, Qureshi R. The absolute lactate levels versus clearance for prognostication of post-cardiotomy patients on veno-arterial ECMO. ESC Heart Fail. Dec 2024;**11**(6):3511-3522. DOI: 10.1002/ehf2.14910. Epub 2024 Jul 9

[43] Laimoud M, Alanazi M. The clinical significance of blood lactate levels in evaluation of adult patients with veno-arterial extracorporeal membrane oxygenation. The Egyptian Heart Journal. 2020;**72**:1-8

[44] Pappalardo F, Scandroglio AM, Latib A. Full percutaneous biventricular support with two impella pumps: The Bi-Pella approach. ESC Heart Failure. 2018;**5**(3):368-371

[45] Tschöpe C, Van Linthout S, Klein O, Mairinger T, Krackhardt F, Potapov EV, et al. Mechanical unloading by fulminant myocarditis: LV-IMPELLA, ECMELLA, BI-PELLA, and PROPELLA concepts. Journal of Cardiovascular Translational Research. 2019;**12**:116-123

[46] Pappalardo F, Schulte C, Pieri M, Schrage B, Contri R, Soeffker G, et al. Concomitant implantation of Impella® on top of veno-arterial extracorporeal membrane oxygenation may improve survival of patients with cardiogenic shock. European Journal of Heart Failure. 2017;**19**(3):404-412

[47] Narain S, Paparcuri G, Fuhrman TM, Silverman RB, Peruzzi WT. Novel combination of impella and extra corporeal membrane oxygenation as a bridge to full recovery in fulminant myocarditis. Case Reports in Critical Care. 2012;**2012**(1):459296

[48] Thiele H, Zeymer U, Neumann FJ, Ferenc M, Olbrich HG, Hausleiter J, et al. Intraaortic balloon support for myocardial infarction with cardiogenic shock. New England Journal of Medicine. 2012;**367**(14):1287-1296

[49] Lee EP, Chu SC, Huang WY, Hsia SH, Chan OW, Lin CY, et al. Factors associated with in-hospital mortality of children with acute fulminant myocarditis on extracorporeal membrane oxygenation. Frontiers in Pediatrics. 2020;**8**:488

[50] Den Uil CA, Akin S, Jewbali LS, dos Reis MD, Brugts JJ, Constantinescu AA, et al. Short-term mechanical circulatory support as a bridge to durable left ventricular assist device implantation in refractory cardiogenic shock: A systematic review and meta-analysis. European Journal of Cardio-Thoracic Surgery. 2017;**52**(1):14-25